Jane Houlton

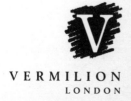

VERMILION

LONDON

First published 1993

© Jane Houlton

Jane Houlton has asserted her right under the Copyright, Designs and Patents Act, 1988 to be identified as the author of this work

First published in the United Kingdom in 1993 by Vermilion
an imprint of Ebury Press
Random House
20 Vauxhall Bridge Road
London SW1 2SA

Random House Australia (Pty) Limited
20 Alfred Street, Milsons Point, Sydney
New South Wales 2061. Australia

Random House New Zealand Limited
18 Poland Road, Glenfield
Auckland 10, New Zealand

Random House South Africa (Pty) Limited
PO Box 337, Bergvlei, South Africa

Random House UK Limited Reg. No. 954009

A CIP catalogue record for this book
is available from the British Library

ISBN 009 177505 1

Printed in Great Britain by Mackays of Chatham Plc Kent
Typeset from author's disc in Century Old Style
by Hope Services (Abingdon) Ltd.

Contents

PART 5: HOW DOES ALLERGY AFFECT MY LIFE? WHAT CAN I DO TO HELP MYSELF?

PART 6: WHAT HELP IS AVAILABLE?

Acknowledgements

I am grateful to many people for their contributions to this book: to Dr Jonathan Maberly and Dr Honor Anthony of the Airedale Allergy Centre (AAC) for all their advice, and for their permission to use material from their book, *Allergy – A Guide to Coping*; to John Collard, Charge Nurse of the AAC for all his support, help and backing over the years, and for his work in checking the typescript; to Janice Thorpe, Dietitian of the AAC for reading and checking material; to Dr Jonathan Brostoff and Linda Gamlin for their permission to use material from their book, *The Complete Guide to Food Allergy and Intolerance*; to Dr Peter Whitehead for his encouragement and humour.

I owe a great debt to many individuals with allergy and sensitivity to whom I have listened and from whom I have learned. In particular, I am grateful to Agnes Moodie for her inspiration, energy and conviction that this book was necessary; to Hilary Dalton, Eva Linnegar, Elaine Maberly and Hazel Megson, and to Arthur, Barbara, Catherine, Colette, Linda, Paul, Sam, Sarah and many others. I would also like to thank the support groups and charities who have allowed me access to their material.

My thanks are also due to Mary Maples, my research assistant, for all her work, and for her thoroughness and perceptiveness; to Gill West and to Superscript for their help with computing and word processing.

I am also grateful to the many experts who advised on specific topics, especially Michael Devenish, Peter Marshall and Ken Rowley, and to all the people, in many organisations, patient enough to give Mary Maples and myself their time to inform and explain.

Finally, my gratitude to my parents for all their love; to Louis for allowing me time off to write, and to Michael who was always there.

Jane Houlton, 1993

Half of the author's profits will be donated to allergy charities.

Foreword

Allergy and intolerance present considerable difficulties to a growing number of people. Unfortunately, few find the help they need to sort out their often-complex problems. Jane Houlton has produced a book which will be of inestimable value to these people. She has indeed achieved her stated purpose in providing a well-researched source of practical guidelines and suppliers, together with a wealth of fundamental self-help advice. Every item of information in her book is easy to find, which is particularly laudable in this complex field.

Anyone who has ever been told to clear house dust mites from a child's bedroom, or wonders why they always feel unwell after the weekly shopping trip, will now be able to gain valuable insight into their problem and learn how to take steps to help themselves.

I sincerely hope that this book finds its market. Many need the help it brings, and will benefit from its contents.

Dr Jonathan Maberly, Consultant Physician, MBBS, MRCP, FRACP
President of the British Society of Allergy and
Environmental Medicine
Medical Director of the Airedale Allergy Centre

Part 1
ABOUT THE SURVIVAL GUIDE

Personal Experience

In May 1985, I was working in London, as a business consultant in the consulting division of a firm of accountants, when my division moved into a newly renovated office. I was then in my early thirties. For most of my adult life, I had had bothersome health problems – arthritis, back trouble, gut pain, diarrhoea, sinusitis, cystitis, vaginal discharges, prolonged viruses, exhaustion. These came and went, sometimes they were minor but at other times they troubled me greatly, particularly when I was tired and run down. I had had one bad period of back trouble which had made me give up work and rest for a few months some years before.

At the time we moved offices, I had been feeling well for some time. I was very happy in my marriage and my career, and had learned to keep myself well through exercise, relaxation, fresh air and a diet which avoided some foods that I knew did not suit me. Some of my old familiar niggles were always there but they did not inconvenience me.

Building work was still going on in the office when we moved, the air conditioning was not working, and the offices were full of brand new materials. I felt suffocated and sick at first, then progressively unwell. After three or four days, I puffed up, my skin came up in red blotches, and I sweated excessively. I had burns and blisters on the backs of my legs from sitting, and I had a horrible burning sensation, like sunburn, just under my skin. I could not breathe; I felt nauseous and could not keep food down. Even when I went home, the effects did not clear. I lay awake for hours at night, my head spinning, feeling sick, giddy and sore.

I saw various specialist doctors at the time and I was diagnosed as having 'allergies to specific chemicals'. No connection was made with my previous health problems; little constructive help and advice was offered; medication was ineffective, and I continued to try to work in That Building for some months. Eventually it defeated me. My firm still occupied the former office building down the road, so I moved back there and found myself a new role within the firm.

For some time after moving out of That Building, I was very well and did not seem to be affected at all elsewhere. When I look back now, however, I can see that from late 1986, my health began steadily to slip away from me. I became sensitive to an ever-wider range of chemicals in everyday use. The choice of foods that I could eat became more and more narrow, and I had obsessive addictions to certain foods that I knew upset me.

By late 1987, I was in constant pain and exhausted. I went to bed at 7.30 in the evening whenever possible; I had diarrhoea or was sick after every meal; I felt as if an elephant was sitting on my chest; I was stiff and arthritic, my joints were sore and throbbing, and my left side was in muscle spasm. I had splitting sinus headaches, and a totally blocked nose. I peed, sweated and discharged constantly. I was bloated with fluid (usually underweight, I had gained over a stone and a half). There was nothing, literally nothing, that I could tolerate on my skin, or for washing or cleaning. I could not wear tights or stockings; all my clothes made me sore. If I sat on certain materials, I got blisters on my vulva.

I did not know what to do about all these problems. My GP was sympathetic but unhelpful and I had given up asking her for advice. I had tried various complementary therapies and they had had no significant impact. At a routine medical for work in December 1987, the company's doctor, concerned but firm, told me that there was no cure for allergy, that I had to learn to live with it, and gave me a prescription for anti-histamines.

I felt desperate and awful, but I just kept going. I have iron willpower, too stubborn and determined perhaps for my own good, and I do not find confessing weakness easy. I held myself together for work, but had little or no social life, and spent most of my free time resting or sleeping. My husband and I were both very worried but could not see a solution.

In 1987 I read an article in *The Guardian* about an allergy specialist, Dr Jonathan Maberly, who had established an environmental unit, the Airedale Allergy Centre (AAC), in Yorkshire. The unit excluded many common allergens, thereby enabling Dr Maberly to test people for sensitivity to chemicals, foods and other allergens in carefully controlled conditions. The article reported that he was able to give advice on how to avoid chemicals and other allergens in everyday life, and that he could treat people with a form of immunotherapy called 'neutralisation', which, although it did not work for everyone, could be effective in preventing or reducing reactions.

By that stage, I did not naturally trust doctors, having had little benefit from them, but I found out a little more about Dr Maberly and, reasonably happy with what I learned, I persuaded my GP to refer me to him, if only to confirm that nothing could be done to help me.

I first saw Dr Maberly for a consultation in early 1988. Nothing I said seemed to surprise him, indeed he laughed in a calming, affection-

ate way, as if it was all very familiar to him and I was one of many –
not weird or unique after all. With his guidance, I began to disentangle
all the possible causes of my symptoms. I went on an elimination diet
and could not find a diet that I tolerated. I tested chemicals at the
Allergy Centre at weekends, while I flew around Europe during the
week on business, carrying exotic foods for testing in my baggage.

Looking back, I think I must have been mad. Either I did not realise
how ill I had become, or I was too stubborn to admit it. Eventually, in
June 1988, having lost an alarming amount of weight, grey and weak, I
went into the Allergy Centre for a full range of in-patient tests. I still
find it difficult to remember much of what happened during those few
weeks. The bare fact is that I tested positive to every substance tried
on me, with the exception of melon and Malvern Water.

My stay at the Centre was emotionally and physically shattering.
The Centre is as free from allergens as possible and at times I had
absolutely no symptoms. I could not remember ever feeling so well,
even as a child. I had got used to pain being my constant companion,
and I had forgotten what it was like not to ache, throb and hurt. It was
extraordinary to know that, for most people, feeling well was normal,
and that I was somehow outside their world.

I had not expected to react to anything other than chemicals, despite
the fact that outside the unit I had been unable to find a diet that
suited me. I thought that I had felt ill on the elimination diet simply
because I was tired, hungry and run down, and that it would all go
away with a bit of rest and if I sorted out the chemicals (few, I
thought) to which I was truly sensitive. I found it almost incomprehen-
sible that I should react to things like house dust mites, moulds, pollens, wool, or cotton, which I had never suspected of upsetting me, or
that I should be allergic to virtually every food. I could not deny the
reality when testing them in controlled conditions gave positive
results and reproduced familiar symptoms, often frightening in their
violence.

Problems I had had for years, and had given up complaining about
– sinusitis, arthritis, gut pain, diarrhoea, muscle spasm, back pain –
were linked to very specific substances and melted away when the
allergens were absent. It turned my world on its head. How could I live
now that I knew the difference between allergic reaction and normality? How could I bear to return to the world of pain of which I was
newly conscious, having once known what it was like to feel well?
Denial had been my strategy for coping – how would I cope now that I
had been forced to confront the truth?

After I came out of the Unit, it was nine months before I really
began to stabilise. Those months are also a blur. I was still reacting

strongly to everything around me, and my husband and I were sorting out our home environment, struggling to find things I could use, wear, sit on, sleep on, or even tolerate in the room with me. Much of those months I spent sitting on a wooden chair in the middle of a room, listening to music, trying to live through it, waiting for my body to learn to work again.

After nine months, the Maberly treatment – the avoidance, the rotation diet, the neutralising vaccines – started to work and I began to feel better and was free of pain much of the time, as long as I stuck to my routines. Most or all of the symptoms I had had for so many years had vanished, and only returned when I could not avoid a specific allergen.

Now, four years later, my life has many constraints but is mostly pain-free. I get tired very fast and struggle to keep my weight up. I do not go into other people's homes much, or into other buildings. I work from home. I rarely travel, and then only a few miles. I do not go into cities. I hardly ever read a newspaper and handle all paper with care. My home life is very carefully planned and managed. I can still only eat a handful of foods and then only with neutralising vaccines. I avoid certain situations totally. Writing this book has been a fight – I have had to rely on other people to do many things that I cannot do myself. I live very much in the present and take each day as it comes.

However, I get stronger and more resilient as time goes on, and my optimism about what I may one day be able to do increases apace. I have a rich and happy life. I have had a child in the middle of all this, and he is a source of constant joy. He is very well himself, though he has many food allergies and I have had to learn more than I wished about caring for a highly allergic baby and child.

I am not a lonely, isolated person, nor do I live in a hermetically sealed cocoon of safe things. I try to lead as normal a life as I can; I work out what I can tolerate and organise my life accordingly. If you met me on the street, or by chance at some gathering, you probably would have no idea of how I live or the precautions I take. Sometimes I forget the power that things have to hurt me and am shocked at how ill I can suddenly become. I am conscious of the healing power of love. I have wise doctors and nurses who care as much with thoughtful love as with technical skill and knowledge. My husband, my child and my family could not be more giving. I have been fortunate in being offered love when I needed it most.

I have learned to accommodate my illness now. I do not fight it, nor deny it, as I once did. I respect it and I allow it its limits, as it allows me mine. We are tolerant neighbours – we both abide by our limits and we have learned to live together in peace.

Why This Book?

This is the book I wish I had had years ago. It would have saved me so much pain, anxiety and money. I have read many books on allergy over the last few years, but none of them ever told me the things I really needed to know.

I wanted a book that would deal with the practical difficulties of daily life; a book that gave me a lot of facts as to how and what and why, so that when I ran into trouble, I had the explanation and resources to dig myself out. I did not want a view of the world, a promise to change my life, nor even an easy cure, but rather open-minded independence and healthy scepticism. I wanted a book written from *my* point of view, not from some doctor's or some expert's, and I wanted product names, telephone numbers and addresses so that I did not have to mess around.

Much of the time, if you have allergies, you are left alone to work things out for yourself. Allergy is so personal – what upsets one person can be well tolerated by another – so how do you find your way through the forest of confusion?

A lot of the advice currently available does not pass the 'Yes, but. . .' test. 'Yes, but what do I actually do?' How do you work out what you react to, when the cause could be so many different things and medical tests are not conclusive? It is fine being advised not to use strong chemicals, but what do you actually do when your oven needs cleaning or your house gets wet rot? You decide to replace your carpets or bedding to get rid of house dust mites, but what do you use instead if you are allergic to various materials, and where can you buy the things you need anyway? How do you cope when you cannot use contact lens solution, contraception, sanitary or incontinence protection, or even toilet paper?

This book answers questions like these. It gives you the information you need when you are on your own, trying to figure out what to do next.

Much of the advice in this book is unique. I have found out an enormous amount about what to do and what to use while sorting out my own life and caring for my child, but it is not just based on my own experience. There is a vast wealth of knowledge among other people in similar situations. I have gathered over the years a hoard of precious information from individuals, from self-help and support groups, and from charities. And I have had extensive access to the knowledge of the doctors and nurses at the Airedale Allergy Centre, who see people with every problem under the sun. All of this information has been carefully checked with other experts, technologists, and manufacturers. However, the people who *really* know how to cope are those who live with allergies each day. They have had to try things for themselves to see if they work. This book draws heavily on their collective experience.

Sometimes, when dealing with allergy, you wish you had someone at your elbow, advising as you work things out, warning of pitfalls ahead. This book can guide you through and help you to learn what others have learned before.

The author welcomes any tips and advice, plus information on products that help. If you would like to send them, there is a cut-out form on page 483 to be returned to:

> The Allergy Survival Guide
> PO Box 37
> Skipton
> North Yorkshire
> BD23 1QX

Also available from this address is information on topics not covered by this *Guide* (for instance, worklife, preconceptual care, footwear, holiday accommodation and gardening). For a full list of information available, send a stamped addressed envelope to the above address.

How to Use the Guide

As you start reading this book, you no doubt have all sorts of questions in your head. *The Allergy Survival Guide* is organised around these questions.

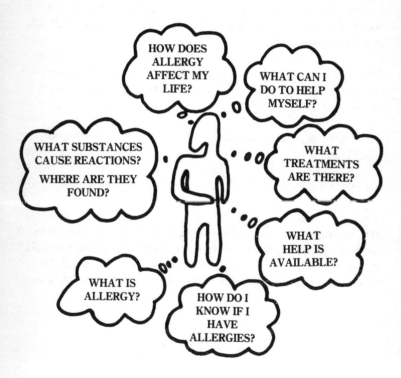

Each Part contains sections which relate to these questions. The following will help you find your way around the *Guide*:

If you don't know where to start
Go to Part 2: WHAT IS ALLERGY? (opposite) and follow the directions into the rest of the *Guide*.

If you are looking for specific advice
Go to the Contents page at the beginning of the book and choose the most relevant Part or section. You can also use the Index at the end of the *Guide* to look for individual topics that interest you.

If you want medical help
For advice on medical treatments, go to the section entitled MEDICAL HELP in Part 6 (page 457). There is also a section on complementary therapy (page 469).

If you have multiple allergies
If you have, or suspect you have, multiple allergies, each section contains within it information on how to detect or deal with multiple sensitivity, and how to make choices. There is a special section on MULTIPLE SENSITIVITY (page 35) and this is a good place to start.

You can choose yourself how far you want to go in using the advice in this book. There are no prescriptions about what you have to do to be well. Living with allergy often involves changing your way of life and your family's habits. The right choice for you is the one that achieves a comfortable balance between how well you want to be and how far you want to adapt your life.

You can use the *Guide* to tell you about a few simple things you can do which will make a real difference, without spending too much time or money. Or, if you are obliged to make major changes, the *Guide* will tell you exactly what you can do to avoid and eliminate allergens.

As you read the *Guide*, each section will refer you to other sections which might interest you. The > symbol, followed by a section name or names, indicates where you will find more advice relevant to your problem. You can choose the level of detail and information you require to meet your needs.

Part 2
WHAT IS ALLERGY?

Defining Allergy

'Allergy' means an abnormal, excessive reaction of the body's defence systems to a substance absorbed from the environment. Allergies now affect 30–40 per cent of the population in the UK and are on the increase; the number of people going to their GPs for treatment for asthma and hay fever doubled in the 1980s. Asthma is responsible for up to 2000 deaths a year in the UK, and one in seven primary school-children carries an inhaler.

There is much controversy over what allergy actually is. Historically, the definition is very broad, encompassing a wide range of illnesses brought about by people reacting to substances in their environment. By the 1960s, scientific research into the workings of the immune system had identified the mechanisms underlying most of the classic allergic diseases – asthma, eczema, hay fever, perennial rhinitis, urticaria, anaphylactic shock (>SYMPTOMS for full details). However, this research left unexplained many disorders that had hitherto come under the umbrella of allergy. Patients with these disorders have symptoms that are not typical of the classic allergic diseases – for example, they may have migraine, arthritis, muscle pains, irritable bowel syndrome, mood swings or other mental symptoms – and their symptoms are often highly variable and difficult to pin down to one specific cause. There is little solid scientific research into the underlying causes of such environmental illness or allergy.

Doctors practising today have been trained in the subject of allergy on the basis of what is scientifically proven – that a range of specific symptoms results from an over-reaction of the immune system, and that objective evidence can be provided by skin and blood tests proving the involvement of the immune system. When doctors use the word 'allergy', this is virtually always what they mean – a much narrower definition than the original one. Most do not accept that illnesses such as migraine, arthritis, colitis and mental symptoms can result from an adverse reaction to something in the environment, apart from certain well-researched kinds of food intolerance, for instance, or exposure to high levels of chemicals.

Some doctors, however, still work with a much broader definition of what allergic disease encompasses. They prefer the term 'allergy and environmental medicine' to describe the field. (In the United States, this is commonly called 'clinical ecology'.) This definition covers a wide range of illnesses and symptoms, including true allergy in the strict immunological sense, but also encompassing food intolerance, chemical sensitivity, and other disorders that respond to avoidance or elimination of specific substances from the individual's environment.

If you know that you react to something in your environment, you may feel that these distinctions do not really matter if the end result for you is the same, i.e. that you react to a given substance and you have to avoid it to stay well. In simple terms, you are right. It doesn't matter, for instance, whether you are 'allergic to chemicals' or 'chemically sensitive' if the outcome is the same in practical terms, that you have to avoid certain chemicals. However, there are differences in the types of therapy and treatment you might find helpful, and in the guidelines on avoidance, so making a distinction does help you to have a greater understanding of what you are asked to do.

It also matters in another important respect. Doctors disagree (sometimes passionately) about what allergy actually is, what its symptoms are and how to treat it. You may get one diagnosis and suggested course of treatment from one doctor, and a totally different approach from another. Many practitioners (on both sides of the argument) make assertions about the nature of allergy when the facts are not fully known, and when the reality is manifestly complex. You need to understand the background to the controversy – and the facts, as far as they are known – in order to be able to make sense of what doctors say to you.

The aim of this book is to steer a path through the controversy, to give you the information you need to make your own choices, and to set out the facts as far as they are known. This book uses the broader definition of allergy and environmental medicine, covering a range of adverse reactions to substances in the environment, particularly true allergy, food intolerance and chemical sensitivity. In some of these disorders, the immune system is clearly involved; in others its role is unproven or other factors are at play.

Terms of definition are used in this book as precisely as possible, so that 'allergy' is used to mean reactions in which the immune system is demonstrably involved. Where other mechanisms, such as chemical sensitivity or food intolerance, are concerned, these terms are used. The following pages outline in detail the specifics of these varying reactions.

Allergy

The symptoms of some allergic diseases have been described since antiquity, and asthma and eczema were named in the mid-first century BC. Foods, inhalants such as feathers or cat fur, and insect stings were recorded as causing reactions in ancient and more recent times.

It was in the early twentieth century that connections between the immune system and the altered reactions of allergy were made. An immune system operating in this way was termed 'hypersensitive'. Experiments in the 1920s showed that hypersensitive reactions to pollen or food could be transferred from one person to another, by injecting a small amount of blood serum from the allergic person into another. The previously unaffected person would show reactions to the allergen, demonstrating the involvement of the immune system.

A further major advance took place in the 1960s when IgE, the antibody particularly associated with allergic reactions, was identified. One of the main lines of attack used by the body's immune system against any substance entering the body is to produce antibodies that bind to the invading substance and activate the rest of the body's defences by chemical reactions. IgE is one such antibody. Its proper function is to defend the body against parasites, such as worms, which could infest the body. The first time such an invader — called an 'antigen' — enters the body, the immune system produces specific IgE antibodies, which then attach themselves to cells in tissues and the bloodstream ready to react should the invader return. There is no reaction as such on the first encounter.

IgE antibodies are primed to bind specifically to the antigen they have already recognised. They are lodged in cells known as 'mast cells' in solid tissues, and in 'basophils' in the bloodstream. Mast cells are especially common in the breathing passages, lungs, gut and digestive tract, and in the skin. There, the antibodies lie in wait for the returning invader. If it returns in the bloodstream, they recognise it and lock on to the molecule of the antigen, thus triggering chemical reactions and the release of chemicals in the body. 'Histamine' is released immediately, while other chemicals — 'leukotrienes' and 'prostaglandins' — are released more slowly. These chemicals are very powerful and stimulate defence mechanisms to expel invading parasites. They have three important effects:

Dilation of small blood vessels

This can lead to hives, fluid retention and swelling, nasal blockage and headaches.

Smooth muscle spasm

This can produce contraction of the airways and gut spasm.

Increased secretions

Mucus flow and discharges increase and are manifest in hay fever, conjunctivitis, asthma and ear complaints.

It is the functioning of this mechanism that goes wrong in most allergic reactions. For some unknown reason, IgE antibodies are produced in response to harmless molecules. Any substance that triggers this abnormal reaction is called an 'allergen'.

Further research into the immune system has shown that there are other mechanisms whereby other antibodies are involved in hypersensitive reactions, such as in delayed contact dermatitis, or when antibodies form immune complexes with invading molecules and are deposited from the bloodstream into tissues. However, the IgE mechanism is the principal one involved in allergy and the most important to understand.

Allergic reactions often happen immediately or within a few hours of encountering an allergen. If you are repeatedly in contact with an allergen, such as a commonly eaten food or house dust mites, you may have continual symptoms which occasionally worsen. You can also get late or delayed reactions, resulting from the on-going chemical changes in your body. These can happen up to several days later in the case of reactions to food.

Most people who display symptoms of the classic allergic diseases (i.e. asthma, eczema, hay fever, urticaria, perennial rhinitis and anaphylactic shock) show raised levels of IgE in laboratory tests. (>DETECTING YOUR ALLERGIES for further details of these tests.) However, this is not true of everybody who suffers from these diseases. Generally speaking, if there is an identifiable trigger (such as pollen, dust mites or animal fur), and the patients display the classic symptoms of allergy, their illness will be diagnosed as allergy even if the tests are negative. Conversely, some people have a positive result to tests for allergens and raised IgE levels but do not actually react and show symptoms.

It is not known why the body's normal defence mechanism goes wrong in this way, although it is known that the tendency for it to happen runs in families and can be inherited. This inherited tendency is known as 'atopy'. This means that if you or your partner suffer from allergies, your children are more likely to suffer from allergies, too, although they may well escape totally. If they do inherit the tendency, however, they will not necessarily inherit your precise symptoms or react to the same specific allergens. For example, you might be allergic to cat fur and get asthma, but they might get perennial rhinitis and be allergic to dust mites. This suggests that the fault in the immune system lies in the controlling or recognising mechanisms.

The Pattern of Allergy

The pattern of disease varies widely. Some people develop allergies very early in life, develop new allergies readily and have wide-ranging problems for most of their lives. Other people can show no sign of trouble, and then develop one or more allergies much later in life, often for no apparent reason. The severity of reaction also varies greatly from individual to individual.

The first time an allergen is encountered, it sets off the primary response from the immune system, to manufacture antibodies to it. No reaction will occur at this first meeting; it is not until the next encounter, or often some time later if you have a particularly heavy exposure to something, that you will react.

Babies in the womb can become sensitised to substances, especially foods, passed from the mother, so they can appear to be born with allergies. Preconceptual and antenatal care can help avoid or minimise this and it is worth taking precautions if you have any history of allergy in the family, not just in the mother (> CHARITIES).

Sensitivity to allergens can vary a great deal. Some people find, for instance, that if they eliminate allergens from their own home or work environment, they can tolerate them reasonably well when they meet them elsewhere. Some people, who live abroad for a while and then return to the UK, find that their level of tolerance to native pollens can change. Other people find, however, that their sensitivity remains very high and lifelong after initial sensitisation, and they have to take extreme care to avoid allergens completely.

The immune system appears to be able to recognise molecules or substances that are related to each other. This means that you are more prone to develop an allergy to something chemically or biologically related to a substance you are already allergic to. In some people, this never happens, but in others, 'cross-reaction' or 'cross-reactivity' is quite a strong phenomenon. You may need to take care to prevent cross-reaction. (>CROSS-REACTION for full details.)

What are Allergens?

In theory, any substance can be an allergen. In practice, some substances are inherently more 'allergenic' (likely to cause allergy) than others and consistently cause more problems. The antibodies of the immune system need a physical handle to grasp on to, and certain chemical structures provide this better than others – proteins, in particular, are more allergenic than other types of molecule. Wool, for instance, is a protein, as are pollens, and these cause allergies more readily than molecules such as cotton, which is not a protein. In the case of foods, proteins are more likely to cause trouble than, say, fats or oils.

A molecule has to be above a certain size for the immune system to react to it. Chemicals are too small to trigger the immune system by themselves, but they can combine with other, larger molecules and form 'haptens', which can then trigger the system.

Anything that can be absorbed into the bloodstream can be an allergen. This means anything inhaled, swallowed, injected or absorbed through the skin or mucosa. It was commonly believed that the place where your symptoms occurred was the site of initial sensitisation. This is not now thought to be the case, since symptoms such as asthma can, in some individuals, be shown to result from substances that have been swallowed rather than inhaled. Allergens are carried by the bloodstream until they meet the place where the mast cells are located, and it is there that the reaction occurs. The most common allergens are shown in Table 1 (see Part 4 for further details). In this book, the word 'allergen' is used wherever possible to mean a substance that causes true allergy. If a food or other substance causes intolerance, or some other sensitivity reaction, they will be called 'substances that cause reactions or sensitivity'.

Inhalants

Allergy to inhalants, particles you can inhale, is usually clearly identified by skin and blood tests. The IgE mechanism appears to be principally responsible for such reactions.

Foods

Food allergy is perhaps less common than most people believe, since many cases of reaction to foods are food intolerance, rather than true allergy. Allergy to foods, rather than intolerance, will show positive results to skin and blood tests. You are likely to react whenever you eat a food to which you are allergic, even if you have not eaten it for a very long time; and you are more likely to have an immediate reaction, even to a small or tiny amount of the food. You may also be able to remember a precise date or occasion when you first reacted to a food. Food intolerance has a different pattern of reaction, and different symptoms (see page 20).

Table 1: **The Most Common Causes of Allergy**

INHALANTS	House dust mites
	Animal and pet hair
	Mould spores
	Pollens
	Feathers
	Wools
	Dusts at work
FOODS	Cow's milk, butter, cheese, yogurt
	Eggs
	Wheat
	Yeast
	Oranges, lemons, grapefruit, satsumas
	Nuts
	Beans, pulses, soya products
CHEMICALS	Formaldehyde
	Perfumes and fragrances
	Paraphenylenediamine (PPDA)
	Rubber
	Phenols and cresols
METALS	Nickel
	Chromates

Chemicals and metals

Allergy to chemicals and metals is sometimes very hard to distinguish from chemical sensitivity. In allergic contact dermatitis, where reactions are often delayed, positive results from patch tests on skin can often establish that an allergic reaction is involved. However, in many cases of asthma, eczema and dermatitis, tests are inconclusive and the dividing line between allergy and sensitivity is unclear. (See page 24 and CHEMICALS for more details.)

Food Intolerance

Food intolerance is, itself, another umbrella term, since it covers a whole range of adverse reactions to foods with a variety of causes, including:

- False food allergy
- Histamine
- Other chemicals in foods
- Enzyme defects
- Other causes

Food intolerance is also found associated with other diseases, such as rheumatoid arthritis, candidiasis, irritable bowel syndrome and Crohn's disease. Some people suffering from these diseases find the conditions improve through changes in diet, although the specific reasons for the links between such diseases and food intolerance are not known.

False Food Allergy

Some foods can trigger reactions directly in susceptible individuals. Chemical components in certain foods bind to mast cells (cells in solid tissue where IgE antibodies lodge in the case of true allergy, see page 15), which then release chemical messengers in the same way as if they had bound to IgE antibodies. However, the immune system is not actually producing antibodies, even if the resulting symptoms are identical to those of true allergy. This is known as 'false food allergy'.

False food allergy can be detected by modified versions of standard laboratory tests for true allergy. It is thought that some genetic defect or underlying nutritional deficiency might be the cause.

The chemicals in foods known to cause false food allergy are:

- *lectins* found in peanuts, beans and pulses, and wheat
- *peptides* found in egg white, shellfish, pork, fish, chocolate, tomatoes and strawberries

Other foods thought to contain substances that cause false food allergy in susceptible people are buckwheat, mango, mustard, papaya, raw pineapple and sunflower seeds. Coeliac disease, a form of wheat and gluten intolerance, is possibly caused by a related mechanism.

For the individual, the symptoms of false food allergy are the same as true allergy, and the treatment will also be much the same. The diagnosis and separate definition is valuable, however, in that it can help in planning diets that avoid potentially harmful foods.

Histamine

Some foods are naturally rich in histamine, one of the chemicals produced by the mast cells (see page 15) and responsible for some of the unpleasant effects of allergic reaction. Histamine is produced in foods that have been allowed to ferment, such as cheese, or in well-ripened foods, such as salami and sausages – especially if they are not kept very cool. Certain fish, particularly those of the mackerel family, also produce histamine if they are kept in too warm conditions. The symptoms that can be caused by histamine include vomiting, nausea, diarrhoea, rashes, headaches and reddening of the skin. These are due to a reaction to high levels of histamine acting directly on the body, not to an allergic reaction.

Other Chemicals in Foods

Histamine is a 'vasoactive amine', a type of chemical that affects the blood vessels. Other vasoactive amines – particularly tyramine, phenylethylamine and octopamine – are found in many foods and can cause direct adverse reactions – notably headaches and migraine, but also flushing and urticaria. Like histamine, tyramine is present in cheeses, and fermented and pickled foods. Other foods high in vasoactive amines include yeast extract, chocolate, bananas, avocados, wine and citrus fruits.

Another, more familiar, chemical, that is present in foods and can cause adverse reactions, is caffeine. It is found in tea and coffee, and in lower doses in chocolate and cola drinks. Some painkillers also contain caffeine. Caffeine can affect some individuals more than others. It is a powerful drug that affects the nervous system and can induce a wide range of symptoms (> SYMPTOMS).

Eating too much fruit can also be the cause of adverse food reactions, such as diarrhoea and stomach pain. Many fruits are naturally laxative. Some are well known, such as prunes, figs or rhubarb, but many others can also have this effect, especially if eaten in large quantity.

Enzyme Defects

The body requires enzymes for many of its chemical reactions. For digestion, many different enzymes are needed to help break down and metabolise foods. Some people are deficient in specific enzymes and simply cannot digest certain foods properly. A number of these defects are well known and have specific symptoms. One of the most common is a deficiency of lactase, an enzyme that breaks down lactose, the sugar found in milk and milk products. The symptoms that result are diarrhoea, wind and a distended abdomen, and this can be a very serious condition in babies. Lactase deficiency can be inherited, or it can develop later in life. Lactase levels are reduced by a stomach upset or gastro-enteritis, and lactose intolerance can follow such an illness for a temporary period. Levels of lactase decrease with age, as well, so adults can also develop the condition.

Some people cannot fully metabolise alcohol, because they lack the specific enzyme required. It is known that up to 40 per cent of Japanese people are deficient in this enzyme, and they can suffer from flushing and other symptoms.

There are other documented enzyme defects besides these, and a specialist doctor may be able to identify them if you have a clear pattern of symptoms.

Other Food Intolerance

As you can see from the above, some adverse food reactions can be explained by a number of specific causes, including allergy, chemicals naturally present in foods, and enzyme defects. However, there is a wide range of other adverse reactions to food which are not explained by the above, nor by psychological factors, and which are increasingly being shown to have a recognisable pattern of disease, and to respond to dietary management. There is no real name for this disorder or range of disorders, but the terms 'food intolerance' or 'food sensitivity' are most commonly used.

A leading specialist in the field, Dr Jonathan Brostoff, has defined such food intolerance as an 'adverse reaction in which the involvement of the immune system is unproven'; immune reactions might yet be shown to be involved and can play a role, but they are not the major factor involved. Diagnosis is difficult because:

- no single set of symptoms characterises the disorder
- symptoms can come and go
- the patient's symptoms often overlap with true food allergy

However, such food sensitivity can be recognised from its history and pattern; and diagnosis can be made from a thorough elimination diet, in which foods are left out of the diet, then reintroduced, with symptoms being carefully monitored. If you have food intolerance or sensitivity of this kind, you will initially feel worse on an elimination diet, then your symptoms should clear after a few days, often leaving you feeling better than you have done for a long time. Looking back over the history of your illness, your pattern of reactions is likely to be much more difficult to identify than that of true allergy described above; you are likely to react more slowly, rather than immediately. You are more likely to be sensitive to foods that you eat regularly, probably at each meal. Another feature of this kind of food sensitivity is that you *can* tolerate the 'problem' food or foods in small amounts; you only react when you eat it in large amounts, or very frequently.

The usual pattern of this disease is that its onset is often hard to identify. Often, people report that their symptoms were mild at first, but then steadily got worse, almost imperceptibly, until they realised that they felt generally very unwell, as well as having specific problems. Symptoms can also disappear for a while, and then come and go. New symptoms can develop over time, as well, which complicates diagnosis.

No specific symptoms characterise this disorder or disorders, which, together with the variability of symptoms, makes many doctors very sceptical of the whole problem. It is very idiosyncratic, and different individuals are affected in different organs or systems of the body.

Dr Brostoff records that the main kinds of symptoms of food intolerance are:

Headache
Migraine
Fatigue
Depression/Anxiety
Hyperactivity in children

Recurrent mouth ulcers

Aching muscles

Vomiting
Nausea
Stomach ulcers
Duodenal ulcers

Diarrhoea
Irritable bowel syndrome
Constipation
Wind, bloating
Crohn's disease

Joint pain
Rheumatoid arthritis

Oedema (water retention)

Many individuals who have sorted out their diets and eliminated trigger foods also report that other vague symptoms (such as earache, vaginal discharge and insomnia) clear up as well as their main presenting symptoms.

The results of scientific trials to identify the pattern of disease have been variable. Some trials have been flawed in their design; others have been better designed and have shown positive responses which have contradicted even the expectations of neutral or sceptical researchers. Clearly, much more work is needed before the mechanisms and causes of food sensitivity can be known.

Estimates from doctors in the field are that up to between 10 and 25 per cent of the population may have food sensitivity of this type; and that usually they are sensitive to more than one common food. Most are sensitive to between one and five foods.

Among the possible causes of food sensitivity of this kind are included the following:

- some involvement of immune system mechanisms, probably limited
- viral infections
- chemicals naturally occurring in foods producing opiates in the body
- enzyme defects causing a failure to metabolise foods
- disturbance of the natural balance of the gut following infection or use of antibiotics
- overload of the system due to chemical exposure, use of antibiotics, decline in breastfeeding and other changes in modern life

For more detailed information on adverse reactions to foods, see SYMPTOMS and FOOD AND DRINK.

Chemical Sensitivity

The field of chemical sensitivity is even less researched, and more hotly disputed, than that of food sensitivity. The dividing line between allergy and intolerance or sensitivity to chemicals is even more blurred and less understood. At the heart of the debate lie the issues of what the underlying mechanisms are, what the symptoms are, and which chemicals cause problems and why.

Chemical sensitivity encompasses a number of types of reactions, namely:

- true allergy
- false chemical allergy
- irritant and toxic reactions
- chemical sensitivity

True Allergy

Chemicals, as discussed above (see page 18), can cause true allergy by combining with other larger molecules and triggering the immune system defences. This kind of reaction can be detected by skin and laboratory tests.

False Chemical Allergy

In susceptible individuals, some chemicals, like certain foods, are able to cause false allergy by binding with mast cells (see page 15) directly and causing histamine release without engaging the immune system at all. This will cause classic allergic symptoms but will not show positive results in skin and laboratory tests.

Irritant and Toxic Reactions

Many chemicals are known to be irritant or toxic at relatively high levels. Many occupational diseases are caused by people handling materials at work, where they have a high exposure to chemicals that are relatively trouble-free at lower concentrations. Breathing problems, asthma, skin rashes and mental symptoms, such as fatigue, malaise, irritability and dizziness, as well as digestive symptoms, can be caused by chemicals at work. Chemicals known to cause such problems include:

Ammonia
Sulphur dioxide
Chlorine
Nitrogen oxide
Enzymes in detergents
Isocyanates
Platinum salts
Solder flux

Workers at, for example, a dry-cleaners, can be affected if high levels of solvents are in use. Fumes from photocopiers or printing presses, and other chemical processes, can also irritate.

Many common chemicals in household use can cause trouble if not handled with care. Washing-up liquids, soap powders, cleaners and bleaches, for instance, can cause direct irritation if you use them in concentrated fashion, inhale them directly and do not rinse well. Most people will react to concentrated doses of such common chemicals; it is not necessarily a sign of an environmental illness. The symptoms resulting will mostly be skin irritation, itchy eyes, breathing problems, and headaches.

Environmental pollution can also cause irritation, particularly to asthmatics. Weather forecasts in the UK now often include reports on 'air quality', that is on levels of sulphur dioxide, nitrogen dioxide, ozone and other chemicals in the air which can trigger reactions. Again, for many people, reactions are caused by *high levels* of chemicals, not by allergy or sensitivity.

Chemical Sensitivity

Chemical sensitivity means adverse reactions to tiny or very low levels of chemicals in the environment, in which the immune system is not demonstrably involved. Susceptible individuals will react when tested with tiny doses under controlled conditions, and they will replicate their symptoms each time they are tested. Like allergy, but unlike irritant reactions, only a tiny amount of chemical is required to trigger a reaction. Reactions usually occur immediately; delayed reactions are rare. They are caused mostly by inhaling chemicals, but also by ingesting them or by absorbing them through the skin or mucosa.

The most commonly reported symptoms of chemical sensitivity are breathing and skin disorders, and mental symptoms very similar to those reported above for toxic and irritant reactions when exposed to high levels of chemicals. Muscle spasm, muscle and joint pains, and nausea and digestive symptoms, are also often reported.

The causes of chemical sensitivity are not known, although a number of factors suggest that some form of enzyme defect or defects may be at work, whereby a susceptible individual simply does not produce the enzymes necessary to detoxify or break down chemicals absorbed into the body. Whereas most individuals can effectively metabolise chemicals at the levels normally encountered in the environment, chemically sensitive people cannot cope with even low levels of chemicals, sometimes even with minute amounts.

Another factor to consider when looking at whether or not chemicals are causing you to react is the so-called 'load effect', also known as the 'cocktail effect', which comes into play when your system is 'overloaded' with chemicals. For details, >CHEMICALS.

Which Chemicals Cause Sensitivity?

There are no hard and fast rules about which chemicals cause sensitivity. Like allergy, almost anything has been known to cause someone somewhere to react at some time, but, like allergy, certain substances are much more troublesome than others and consistently cause problems. For more detailed information and a list of chemicals that commonly cause chemical sensitivity, >CHEMICALS.

Other Environmental Illnesses

There is a range of environmental illnesses that can respond to treatment for allergy, food intolerance and chemical sensitivity, and some doctors of environmental medicine include them in their practice, the principal ones being:

- sensitivity to electro-magnetism
- seasonal affective disorder (SAD)
- occupational sensitivity (such as reactions to VDU use)
- sick building syndrome

These illnesses are beyond the scope of this book. Other such illnesses include Candidiasis (overgrowth of Candida) and Myalgo-encephalitis (ME), which are disorders that sometimes respond to treatment for allergy, food intolerance and chemical sensitivity. These conditions are included in the *Guide* wherever relevant. If you want to know more about the subject of allergy and environmental medicine, >FURTHER READING.

If You Want To Know More

If you want to know about likely symptoms, >SYMPTOMS

If you want to know if you have allergies or other forms of sensitivity, >DETECTING YOUR ALLERGIES.

If you want to know more about allergens or things that cause reactions, >CHEMICALS, FIBRES, FOOD AND DRINK, HOUSE DUST MITES, MOULDS, PETS AND OTHER ANIMALS, PLANTS AND TREES, POLLENS and MISCELLANEOUS ALLERGENS.

If you want to know how to sort out a particular area of your life, >INDEX

If you want to know what treatments there are, >MEDICAL HELP and COMPLEMENTARY THERAPY.

If you want to know who can help, >CHARITIES, SUPPORT GROUPS and FINANCIAL HELP.

Cross-Reaction

What is Cross-Reaction?

Cross-reaction, or cross-reactivity, is a phenomenon whereby if you react to a particular allergen or substance, you are prone to react to other substances that are closely related to it, biologically or chemically. In true allergy, the immune system has an ability to recognise and produce antibodies to allergens that are related. In food intolerance and chemical sensitivity, the body also seems able to recognise and react to related substances; the mechanisms for this are not known, although one hypothesis is that it is caused by enzyme defects that result in the body being unable to metabolise or detoxify specific (and related) foods or chemicals.

Only some people with allergies and related disorders are prone to cross-reaction, and people who do cross-react do not always do so; they are most susceptible when they are run down, reacting badly to another allergen, or under physical or mental stress. So you should not assume that, because you react to one thing, you will automatically react to closely-related substances. Cross-reaction is not inevitable.

An understanding of cross-reaction is only really useful in three situations, namely where:

- you know already that you cross-react to specific things;
- you have problems in working out a pattern to your reactions and suspect cross-reaction as a cause;
- you have multiple sensitivities and need to know substances are related in order to manage your condition.

ONLY READ ON if any of these three apply to you.

Which Substances Cross-React?

Certain allergens or substances are more likely to cause cross-reaction than others. Moulds, for instance, have a high degree of cross-reactivity and if you react to one particular mould, you are more likely to react to other moulds or yeasts. Grass pollens cross-react with other grass pollens. Foods are also prone to cause cross-reaction, especially between closely related foods within the same biological classification. Certain chemicals, natural and synthetic, are known to cross-react with other chemicals, drugs or foods – the active chemical in aspirin is a specific example.

Some pollens cause cross-reaction to nuts and fruits that are related to them, but, by and large, if you react to one species of pollen, there is no reason why you should cross-react to other pollens. Being allergic to grass pollen, for instance, does not pre-dispose you to react to tree pollens, say, or any other species of pollen. Similarly, being allergic to one species of animal should not make you cross-react to another species of animal, though you can react to related animals; people known to be allergic to horses have cross-reacted to donkeys, mules and zebras, which are of the same species.

Aspirin

Acetylsalicylic acid is the active chemical in aspirin. It was originally extracted from the bark of willow trees and occurs naturally as methyl salicylate, oil of wintergreen. Synonyms for acetylsalicylic acid are salicylate and salicylic acid. If you react to aspirin, you may cross-react to other drugs and painkillers containing salicylates. Your doctor or pharmacist will be able to advise you on what to avoid.

Oil of wintergreen (methyl salicylate) is used in many over-the-counter liniments, antiseptics and medicines (including sinus decongestants, sinus inhalers and rectal suppositories). Your pharmacist will be able to tell you whether a product you are using contains oil of wintergreen. It is also used as a flavouring in some toothpastes. Contact the manufacturer if you want to check any toothpaste you use.

Many foods naturally contain salicylates, especially certain fruits, spices, herbs and nuts. If you react strongly to aspirin, and still have reactions after avoiding it, it may be worth trying a diet that avoids foods rich in salicylates. However, such a diet would need to be very restrictive so it is only worth doing if you have strong motivation. It should only be undertaken with medical supervision. The foods shown in Table 2 (overleaf) are low in salicylates and should form the core of a low-salicylate diet. Those listed in Table 3 are high in salicylates and should be avoided if possible.

Chemicals

Apart from the salicylate in aspirin (see above), there are other examples of chemicals in drugs and medicines that cross-react with other

Table 2: Foods Low in Salicylates

Meat	Gin	Cabbage
Fish	Vodka	Brussels sprouts
Shellfish		Bean sprouts
	Bananas	Celery
Milk	Pears (without peel)	Leeks
Cheese	Pomegranates	Lettuce
Eggs	Mangoes	Peas
	Papaya	Potatoes (without skin)
Wheat		
Rye		
Oats		
Barley		
Rice		

(From *The Complete Guide to Food Allergy and Intolerance* by Dr Jonathan Brostoff and Linda Gamlin.)

Table 3: Foods High in Salicylates

HERBS	Mint, thyme, tarragon, rosemary, dill, sage, oregano, marjoram and basil. Also celery seed and sesame seed.
SPICES	Aniseed, cayenne, cinnamon, cumin, curry powder, fenugreek, mace, mustard, paprika and turmeric.
FRUITS AND FRUIT JUICES	
VEGETABLES	Cucumbers, gherkins, olives and endive.
NUTS	Almonds, brazil nuts, macadamia nuts, peanuts, pine nuts, pistachios, walnuts, coconuts and water chestnuts.
BEVERAGES	Coffee, tea, cola drinks and peppermint tea.
ALCOHOLIC DRINKS	
MISCELLANEOUS	Honey, liquorice, peppermint; yeast extract, stock cubes and yeast products; tomato sauce; many processed foods and instant meals.

(From *The Complete Guide to Food Allergy and Intolerance* by Dr Jonathan Brostoff and Linda Gamlin.)

substances. Your doctor or pharmacist will be able to advise you on possible cross-reactions to drugs, but the following gives details of the most common.

If you are sensitive to mould-based antibiotics, such as the penicillins or the cephalosporins, you may also be sensitive to inhalant moulds or moulds in food. Not all antibiotics are synthesised from moulds, however, so this does not mean you will react to all antibiotics (>MOULDS for more details). Moreover, you can be sensitive to one type of penicillin without reacting to every penicillin.

Ethylenediamine is a solvent and emulsifying chemical that is used in topical preparations (for instance, in Mycolog or Nystatin). People with dermatitis have been known to cross-react to ethylenediamine if they use some topical anti-histamines that are chemically related.

Phenothiazine drugs are known to produce dermatitis and photosensitivity reactions (in which reactions are triggered in the presence of certain kinds of light, >FURTHER READING). Phenothiazine is used as an anti-parasite drug and as an insecticide. Its derivative, chlorpromazine, is a tranquilliser. These drugs are also known to cross-react with phenothiazine-based anti-histamines such as Phenergan.

A drug called Antabuse (given as an aid in the treatment of alcoholism) cross-reacts with thiram, a chemical used as a rubber accelerator, and found commonly in footwear, gloves and condoms. Thiram is also used as a fungicide, an insecticide and a germicide.

Of other widely used chemicals, paraphenylenediamine (PPDA) is well known to cause allergic reactions, and has a wide range of cross-reactions. PPDA itself is found in hair dyes, elastic, shoes, printers' ink and photographic developing agents. It cross-reacts with azo dyes, which comprise a significant share of all textile dyes, and are used almost entirely on synthetic fibres. It also cross-reacts with benzocaine, a topical anaesthetic, and procaine, an injectable local anaesthetic, as well as to sulphonamide drugs which inhibit bacterial growth. It also cross-reacts with isopropyl-n-phenyl paraphenylenediamine (IPPD), an antioxidant found in black rubber.

Foods

Opinion among doctors and experts as to the degree of cross-reaction between foods varies widely; you will often encounter differing (sometimes conflicting) advice on which foods cross-react.

Foods, as all living things, are classified biologically into groups and sub-groups according to their inter-relationships. These categories include 'family' and 'sub-family' groupings. It is argued that cross-reaction is more likely to occur within a food family, and diets may be planned and managed on this basis. If you are on a rotation diet (see page 148), for instance, you will often be advised to leave an interval of two days or more between eating foods that belong to the same family. This can be quite restrictive.

In practice, the family model is not always helpful. Some families, such as the legume family, which includes peas, beans, pulses and peanuts, are very broad. Some foods within such a family are very distantly related, and cross-reaction can be rare. Sometimes cross-reaction only occurs consistently within sub-families. The grass family includes the wheat sub-family, the corn sub-family, and the rice sub-family, and cross-reaction often occurs within the sub-families, but less commonly between them. If you react to wheat, for example, you are more likely to cross-react to oats, which is part of its sub-family, than to rice, which is related but belongs to a separate sub-family.

Moreover, in the case of some highly allergenic foods, such as fish, birds' eggs, birds and nuts, some people appear to react to *all* types of the food, irrespective of the family from which they come, and managing the families of these food types has no relevance at all for these individuals.

Like many aspects of allergy and sensitivity, the cross-reaction of foods can be very confusing, and you will probably have to work out for yourself, with expert guidance, what you tolerate and what causes cross-reaction in *you*.

The best way to deal with the question of food cross-reaction is probably to adopt a strict and conservative approach initially, when you are first working out what you react to. On an elimination diet (or on a rotation diet, if this is advised), start by being careful about the food families, and then relax gradually in order to find out what you can tolerate. You may not need to observe the families at all eventually. (For full advice on planning diets, >FOOD AND DRINK; for a full list of food families, >FURTHER READING.)

Some foods contain moulds and can cause cross-reaction (see **Moulds**, below). Oils and terpenes in foods can also cause cross-reaction (see **Plants**, below). Some foods cross-react with pollen (see **Tree Pollens**, below).

Moulds

Moulds have a high degree of cross-reactivity and if you know you are allergic to one mould, you are likely to react to other moulds or yeasts. Some foods *are* moulds or yeasts (fungi), such as mushrooms and yeast, and other foods *contain* moulds or yeasts, although they are not fungi by biological classification. These foods include, among others, all cheeses (except cottage cheese), yeast bakery, vinegar, alcohol and malt.

Moulds in foods can explain cross-reaction to foods. Following a mould-free diet, and following the advice for eliminating moulds from your environment, may help control reactions (>MOULDS).

If you suffer from candidiasis (overgrowth of Candida), you can be allergic to the yeast Candida itself, as well as experiencing symptoms specific to candidiasis (>SYMPTOMS). Candida can also cross-react with moulds; following the mould-free diet and elimination programme (>MOULDS) can sometimes help. The mould-free diet is distinct from the anti-Candida diet which eliminates foods which feed the yeast (>FOOD AND DRINK).

For information on *mould-based antibiotics*, see **Chemicals** (above) and MOULDS (page 201).

Plants

Sensitivity to plants can cause cross-reaction to other plants, foods or chemicals. The cause is thought to be closely related chemicals that occur naturally within them. Some of the principal plants and plant products known to cause cross-reaction in people with dermatitis are:

Turpentine

This is a natural resin derived from pines, but it can also be produced synthetically. In cases of dermatitis, it is known to cross-react with Balsam of Peru (see below), benzoin (found in tinctures, creams and many home medicines), and the chrysanthemum family (see below). It may cross react with orange and lemon peel. Turpentine is widely used in cosmetics, polishes, varnishes, paint thinners and anything pine-scented.

Balsam of Peru

Produced by cutting wounds in the bark of a Latin American tree, this balsam has an aromatic smell, resembling cinnamon. It contains a number of chemicals known to cause allergy, including cinnamic acid. It is used widely in perfumery and cosmetics, and as a flavouring agent in confectionery, preserves and bakery. It is also used in topical medications and in suppositories.

Balsam of Peru cross-reacts with benzoin (see **Turpentine**, above), numerous essential oils, orange peel, cinnamon, cloves, turpentine, wood tars and eugenol (found in many spice oils, perfumes, and as a flavouring agent in foods and toothpastes). It also cross-reacts with rosin (used in adhesive tapes, paper coating and size, glues, adhesives, varnishes, depilatory wax, cosmetics, cements and chewing-gum, and many other items). Balsam of Peru also cross-reacts with resorcinal monobenzoate (RMB), a chemical used in the production of plastic resins and adhesives.

Chrysanthemum and pyrethrum

Chrysanthemum and pyrethrum (often used as an insecticide in organic gardening) are members of the *Chrysanthemum* genus and are thought to cause dermatitis by cross-reaction. They may also cross-react with turpentine (see above) and with arnica and camomile, both members of the same biological family.

Cashew nut and mango

These are members of the same family as poison ivy, which is probably the single largest cause of dermatitis in the United States. They can cross-react with each other, and with other members of their family, including the Japanese lacquer-tree (used to produce furniture lacquer) and the marking nut tree of India (producing black marking ink for laundry). Cashew oil is used in producing some phenol formaldehyde resins for clothing (>CLOTHING), in printers' ink and in varnishes.

Tree Pollens

Some tree pollens cross-react with certain nuts and fruits. You may get a reaction when you eat these foods if you are allergic to the relevant pollens.

Allergy to beech pollen can make you cross-react to hazelnuts. Allergy to walnut pollen can make you cross-react to walnuts. Allergy to birch pollen can cause cross-reaction to hazelnuts, to apples, and to peaches, cherries, pears and carrots.

For more information on tree pollens, >POLLENS.

Multiple Sensitivity

This section deals with the areas of 'multiple allergies' and 'multiple sensitivity'. It covers issues such as why some people have a tendency to develop many and multiple sensitivities; how you can work out what is upsetting you if you have multiple sensitivity; how to live and cope with your situation.

What is Multiple Sensitivity?

If you have an allergy to something specific (a food, chemical or inhalant, for instance), it is common to develop allergies to other substances, especially if you have a high level of exposure to them. This pre-disposition to develop further allergies is well documented and runs in families. Some people with a specific allergy never develop an allergy to anything else, but many do.

People suffering from chemical sensitivity and food intolerance, which are disorders in which your system reacts to chemicals and foods without the involvement of the immune system (>DEFINING ALLERGY for a full description), also show a marked tendency to develop further sensitivities. Furthermore, there is in some people an apparent link between all three – allergy, chemical sensitivity and food intolerance. These individuals develop very widespread multiple sensitivity to all kinds of things, which seem to aggravate each other. In some cases, people appear to become sensitive to virtually everything around them. This type of reaction has been given various titles, including 'multiple sensitivity', 'multiple allergy syndrome' and 'total allergy syndrome'. People who react in this way are sometimes called 'universal reactors'.

In some cases, this condition can be disabling and severe in its impact. In other cases, even though the person has widespread intolerance and sensitivity, the symptoms can be managed and people can live reasonably normal lives.

Why some people should develop multiple allergies or sensitivity (however widespread or severe) is not fully understood, although it is well observed. One theory, for which there is some supporting evidence, is that the people concerned have enzyme defects as well as the hypersensitivity of the immune system characteristic of true allergy.

This, it is argued, leads to far-reaching intolerance; failure to metabolise many substances eaten, absorbed, or inhaled; and competition for vitamins and minerals which act as catalysts or essential components in the body's detoxifying systems. Demand for vitamins and minerals can then be further undermined by poor nutrition resulting from a restricted diet, if people have food sensitivity, or from malabsorption. Other theories suggest that some parasite, unresolved virus or infection may contribute, or be the fundamental cause.

How to Avoid Multiple Sensitivity

Whatever the cause of multiple sensitivity, the advice that doctors give on the need to avoid allergens and other substances is based upon the value of avoidance measures in preventing and controlling multiple sensitivity. Avoidance can help prevent you developing new sensitivities, and can control and help you live with multiple sensitivity if you know you are already prone to it.

Managing Your Load

The term that is commonly used is 'managing your load'. Most people with multiple allergies or sensitivity find that they get worse at times when their load of allergens or other substances is high. For instance, people allergic to pollens sometimes find that their other allergies (such as to foods, house dust mites or pets) become noticeable or worse during the pollen season, whereas they cause no trouble or can be controlled at other times of the year. People who have food allergy or intolerance usually find they start reacting badly to multiple foods or chemicals, or other allergens, if they are eating a lot of the foods that upset them, but that the severity of the reactions declines, or they disappear altogether, if they keep to a strict diet. People sensitive to chemicals find they start reacting to many things if they have high levels of exposure – say, after a long car journey, or after decorating – but that their system calms down again if they keep their general exposure low.

You can use the avoidance process to manage your sensitivity if you know you react to many things. It can sometimes be hard to sort things out and to adapt your life, but avoidance actually works. It can prevent, especially with babies and children, and it can alleviate and cure. For some severely ill people, it is their only route to improvement in symptoms. It can mean a substantial reduction in the drugs that they take, and a return to something close to a tolerable life.

Even if you are not severely ill, you are likely to benefit from avoidance if you have any tendency to multiple sensitivity. The best route is to reduce your overall load of allergens and things that cause you to react.

Reducing Your Load

Reducing your load of common allergens, taking certain precautions with general diet, and limiting your exposure to chemicals can help generally in managing multiple sensitivity, and in preventing further allergies developing if you or your family have the tendency.

House dust mites and moulds both thrive in damp, poorly aired environments. Keep your surroundings as dry, warm, and aired as you are able to help keep them at bay. Ventilate properly and, in particular, keep beds and bedding (which harbour mites and moulds) aired and dry. Dry laundry (and anything else damp) outside the home and avoid creating damp and steam where possible. Gas and paraffin fires, heaters and cookers create damp when burning and it is best either to avoid their use altogether, or to take extra care in ventilating and removing condensation if you do use them.

To remove allergens, and to avoid dispersing them when cleaning, use filters on a vacuum cleaner or a special vacuum cleaner. This helps enormously to protect against all kinds of allergen which are usually blown back into a room by the exhaust. Over time, vacuuming with filters helps to remove allergens already lodged in furniture, flooring and furnishings. (>VACUUM CLEANERS for full advice). Also 'damp dust' – do the dusting with a cloth that is slightly damp, so that dust and allergens do not disperse into the air.

Avoid keeping pets and animals if you can. If you do have pets, make sure that they sleep outside the home, if possible. Above all, do not let them sleep on beds or in bedrooms (even during the day).

If you are allergic to pollen or mould spores, take care about going out at seasons when they are present at a high level in the air (>POLLENS and MOULDS for details). Keep windows and doors closed as much as you can during peak periods.

To help prevent food sensitivity, vary your diet and limit the frequency at which you eat the most allergenic foods – wheat, eggs, corn, cow's milk, nuts, citrus fruit, yeast, fish, beans and pulses. With other foods, do not eat the same foods repeatedly each day; keep the whole diet full of choice and variety. Eat fresh and wholesome food and keep your use of processed food to a minimum. Sort out your diet properly if you need to, and avoid any foods that clearly upset you – even if you love and crave them. Variety plus avoidance of trouble-makers will do more than anything to reduce your tendency to react generally.

Keep your use of any chemicals to the absolute minimum. Think before you use anything on yourself, your home, or at work or school. Do you really need it or is there a less aggressive alternative? Stop smoking and avoid smoky atmospheres. Take care with perfumed products of any kind. Air and wash anything new, and avoid situations or places where chemical fumes are high.

If You Want To Go Further

If you know that you react to many things and that basic avoidance has not helped very much, you will probably need specialist help and advice. If you need advice on medical treatments, >MEDICAL HELP. >also COMPLEMENTARY THERAPY.

Skin and laboratory tests can help to identify what substances you are allergic to, although they will not help with chemical sensitivity or food intolerance. >DETECTING YOUR ALLERGIES, which will also help you work out what might cause your problems in different areas of your life, and help identify patterns of symptoms.

If you want to take the process of elimination and avoidance much further, and clear your environment of the things that cause you to react, use the other sections of this *Guide* to help you with thorough avoidance. Choose *either* an area of life where you have the most pressing problems (for instance, BEDDING or CLOTHING), *or* a type of allergen or substance that seems to be particularly troublesome. Only investigate *one* area or type of allergen at a time – you will get very confused results if you are eliminating many things at once and you do indeed have multiple sensitivity. You may find the process compli-cated in that your symptoms may not totally disappear when you remove only one cause from around you, but you should always notice some difference, and usually some improvement, when you avoid one thing, as long as it is something that causes you to react. If you notice no change or disturbance at all in your symptoms, then you are unlikely to be sensitive to the one thing you have chosen to avoid.

This phenomenon of 'masking', or the symptoms of multiple sensitivities hiding or blurring each other, is one of the most difficult things to untangle when you start avoiding things. Often, when you avoid and eliminate one allergen or substance, you find that another starts to bother you more intensely than before, as if its effects have been unmasked by the removal of the first substance.

Some people also find, when unravelling multiple sensitivity, that they become *unusually* sensitive and react very intensely to things around them, as if their systems have been stressed or de-stabilised. It is common to appear to be sensitive to many things while eliminating and unmasking, but your system will eventually settle down and tolerate things again, once you have sorted out the true troublemakers and are avoiding them.

If this happens to you while in the process of sorting yourself out, take a deep breath and *do not panic*. Some of the things you are reacting to (especially foods and chemicals) may well be temporary intolerances and could go away with time. *Concentrate on avoiding the things that upset you particularly badly* – reduce your overall load of allergens and substances generally and do not assume that you will be hypersensitive for ever more. Many reactions will be just temporary. Multiple sensitivity is not an automatic life sentence and it is rarely crippling. Stay calm and you will come through. *Never throw anything away* until you are absolutely sure that you do not tolerate it permanently. It is common to find that you can use or wear something for a while and then become sensitive to it again. If you leave it off for a time and then try once more, often you can tolerate it after the break. Some people use this process to help them cope with multiple sensitivity – rotating the fibres of the clothes or bedding they use, or keeping curtains, rugs or pieces of furniture in a spare room and bringing them out for short periods. So, put things away in a spare room, outhouse or attic, and give them a rest before you test them again.

TIP

Borrow whatever you can to save money when you are testing things out, but take care that anything you borrow is not washed or treated with any product you do not tolerate. Watch out for dust mites, moulds, pet debris or tobacco smoke. Air, vacuum and wash anything you can before using it.

How to Cope with Multiple Sensitivity

Managing your load is the main principle, again, of coping with multiple sensitivity. Keep the load of allergens and substances that upset you as low as you are reasonably able. Keep other stresses as low as you can, as well – multiple allergies and sensitivity can be noticeably aggravated by unhappiness, loneliness, worry, grief, conflict, family troubles and other stresses.

Your attitude to your own situation can also help. The terms 'total allergy syndrome' or 'universal reactor' dramatise the situation and are not always helpful. By themselves, they can make you feel depressed and demotivated. Many people with multiple sensitivity have days (or even weeks) when they feel they react to absolutely everything – when *nothing* is safe and everything seems to upset. These times can be very hard to bear (and very scaring), but they usually pass or things get much better – they virtually never persist. In many situations, you will be able to tolerate reasonably well things that at other times lay you completely low. Psychologically, it helps a great deal, therefore, to avoid talking about 'being allergic to everything', 'being a universal reactor' or of 'nothing being safe', and to use a different vocabulary and to see the world in terms of things that you do tolerate and things that you do not tolerate. You will probably *tolerate* quite well something to which you are strictly speaking allergic or sensitive, if you avoid it much of the time, or avoid situations in which it is at its peak. That particular thing is not totally 'safe' for you, but it can be 'tolerable' and you may be able to live with it quite well. This type of approach helps you to perceive the world as a less hostile, aggressive place and to deal better with your situation.

If you are very severely affected by multiple sensitivity, reaching a balance in your life may mean major changes and upheavals – giving up things that you enjoy, changing things that you do. You will inevitably have to make compromises in order to make a living or meet the requirements of your job or home life.

It is easy to become very isolated and confined if your life is restricted by your sensitivities, particularly if you cannot go out or mix easily with other people. Support and counselling can help: ask your doctor, or contact an allergy charity or support group. Some of these have telephone networks for people who are confined to home (>CHARITIES and SUPPORT GROUPS).

If you can manage it, it also helps to develop interests or contacts outside your illness. So few people understand how severe multiple allergy and sensitivity can be that it becomes easier to mix only with people who understand, but this in itself can be confining and cut you off from the world. You may be better mixing more widely, even doing things that upset you, in order to stay in touch and lead as close to a normal life as possible. It can help to keep you happy and sane.

Part 3
HOW DO I KNOW IF I HAVE ALLERGIES?

Symptoms

This section describes the symptoms of:

- allergy
- food intolerance
- chemical sensitivity

For definitions of these conditions, >DEFINING ALLERGY.

Before You Read On

You should take medical advice before trying to identify for yourself the cause of symptoms you think are related to an allergic or sensitivity reaction. Many symptoms – such as headache, breathlessness, gut pain and diarrhoea – can be caused by other diseases and you need to be sure that other possible causes have been ruled out.

Some reactions to things you inhale, swallow or touch are entirely normal. The body has normal defence mechanisms to protect it. It is usual for anyone to sneeze or cough, or for your eyes to run, if you encounter a lot of dust and particles. Most people also find that strong household chemicals or DIY materials irritate their breathing passages, give them a sore throat or headache, or make their hands sore. Only if your reactions make you feel very unwell, and affect your system for quite a while afterwards, or if you are affected by minute amounts, should you suspect sensitivity or allergy. If your symptoms are not severe or long-term, they are probably a natural response.

Hyperventilation and withdrawal symptoms often accompany reactions, or follow soon afterwards. The symptoms of these can be confused with true reactions. See page 50 for detailed descriptions of the symptoms of hyperventilation and withdrawal.

Allergy

The main symptoms of true allergy are shown in Diagram 2 (overleaf). Allergy can be caused by any kind of substance, but inhaled particles, such as dust mites, pollens and moulds, are the most common. Foods and chemicals can also cause allergy. The symptoms are caused by

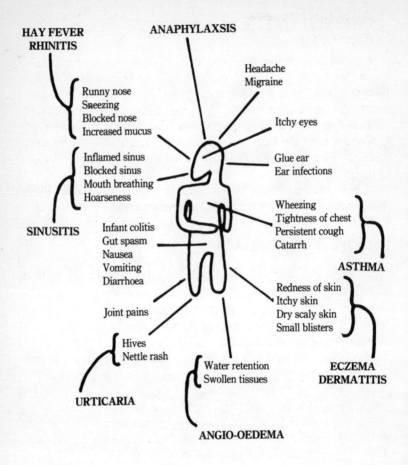

Diagram 2: **The Symptoms of Allergy**

the release of chemical messengers in the body which bring about (either immediately, or after some delay):

- dilating of small blood vessels
- spasm or contraction of smooth muscle
- an increase in secretions, such as mucus

The classic allergic diseases are:

- angio-oedema
- asthma
- eczema
- dermatitis

- hay fever
- rhinitis
- urticaria

Allergic Diseases

Angio-Oedema

Angio-oedema (water retention) is characterised by puffiness and swelling of the tissues and deeper levels of skin. As small blood vessels enlarge in an allergic reaction, fluid escapes from them into the surrounding tissues and causes the swelling. This can be painful and give a burning sensation. The swelling is commonly found around the face, lips, tongue, eyes, and also in the hands, feet and legs. Occasionally, it can be dangerous if it causes blockage of the airways.

Angio-oedema often accompanies urticaria (see below); like urticaria, it can be caused by false allergy reactions (see pages 20 and 25) to foods and chemicals. Aspirin is a common trigger.

Asthma

If you have asthma, you may experience one or more of the following symptoms:

- wheezing
- shortness of breath
- constriction of the chest
- cough

These symptoms can also be caused by other diseases, such as bronchitis or heart disease; asthma can be distinguished by measuring changes in the diameter of the airways of the lungs. Severe asthma is readily recognised, but mild asthma can go unidentified. Tightness of the chest, and shortness of breath are often accepted as normal, or go unperceived. A dry, persistent cough, especially in children, can often be a symptom of mild asthma. In a severe attack, a dry cough often becomes productive as phlegm is produced.

Asthma can occur immediately on meeting an allergen, or as a late phase reaction several hours later. Attacks are often bad late at night; this is linked to changes in the blood levels of a hormone, adrenalin.

Asthma is not always caused by an allergic reaction. It can be triggered by irritants, such as smoke or fumes. Cold air, exercise, or a viral infection can all cause asthma without allergy being involved. Stress, particularly emotional stress and anxiety, can also trigger or aggravate asthma.

Asthma can also be a symptom of food intolerance, chemical sensitivity, or of false allergy reactions to foods and chemicals.

Eczema and Dermatitis

Atopic eczema is principally a disease of infancy and childhood. 'Atopic' means the condition is likely to have been inherited; the disease often runs in families. Red itchy patches show first on the skin on the chin and cheeks, spreading next to the trunk. The creases around knees, wrists and ankles are also vulnerable. The skin is very itchy and the redness increases. Vesicles (blisters) can form which weep and bleed if scratched, and the skin can become infected, causing further complications. As children age, the skin can become thickened and leathery. In adults, the skin does not generally ooze but the skin is thickened. The condition in adults is often called dermatitis rather than eczema. Skin and blood tests for allergy are often negative in cases of eczema, but if there is a family history of allergy, and clear trigger factors are identified, allergy will be diagnosed.

In atopic contact dermatitis, the symptoms are very similar to those of atopic eczema, but they occur on the skin in the places where it has come into contact with the allergen. This is a different type of allergic reaction from the principal IgE reaction (see page 15); it is often a delayed reaction, and can be reliably detected by patch testing.

In irritant eczema, the symptoms are again similar to atopic eczema and are caused by contact with substances such as washing powder, detergents, or occupational chemicals. In people with atopic eczema, such irritants can exacerbate their basic disease and need to be avoided even though they do not cause allergy. Like atopic eczema, irritant eczema will respond to treatment with moisturising creams and topical medication, whereas contact dermatitis invariably will not.

Hay Fever and Rhinitis

Rhinitis means inflammation of the nose. Allergic rhinitis can occur seasonally (hay fever) or all year round (perennial). The most obvious symptoms of rhinitis are sneezing, a runny nose and itchy eyes. The tissues of the upper breathing passages, the nose and the eyes become swollen and inflamed; wider effects can be caused in the sinuses and ears. Symptoms also include a blocked nose with swollen tissues; blowing the nose does not relieve symptoms at all. Blocked passages can lead to headaches, disturbed sleep and puffiness around the eyes. Another characteristic sign of rhinitis are so-called 'allergy shiners', big black rings under the eyes where the nasal passages are chronically inflamed.

In babies, a persistent snuffle, breathing through the mouth, and difficulty in sucking, can sometimes be an early sign of rhinitis. In children, typical signs of rhinitis are recurrent head colds, mouth breathing, and habitual rubbing of the nose. Glue ear, and recurrent ear infections, can also be a complication of rhinitis.

Rhinitis can also be caused by food intolerance, chemical sensitivity and false allergy reactions to foods and chemicals.

Urticaria

Also known as nettle rash or hives, this is an acute eruption of groups of pale blisters, surrounded by a red itchy flare, similar to a nettle sting. Usually, the blisters are small, but sometimes a few very large blisters can appear. Only the upper layer of the skin is affected. Urticaria appears suddenly and seldom lasts for more than a few hours, though it can last for up to 48 hours. The condition may be accompanied by fever, faintness and nausea.

Acute urticaria can be triggered by non-allergic causes, such as exercise, cold, sunlight, and sudden shock or nervous strain. It is also commonly caused by false food and chemical allergy – aspirin and some food additives are often associated with triggering non-allergic urticaria. Chronic or long-lasting urticaria is rarely caused by allergy.

Other allergic symptoms are headache or migraine; itchy eyes or conjunctivitis; gut spasm, nausea, vomiting and diarrhoea. Infant colic can sometimes be caused by allergy (>BABYCARE). Joint pains sometimes accompany other allergic symptoms. Allergy is also among the possible causes of persistent coughs, sinusitis, and of glue ear and chronic infections of the middle ear – resulting from inflammation and swelling of tissues and the collection of mucus.

Anaphylaxsis, sometimes called anaphylactic shock, is the most severe type of allergic reaction, and extremely rare. It is most unlikely ever to happen to you. It is a violent, massive reaction to an allergen – often immediate, and usually in response to something swallowed or injected – a food, a drug or an insect sting. Its symptoms can include urticaria; swelling of the tongue, mouth, throat and breathing passages; nausea, vomiting, gut pain and diarrhoea; a sudden drop in blood pressure. Unconsciousness and even death can follow. Urgent medical attention is required. (>EMERGENCY INFORMATION for more advice on how to be prepared.)

The symptoms of allergy overlap to some degree with those of food intolerance and chemical sensitivity. Skin and blood tests can go some way to identifying allergy, but understanding the pattern of your symptoms, and knowing where allergens and other substances causing reactions are found, can often help you better to identify the cause of trouble. (>DETECTING YOUR ALLERGIES for more information.) The conditions are not mutually exclusive; you can have an allergy as well as having intolerance or sensitivity.

For information on treatment and therapy to help with the symptoms of allergy, >MEDICAL HELP.

Food Intolerance

Some reactions to food are caused by false food allergy and by reactions to chemicals, such as histamine and tyramine, that occur naturally in food (>FOOD INTOLERANCE, page 20).

The main symptoms caused by the principal types of food intolerance are shown in Diagram 3. You may find you suffer from one or more of these symptoms. Symptoms can come and go, or you may only react to a food if you eat large amounts of it, or if you eat it regularly.

Another characteristic of the symptoms of food intolerance is that if you leave out a food that you eat regularly for a while, and then reintroduce it, you can experience different, often intense, symptoms. This is the result of a phenomenon known as 'masking'. People who are intolerant of a food they eat regularly, even several times a day, often complain of constant, background symptoms, such as exhaustion, muscle aches, indigestion and headaches, that they have learned to live with. These symptoms disappear when they leave out the food causing the trouble. On reintroduction of the food, some people, *not all*, find they experience symptoms that are not the same as the background, masked symptoms they were used to, but which are quite clearly linked to the reintroduced food. These unmasked reactions can be very strong. Conversely, it is also common that, if people with food intolerance of this kind leave the offending food out of their diet for some time, they can then eat it again without problems. Masking is also common in people with multiple sensitivities. (>MULTIPLE SENSITIVITY for more details.)

Withdrawal symptoms can result if you stop eating a food that you eat regularly, or the day after you eat a food that you only have every so often (see box, on page 50).

Hyperventilation is common in some people with food intolerance,

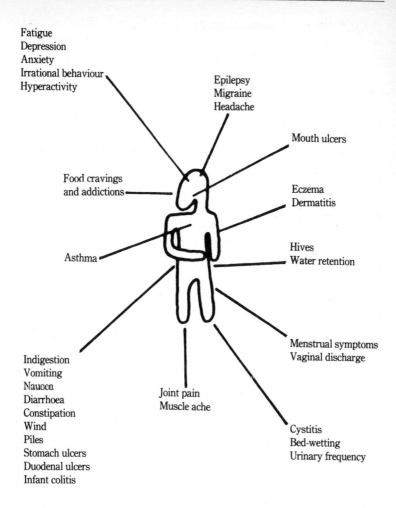

Fatigue
Depression
Anxiety
Irrational behaviour
Hyperactivity

Epilepsy
Migraine
Headache

Mouth ulcers

Food cravings
and addictions

Eczema
Dermatitis

Hives
Water retention

Asthma

Indigestion
Vomiting
Nausea
Diarrhoea
Constipation
Wind
Piles
Stomach ulcers
Duodenal ulcers
Infant colitis

Joint pain
Muscle ache

Menstrual symptoms
Vaginal discharge

Cystitis
Bed-wetting
Urinary frequency

Diagram 3: **The Symptoms of Food Intolerance**

or sometimes accompanies a food intolerance reaction. This can be
mistaken for the symptoms of a reaction itself (see box on page 50).

Some people develop food intolerance in association with other diseases, such as candidiasis, Crohn's disease, irritable bowel syndrome
and rheumatoid arthritis (see box on page 51).

Coeliac disease is a disease caused by intolerance of gluten (found in
wheat, rye, barley and oats), which damages the lining membrane of
the small intestine, and thus interferes with the absorption of fat. Its
symptoms are distinctive and usually occur in infants soon after the
foods are introduced into their diet. These babies have wind, bloating,

Withdrawal Symptoms

These can occur when you totally avoid something to which you are sensitive or allergic. You may notice them, for instance, after you eat a food that you rarely eat, or after an unusual exposure to chemicals, e.g. the day after decorating, or after a long car or train journey.

If you go on an elimination diet to identify trigger foods, or if you fast totally, you will have no withdrawal symptoms if you have no food sensitivities. If you are food sensitive, you may well experience withdrawal symptoms for a few days, or even up to 14 days.

Withdrawal symptoms can be mild or quite severe. They are not dissimilar from a hangover, or from withdrawal from addictive drugs. The most commonly reported are aches in the hips, thighs and legs; headaches; insomnia or sleepiness; fatigue; lethargy; irritability; restlessness; nausea; sweating; shivering; palpitations; racing pulse; skin rashes; muscle and joint aches.

Hyperventilation

Hyperventilation, or overbreathing, is sometimes found in people who are sensitive to foods and chemicals. If you breathe too fast, this causes the levels of carbon dioxide in the blood to drop, and increases the acidity of the blood. This induces a wide range of symptoms including choking, chest pains, palpitations, dizziness, aching muscles, tremors and cramps, numbness, pins and needles, a sense of unreality, and panic attacks. These symptoms can be mistaken for symptoms of allergy and other sensitivities.

To see if you are hyperventilating, hold a paper or cloth bag over your nose and mouth, and breathe in and out for some time. If you inhale the air in the bag, you are breathing carbon dioxide back in, raising the level in your blood. If this improves your symptoms, then hyperventilation may be their cause.

Hyperventilation can clear up of its own accord if you identify and avoid substances that cause your reactions. Alternatively, breathing exercises can help you learn to breathe properly again. Your doctor can refer you to a physiotherapist for help with this.

Diseases Associated with Food Intolerance

Candidiasis

Candida is a yeast that is found naturally in the gut. In some people, the natural balance of the gut is disturbed and candida overgrows. This is called candidiasis and can cause various symptoms, sometimes severe. Some people with food sensitivity and chemical sensitivity have candidiasis as well and the symptoms can be confused. In some people, treating the Candida overgrowth can improve their tolerance of foods and chemicals.

Candida infections are found in the gut, throat, mouth, anal passages, vagina and in damp areas of the skin. Thrush is the name for candida infections in the mouth and vagina.

The principal symptoms of candidiasis are thrush, itchy anus, cystitis, bloating, diarrhoea, recurrent fungal infections of the skin, headache, migraine, joint pains, aching muscles, eczema, psoriasis, sinusitis and nappy rash in babies. Craving for sweet foods is also a primary characteristic. You can be allergic to the yeast Candida itself, in which case you will experience the usual symptoms of allergy.

Crohn's Disease

This is a serious and unpleasant illness in which there is inflammation of an area of the small intestine. This induces cramps, diarrhoea, abdominal pain, irregularity of the bowels, slight fever and malaise. Weight loss and malabsorption of food follow. Some doctors have found that people with Crohn's disease respond well to treatment for food intolerance.

Irritable Bowel Syndrome (IBS)

This covers a range of minor disorders of the gut, characterised by abnormal bowel function. Although the disease is not serious, its effects can be distressing and debilitating. Some people with IBS suffer mild diarrhoea, with gut pain and occasional constipation. Others suffer constipation frequently, with bloating and wind, and occasionally have diarrhoea. The symptoms often start after an intestinal infection. They rarely affect general health, and do not get worse or produce other symptoms as time goes by.

Rheumatoid Arthritis

This is a disease in which the joints and the surrounding tissues become inflamed and painful. It usually manifests itself first in the small joints of the hand, and is gradual in onset. The joints are painful, red, swollen and warm to the touch. Symptoms are usually worse in the morning. The normal course of the disease is to spread slowly to other joints, reaching the larger ones, such as the hip or shoulder, last of all. The joints become fixed and more swollen over time with wasting of the muscles and show characteristic changes under X-ray. The diagnosis of rheumatoid arthritis is confirmed by specific blood tests. Some people with rheumatoid arthritis respond to treatment for food intolerance.

and their stools are pale and smelly; the babies usually fail to grow. If the disease develops in adulthood, the symptoms are diarrhoea, gut pain, bloating, weakness and weight loss.

Hyperactivity in children has been linked to food intolerance and to chemical sensitivity (>CHILDCARE).

People with food intolerance who have sorted out their diets often report that a number of symptoms other than the main ones clear up once they exclude their problem foods. These are not formally recognised as symptoms of food intolerance, but they are so commonly reported by people that they are taken seriously as indicators of food intolerance. These can include excessive weight swings (more than 0.5 kg/1 lb gain or loss per day); irritability and mood swings; body odour; flushing and excessive sweating; difficulty in controlling body temperature; feeling too cold or too hot; food cravings; excessive thirst; insomnia.

So-called 'allergy shiners', big black rings under the eyes, are often typical of the allergy or intolerance sufferer. These often disappear once problem foods are removed from the diet.

Chemical Sensitivity

Some reactions to chemicals, especially contact dermatitis, are caused by allergy (see box on page 46, for details). Other reactions can be caused by false allergy, whereby chemicals can directly trigger the release of chemical messengers and cause symptoms (see **Food Intolerance**, page 20).

The principal symptoms of chemical sensitivity are shown in Diagram 4. Most reactions are caused by *inhaling* traces of chemicals, and are usually immediate. As with food intolerance, hyperventilation and withdrawal symptoms are common with chemical sensitivity (see boxes on page 50).

Other indicators of chemical sensitivity include an abnormal sense

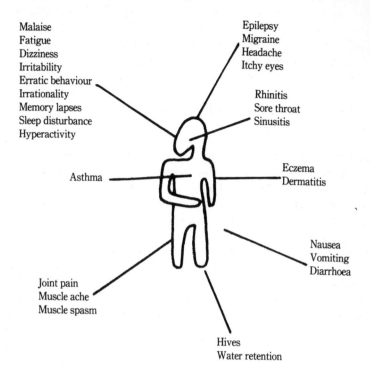

Malaise
Fatigue
Dizziness
Irritability
Erratic behaviour
Irrationality
Memory lapses
Sleep disturbance
Hyperactivity

Epilepsy
Migraine
Headache
Itchy eyes

Rhinitis
Sore throat
Sinusitis

Asthma

Eczema
Dermatitis

Nausea
Vomiting
Diarrhoea

Joint pain
Muscle ache
Muscle spasm

Hives
Water retention

Diagram 4: **The Symptoms of Chemical Sensitivity**

of smell – either peculiarly heightened or totally absent. People also report addictions or aversions to the smell of chemicals to which they are sensitive. 'Allergy shiners', big black rings under the eyes, are also a frequent indicator of chemical sensitivity. Poor tolerance of alcohol is often common in chemically sensitive people.

Trigger Factors

Certain factors can trigger allergic and sensitivity reactions. Stress on your system can set off a reaction where normally you would be fine. Physical trigger factors can include getting too hot or cold, excessive exercise, a viral infection, and allowing blood sugar levels to get too low or too high. Many women find their symptoms only appear, or get worse, at times of hormonal change – at menstruation, at ovulation in mid-cycle, after childbirth. A significant number find they develop symptoms for the first time at the menopause, or after hysterectomy.

Emotional or mental stress can also play a part in setting things off. Overwork, anxiety, bereavement, money worries, depression – all of these can trigger reactions.

The use of certain drugs can also cause onset of allergic disease and sensitivity for the first time. Some people can link the beginning of their problems to a course of antibiotics or, in some women, to use of the contraceptive Pill. An accident or injury may also bring on allergy and sensitivities. In some people, chemical sensitivity follows an episode of overexposure to chemicals – such as accidental contamination, occupational exposure, or exposure to building, DIY or gardening chemicals. Sunlight can trigger symptoms in certain individuals, while others with allergies may also be sensitive to electrical fields or to the lack of sunlight in winter. (For information on photosensitivity, >FURTHER READING.)

People with multiple allergies are often also sensitive to the level of 'overall load' on their systems. They may have few problems most of the time, but will start to react to things they normally tolerate when they come into contact with other allergens or substances to which they are sensitive. Thus some people find they only suffer from food sensitivity in the summer, when they are reacting to pollens, or in the autumn when the concentration of mould spores is high. Other people discover that they only react to chemicals if they eat a food to which they are sensitive, or if they get a viral infection. (>MULTIPLE SENSITIVITY)

TIP

Be careful with any product that claims to be low-allergen, allergen-free or hypoallergenic. These terms mean that products are free of the most potent of possible allergens, that they have been more rigorously tested and that they will rarely cause problems. It does *not* mean that they are totally 'safe'. You may possibly (although rarely) have problems with them. So take care when trying, as you would with anything else. Allergy is highly idiosyncratic –what works for one person may not work at all for another –so treat these descriptions with care.

Detecting Your Allergies

There are three basic methods of detecting whether or not you have allergies, or other kinds of intolerance or sensitivity, and of identifying the cause of your reactions. These are:

- analysing the pattern of your reactions to identify suspects
- medical and laboratory tests
- undertaking an elimination programme to see if symptoms improve

This section describes the basic methodology and refers you on where necessary to other sections in this book that will guide you, step by step.

This section is written from the point of view of you, the individual, analysing your own symptoms. However, if you are trying to work out what is upsetting someone else – your child, for instance – you can use it as a questionnaire for another person. If you need more specialised advice on babies and children, you should read this section in conjunction with BABYCARE and CHILDCARE.

Symptoms As A Guide

Symptoms are only partly helpful as an indicator of the cause of reactions. It used to be thought that the site where your symptoms occurred was the route or the place where the substance causing the reactions had entered the body. On this basis, only things you inhaled could cause nasal and breathing symptoms; only things you swallowed could cause gut symptoms; only things you touched could cause skin symptoms, and so on. Many doctors no longer accept this, since there is evidence that molecules travel in the bloodstream and can trigger allergic and other reactions at sites in the body other than those where the substance entered. Some doctors, however, still hold firmly to the original belief that symptom = site of reaction = cause of reaction. (>DEFINING ALLERGY and SYMPTOMS for more information.)

Nonetheless, it is true to say that certain symptoms do have prime suspects as causes, and they are a good place to start. Nasal and breathing symptoms *are* most likely to be caused by things you breathe in, especially house dust mites, pollens, moulds, fibres, feathers, animal hair and chemicals. Start with these, perhaps, but remember that other things, such as foods, do cause such symptoms. Gut and digestive symptoms *are* most commonly caused by things you eat or swallow, such as foods, drinks and drugs, but they are also very often caused by chemicals you inhale. Mental symptoms are most likely to be caused by inhaling chemicals, but are often caused by intolerance of foods, drinks or drugs.

Skin symptoms *are* commonly caused by things you touch, such as chemicals, but they are equally likely to be caused by things you eat or swallow, such as foods, drinks and drugs; or by things you inhale, such as house dust mites, pollens, moulds, fibres, feathers, animal hair or chemicals. Itchy eyes, headaches, joint pain, nettle rash and water retention have no real prime suspects as cause.

So use the nature of your symptoms as a partial guide only. The *pattern* of your symptoms – when and where they occur – is a much better guide.

Where to Start

Medical and laboratory tests for allergy and intolerance can be very helpful in identifying what you react to. To be most effective, however, they need to be done in conjunction with knowledge of the history of your symptoms, and their pattern. For details of tests that can be carried out, see page 65.

Analysing the Pattern of Symptoms

Do you have an obvious suspect?

Now the detective work starts. If you have an obvious suspect, you may not need to read the rest of this section. If you feel ill after you eat a particular food that you eat only seldom – say on holiday or if you go out to eat – then you could go straight for that. Do you feel ill during or after visiting friends or family? If so, it could be something in their house – their pet, their gas fire, their carpet, their soap powder.

Do you feel unwell only if you wear certain clothes, or if you dress up to go out? If so, it could be the fibres or the clothes, or it could be toiletries or cosmetics that you do not usually wear. Do you get symptoms after doing DIY, doing a particular hobby, after specific lessons or activities at school? Think hard about when and where your symptoms occur.

You can also keep a symptoms diary. For a week or longer, note down whenever you feel particularly bad. Look and see if there's any pattern. Do it for a few weeks, or longer if you need to.

Symptoms can be delayed

Remember that you can get delayed reactions, due to late phase reactions in the body, that usually occur within five or six hours of meeting a substance to which you react, but sometimes not until the next day. Less commonly, reactions can happen up to a few days later; these very late reactions are more likely to be caused by foods than by other allergens.

A more common pattern is that you will feel worse in the evening or night after encountering an allergen, or the morning after. In babies and children, wakefulness at night can often be caused by reactions to substances, especially foods, encountered during the day. So look back at the previous 12 hours and see what has happened.

Can you identify a trigger?

It may help to identify a date or time where you first noticed your symptoms, even if it was some time ago. Did anything particular change in your life around that time? Did you get a new pet? Did you change jobs, schools, or move house? Did the season change? Did you start using a new soap powder or change your carpet? Did you redecorate or have building work done? Did you change your hairstyle? Did you take a specific drug or have an operation? Is there anything at all you can pinpoint that might indicate a suspect?

Do your symptoms have a pattern?

Now that your thoughts are flowing, think about the *pattern* of your symptoms. Do you get them

- continually or intermittently?
- only in certain seasons?
- mainly at home?
- in a highly variable, random pattern?

Look at the flow-chart (Diagram 5) on page 58 and follow it through according to your answers to these questions.

Once you have identified your prime suspects, go to page 69 for general advice on how to run an elimination programme to detect things causing your reactions. *Read this general advice* before you move further into the *Guide*.

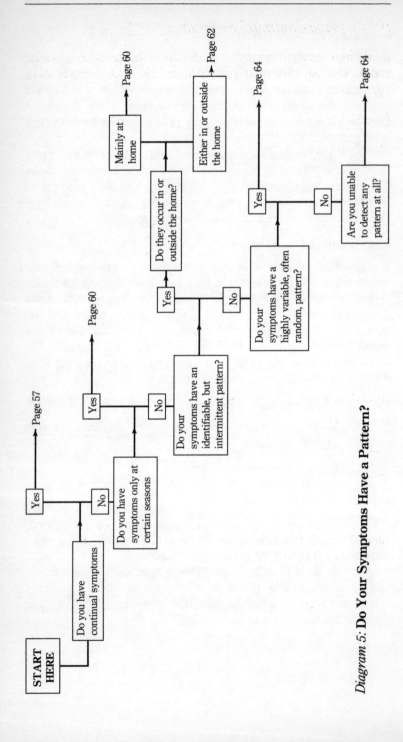

Diagram 5: **Do Your Symptoms Have a Pattern?**

If You Have Continual Symptoms

If you have constant symptoms with little or no variation whatever you do, in or out of home, day or night, then the most likely causes of your reactions are:

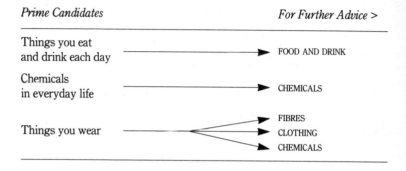

Prime Candidates	*For Further Advice >*
Things you eat and drink each day	FOOD AND DRINK
Chemicals in everyday life	CHEMICALS
Things you wear	FIBRES CLOTHING CHEMICALS

Also consider the following questions:

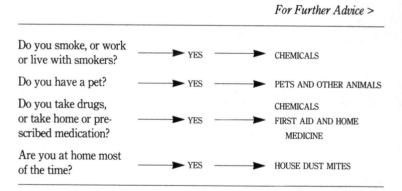

For Further Advice >

Do you smoke, or work or live with smokers?	YES	CHEMICALS
Do you have a pet?	YES	PETS AND OTHER ANIMALS
Do you take drugs, or take home or pre-scribed medication?	YES	CHEMICALS FIRST AID AND HOME MEDICINE
Are you at home most of the time?	YES	HOUSE DUST MITES

Continual symptoms, with occasional peaks and troughs, can sometimes be a sign of multiple sensitivity (>**MULTIPLE SENSITIVITY**).
NOW GO TO PAGE 69.

If Your Symptoms Have a Seasonal Pattern

If you have symptoms at specific times of year in the UK, the most likely causes of reaction are:

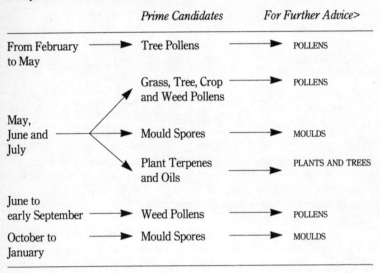

	Prime Candidates	For Further Advice>
From February to May	Tree Pollens	POLLENS
May, June and July	Grass, Tree, Crop and Weed Pollens	POLLENS
	Mould Spores	MOULDS
	Plant Terpenes and Oils	PLANTS AND TREES
June to early September	Weed Pollens	POLLENS
October to January	Mould Spores	MOULDS

Most people with seasonal allergies feel better in late August and September. Particular climatic conditions – hot, humid weather – can favour early mould spore production in August and September, and may affect you some years but not in others.

NOW GO TO PAGE 69.

If You Have Intermittent Symptoms, Mainly When You Are At Home

If your symptoms have an identifiable pattern, but are not continual, and occur mainly when you are at home or in other people's homes, consider first of all:

	Suspect	For Further Advice>
Do you smoke or live with smokers?	Tobacco smoke	CHEMICALS
Do you have a pet?	Pets	PETS AND OTHER ANIMALS

Diagram 6: Identifying the Cause of Intermittent Symptoms at Home

PRIME CANDIDATES
For Further Advice >

DO YOU GET SYMPTOMS...?	Tick for yes	House dust mites	Chemicals	Moulds	Food and drink	Water and water filters	Fibres	Plants and trees	Bedding	Clothing
First thing on waking		•							•	
Using household cleaners			•							
Near wet laundry				•						
When gardening			•	•				•		
When heating or fires are on		•	•	•						
Doing repairs or DIY			•							
When doing the ironing or folding laundry			•	•			•			•
In dusty rooms or attics		•		•						
Having a bath or shower			•	•		•				
Vacuuming or dusting		•								
Doing car repairs			•							
In damp rooms or cellars				•						
Making the beds		•					•			
Sitting on a particular piece of furniture		•	•				•			
When cooking			•		•					
Doing the washing-up			•			•				

Next, look at Diagram 6 and consider the list of possible situations in which you might get symptoms. If you get symptoms in any of those situations, put a tick in the empty column. Look across the columns to where the prime suspects in each case are marked. For further advice, go on to the section or sections that seem most relevant to you. If the situations do not relate at all to your symptoms, see below, where patterns of intermittent symptoms in or outside the home are discussed.

NOW GO TO PAGE 69.

If You Have Intermittent Symptoms, Either at Home or Outside

If you can identify a pattern to symptoms, but they are not continual, and they occur either inside or outside the home, consider first the following:

For Further Advice>

Do you get	AT SCHOOL	⟶	CHILDCARE
symptoms ... ?			
	AT LEISURE,		
	SPORTS OR	⟶	CHEMICALS
	SOCIAL EVENTS		

Next go to Diagram 7. Look at the list of possible situations in which you might get symptoms. If you get symptoms in any of these situations, put a tick in the empty column. Then look across the columns to where the prime suspects in each case are marked. For further advice, go on to the section or sections that seem most relevant to you. If you have many potential causes, >MULTIPLE SENSITIVITY. If the situations do not relate at all to your symptoms, see page 64 for further advice.

NOW GO TO PAGE 69.

Diagram 7: Identifying the Causes of Intermittent Symptoms at Home and Outside

PRIME CANDIDATES
For Further Advice >

DO YOU GET SYMPTOMS...?	Tick for yes	Chemicals	Moulds	Multiple sensitivity	Sex and contraception	Travel	Food and drink	Miscellaneous allergens
In damp, cloudy weather		●	●					
When air pollution is high		●						
During or after making love		●			●			
If you take drugs or home medication		●						
Linked to your menstrual cycle				●				●
In public places like shops, banks, hospitals, doctors' surgeries		●						
During or after travelling		●				●		
Before thunderstorms			●					
When handling paper		●						
In damp places			●					
In busy traffic		●						
Near woods or undergrowth			●					
After drinking alcohol		●					●	
Near cigarette smoke		●						
At the hairdresser or barber		●	●					
In or after exposure to sunlight		●		●				

If You Have a Highly Variable Pattern to Your Symptoms

If your symptoms come and go with no regular pattern, and often appear to be capricious, the most likely causes of reactions could be:

Prime Candidates   *For Further Advice >*

Food Intolerance —————————<   DEFINING ALLERGY
                                                       SYMPTOMS
                                                       FOOD AND DRINK

Weather and climate
changes affecting   ————————————▶   MOULDS
mould spore production

The effect of multiple
load on your system   ————————————▶   MULTIPLE SENSITIVITY

Cross-reactivity   ————————————▶   CROSS-REACTION

If you still see no pattern to your symptoms, go back to **Intermittent Symptoms,** page 60, and see if this helps you detect a pattern.

NOW GO TO PAGE 69.

If You Are Unable to Detect Any Pattern At All

If, after going through the previous steps, you can identify no pattern at all that corresponds to your symptoms, it is possible that you have no allergies or sensitivities. It could be a waste of time investigating further.

If you want to read some more of this book just to be fully sure, have a look at the following sections:

CHEMICALS

FOOD AND DRINK

MOULDS

MULTIPLE SENSITIVITY

You may also find the section on MISCELLANEOUS ALLERGENS helpful, where the causes of specific reactions are described.

NOW GO TO PAGE 69.

Medical, Laboratory and Other Tests

Formal tests for allergy and intolerance fall into two basic types. The first are skin and laboratory tests; the second are challenge tests. Skin and laboratory tests can help in identifying true allergy; they are not helpful in identifying food intolerance or chemical sensitivity. Challenge tests can help in identifying all three.

Skin and Laboratory Tests

The main skin tests to identify allergies are:

- skin-prick test
- intra-dermal test
- patch test

The main laboratory tests are:

- eosinophil test
- RAST test

In skin-prick tests, extracts of a number of allergens are placed on the skin, usually on the inner skin of the forearm. The skin is then pricked or scratched, allowing the allergen to enter the skin. The skin is marked with a pen to show the site of each allergen; the individual being tested is not told what is being tested. If you are sensitive to the allergen, there will be a positive reaction, usually starting as an intense itching within a couple of minutes. Within 10–15 minutes, a raised blister-like weal will form, surrounded by a flare – an area of red itchiness around the weal. There are no side-effects or further symptoms.

The skin-prick test is most reliable at confirming allergy to things you inhale, such as house dust mites, moulds or animal hair, but it can be used to confirm sensitivity to foods or insect stings. It can, however, be misleading. You can have a positive result to a skin-prick test without actually having any symptoms. You can also get a false negative reaction to something to which you are clearly allergic, particularly with foods. As a result, most doctors use skin-prick tests as an aid to *confirm* a case history, not as a stand-alone test.

In intra-dermal tests, a higher dose of allergen extract is introduced just under the outer skin using a syringe. A similar weal and flare response within 10–15 minutes indicates a positive reaction. In addition, you may get a late skin reaction – a raised red swollen bump around the test site – about five or six hours later. Sometimes there may be a late skin reaction on the following day.

The intra-dermal test is much less commonly used in the UK than the skin-prick test. It can be painful, it has a slight risk of adverse reaction, and some people feel unwell on testing. It can, however, be useful in that it can detect positive reactions where skin-prick tests have previously been negative.

Patch tests are used to confirm a diagnosis of contact dermatitis – a delayed allergic skin reaction to something you have touched. Patch tests can be very useful in identifying specific things that you can then avoid. Small patches containing a range of common allergens, mostly chemicals, are attached to the skin, usually to the upper back. The sites of the tests are marked on the skin. The patches are left there for 48 hours, and then removed. The sites are examined for reaction and then left unwashed for a further 48 hours, when the sites are examined once more. A raised red bump at the site of the allergen is an indication of positive reaction. False positives and false negatives can result, so once again patch tests are used mainly to corroborate a case history. You can use patch tests to test specific things you suspect – for instance, a fabric, a leaf or a chemical you use at work or school. You can also do a home version of the patch test for yourself (>COSMETICS, TOILETRIES AND SKINCARE for details).

Anti-histamine drugs block the release of histamine and can interfere with skin test results. Such drugs should not be taken for several days before testing.

Laboratory tests for allergy include the eosinophil test. Eosinophils are white blood cells always present at the place where an allergic reaction takes place. Samples of blood, or of sputum, or of secretions from nose or eye, are taken. The cells are stained with a red dye, eosin, and are counted under a microscope. A high count indicates an allergic reaction is taking place, but it can be an indication of other diseases as well, and it can also be found in symptom-free individuals. Steroid tablets suppress the level of eosinophils and can cause misleading results. The eosinophil test cannot identify allergy to specific substances.

A useful but expensive laboratory test for allergy is the radio-allergosorbent test, or RAST test. It can measure the levels of IgE antibodies in the blood specific to a particular allergen, such as pollens, house dust mites or food proteins. The blood sample is passed over an extract of the allergen attached to an inert substance. The IgE antibodies will bind to the allergen if they are present in the blood, as during an allergic reaction. Then another liquid, containing anti-IgE antibodies marked with radioactivity or colour, is passed over the sample. These will adhere to any IgE bound to the allergen, or will simply wash away if none is there. The level of IgE in the sample can then be taken by measuring the level of the marked anti-IgE that does not adhere.

The RAST test is more helpful than skin tests in cases of food allergy, and its results are not influenced by medication. However, results can vary – some people allergic to seasonal allergens, such as moulds or pollens, will have negative results outside the season, but positive results when exposed to their allergen. Similarly, if you have not eaten a problem food for some time, you may get a negative result, whereas you could get a positive result if you eat it regularly.

A modified version of the RAST test can identify false food allergy, as well as true allergy.

Challenge Tests

Challenge or provocation tests are tests in which the individual is exposed in various ways to a potential allergen and any reactions are recorded.

Nasal and bronchial challenge tests are used most commonly to test inhaled allergens such as pollens or house dust mites. In the nasal challenge test, a tiny amount of a suspected allergen is applied to the lining of the nose and reactions are recorded. The results are measured by counting sneezes in the first 15 minutes, measuring nasal discharge and by examining the inside of the nose. Instruments measuring nasal airflow can also be used.

In the bronchial challenge test, more sophisticated techniques are used, involving inhaling measured quantities of suspect substances, and then recording reactions and measuring lung function. There is a risk of adverse reaction and these tests are usually done in hospital as an in-patient, in case adverse or delayed reactions occur. Tests of this kind are time-consuming and can be risky.

Oral challenge tests are used to identify food allergy or food intolerance. There are a number of ways to undertake these; and unless you are seriously ill, or have severe multiple allergies, you will be able to do them at home yourself in the form of an elimination diet under medical guidance.

The main principle of an elimination diet is to go on a low-allergen diet, or to fast for some time, and then reintroduce and eat suspect or problem foods, monitoring your symptoms. >FOOD AND DRINK for more information on how to run an elimination diet.

Oral challenge tests can be organised on a double-blind basis, so that the food eaten is disguised and neither the person testing the food, nor the doctor or nurse supervising the test, knows what food is being tested. This is expensive and not always easy to arrange – you can disguise lentils easily, but not carrots or beetroot, for instance – so it is not commonly used.

The sublingual challenge test can be used for testing for food allergy or intolerance, or for chemical sensitivity. In each, a dilute solution of extract of a suspect substance is placed under the tongue and symptoms are monitored for 10 minutes. Testing is usually done blind so that the patient does not know what is being tested.

Sublingual testing for food sensitivity can be ineffective, especially if the food concerned has not been consumed within the previous 48 hours, so it is rarely used. Sublingual testing for chemical sensitivity, however, is more effective and can be useful in identifying chemicals to which you react. It is less effective when carried out in an environment with a high level of chemicals in the air, which can affect results. Best results are obtained in a chemical-free or carefully controlled environment.

Your doctor can refer you to have any of the above medical and laboratory tests if you ask for them, but they may not be available on the National Health Service, or in the area where you live. If you want further advice on where to go for testing, the British Society for Allergy and Environmental Medicine and The British Society for Allergy and Clinical Immunology can give you the names of doctors (>MEDICAL HELP for addresses).

Other Tests

There are other tests available that, it is claimed, can identify allergies and other sensitivities. These include the cytotoxic test, in which white blood cells are exposed to allergens. This has been shown to be a valid test, but accurate only in up to 70 per cent of cases. Until its accuracy can be improved, it may mislead you dangerously.

Hair analysis is inaccurate in diagnosing allergies and sensitivity and has little value. Other diagnostic tests available often involve measuring energy flow or electro-magnetic fields, such as dowsing, Vegatest electrical devices, or energy boxes. Applied kinesiology is based on measuring muscle strength. Such tests are often attractive as a means of diagnosing allergy or sensitivity, in that they are relatively quick and easy and it is tempting to think that they can do no harm, but they *can* do harm in that they are often inaccurate.

People whose allergies have already been identified and who know what they react to, report that they get different or varying results from such methods and that they do not find them reliable. So, if you use any of these methods, keep an open mind, use them to corroborate

TIP

There are a number of practical tests that you can do yourself at home to help you work out what you react to. These include the

- Iron Test (page 346)
- Sniff Test (page 88)
- Pillow Test (page 110)
- Home Patch Test (page 88)
- Tile Test (page 297)

your own detection work, but do not allow them to send you off on wild goose chases.

Undertaking an Elimination Programme

If you have identified your prime suspects, you will be ready to move on to the relevant sections of the *Guide* to learn more about what you can do to avoid and eliminate them. Before you move on, here is some general advice about how to approach an elimination programme.

The basic principle of an elimination programme is to remove from your environment, as far as is practicable, the things that you suspect of causing reactions. You then monitor your symptoms and see if they improve after a period of time. If you want to confirm the results of the trial, you can then reintroduce the substances or start using them again. You do this with care, monitoring your symptoms as you do it.

To make the programme work, you have to be thorough and you have to be systematic. You also have to be patient and to give things time to settle before you make a judgement. It is better to eliminate only one group of substances at a time, say only foods, only house dust mites, or only chemicals, and do it thoroughly, rather than to try several things at once and only do each partially. People often start by doing the latter because it seems less work and they hope it will be sufficient to make them feel better.

If you have only mild allergies or sensitivities, a partial approach will work well. However, if you are significantly affected by your reactions or if you have multiple sensitivity, most people find that the only way to work out what affects them is to eliminate one thing at a time, and to do it wholeheartedly. Although it appears more work, it is shorter in the long run and less confusing.

In each section of the *Guide*, there are suggestions for helpful things

to do if you do not think you need to do a thorough elimination programme, as well as guidance on a comprehensive approach. Choose
yourself which approach you will adopt. Whichever way you go, keep
an open mind as you go along, monitor symptoms carefully and retest
things whenever you are not sure.

Part 4

WHAT SUBSTANCES CAUSE REACTIONS? WHERE ARE THEY FOUND?

Chemicals

What is Chemical Sensitivity?

As discussed in Part 2 (see page 24), allergy and sensitivity to chemicals is a contentious and highly controversial area. Many doctors and scientists would agree that they have an inadequate understanding of many people's apparent reactions to chemicals in their environment. There is little research data to explain what chemicals cause reactions, what symptoms result, and what the underlying mechanisms in the body actually are.

The areas that are best documented, and where most doctors and scientists agree, are those of allergy to chemicals (where the immune system is involved, and which can be detected by skin and laboratory tests), and irritant and toxic reactions, where exposure to high levels of chemicals, usually at work, causes symptoms and disease.

The area that is most disputed and under-researched is the one which some doctors call 'chemical sensitivity'. The definition of chemical sensitivity is substantially empirical, based on clinical practice and observation of large numbers of people with a common history of disease and presenting symptoms. In this definition, chemical sensitivity means *adverse reactions to tiny or very low levels of chemicals in the environment*, in which the immune system is *not* demonstrably involved.

It may appear to you, if you react to chemicals, that this controversy over allergy versus toxic reactions versus sensitivity has very little relevance for you. However, it is important in that it conditions the response of any doctor who may treat you. You will get very widely differing diagnoses, sympathy and treatment, according to the individual doctor's own beliefs and attitudes. For information on treatments, >MEDICAL HELP.

No objective measure of chemical sensitivity exists, other than challenge tests (when individuals are 'challenged' with chemicals to provoke a reaction) in controlled conditions. Doctors are largely dependent for diagnosis on symptoms reported by patients, and because of this, many of them do not believe that it is a real disorder. Furthermore, because many of the symptoms people typically complain of are mental symptoms, many doctors commonly diagnose a psychiatric or psychosomatic illness, saying that the individual's problems are all in his or her mind, that no-one can be made unwell by tiny doses of chemicals, that the illness is a stratagem, probably unconscious, for dealing with personal or psychiatric problems.

Psychosomatic illnesses clearly exist – the link between mind and body is strong – and there will be in the field of allergy and sensitivity, as in any other area of medicine, cases where underlying psychiatric disorder is a component, perhaps an important component, of the individual's ill-health. However, the fact that psychosomatic illness exists should not lead to the common bias that people claiming that tiny doses of chemicals make them ill must be suffering from psychiatric problems.

The evidence from clinical practice of doctors who treat people who have positive results from controlled testing with chemicals is that the vast majority of their patients are average, happy, sane people whose abnormal symptoms (psychiatric or otherwise) appear when they are exposed to certain chemicals, and disappear when they are not. The level of improvement in symptoms in clinical practice is significantly above that expected from the placebo effect. (In medical trials, it has been found that, on average, one-third of patients – or more in the case of psychiatric patients – respond to being given dummy or inactive therapy or medication – a placebo. Only improvement in excess of expected placebo results is taken as serious evidence of the effectiveness of any therapy.)

Which Chemicals Cause Reactions?

The chemicals commonly implicated in allergy and sensitivity are broadly the same, although allergic reactions are most commonly associated with contact – touching and handling chemicals – while sensitivity is more linked to inhaling chemicals, as well as contact or absorption through the skin or mucosa. Table 4 shows a list of common chemicals causing reactions. If you react to chemicals and have to organise your daily life around avoidance, a list of this kind begs more questions than it answers. Why those chemicals and not others? Where are they found and how do I know? What can I actually use?

If you are not interested in the whys or wherefores, and simply want to know how to detect what upsets you, and how to avoid problems, turn to page 87 for practical advice. If you want to know more about which chemicals cause reactions and why, read on from here. The term 'sensitivity' in the remainder of this section includes both allergy and sensitivity.

Table 4: **Chemicals Commonly Causing Chemical Sensitivity**

Coal tar and derivatives	Fragrances (synthetic and natural)
Asphalt	Natural oils and terpenes
Benzene	Essential oils
Creosote	Latex
Phenol	Plant terpenes
Some food additives	Turpentine
Common chemicals	Organic solvents
Ammonia	Alcohol (ethanol)
Chlorine	Glycerol
Formaldehyde	Methylated spirits
Sulphur dioxide	Phenols
Contaminants in food and water	Styrene
Herbicides	Toluene
Insecticides	Trichloroethylene
Organic solvents	White spirits
Pesticides	Synthetic fibres, fabrics and materials
Environmental pollutants	
Gas fumes	
Industrial discharges	
Paraffin fumes	
Tobacco smoke	
Vehicle exhausts	

Which Chemicals and Why?

It is worth taking time to sort out some preconceptions about chemicals and to make clear the terms of this discussion. A 'chemical', according to the Oxford English Dictionary, is 'a substance obtained by, or used in a chemical process'. The adjective 'chemical' means 'relating to the science of the elements and compounds and their laws of combination and change'. So, the element oxygen, which humans need to breathe and survive, is a chemical. So is water, which is a combination of hydrogen and oxygen.

When people use the word 'chemical' in everyday life, however, they mostly do not use it in this neutral sense, but rather with overlays of values and attitudes. Most people use it to mean chemicals that are potentially harmful or toxic (to the environment or individuals), or wasteful of natural resources; and often also to signify synthetic chemicals, rather than natural.

To understand chemical sensitivity, you need to be as objective as you can and to clear your mind as far as possible of your preconceptions about 'good' and 'bad' chemicals. The concern of this section, and the book as a whole, is with *any chemicals that are potentially harmful to individuals at low levels*.

Some environmentally friendly chemicals can be harmful to chemically sensitive or allergic individuals, as can some natural chemicals from plants or trees, while some synthetic chemicals are fairly harmless. Some chemicals never cause reactions, and these are the building blocks of life – oxygen, pure uncontaminated water and carbon. Some people apparently react to water and to activated carbon (for instance in water or air filters) but this is more likely due to minute contaminants (>AIR FILTERS and WATER AND WATER FILTERS for more information).

Some chemicals are very inert, and do not cause reactions. They do not give off vapours at all. Substances such as glass, china clay, cement, ceramics, clay, stone, marble, cork and non-resinous woods (>PLANTS AND TREES) do not cause reactions. If other chemicals (such as varnishes) are used on them, then they can cause reactions, or if you are exposed to heavy levels of dust, you can get irritant reactions, but they virtually never cause sensitivity.

Metals can cause allergy, but do not cause sensitivity. (>MISCELLANEOUS ALLERGENS for more information on metals.)

Some chemicals are extremely simple in their chemical structure, as well as being inert, and again do not cause reactions – for instance, sodium chloride (ordinary salt), sodium bicarbonate, Borax and washing soda. Additives in table salt sometimes cause reactions, but pure sodium chloride does not.

There are three prime characteristics of those chemicals that commonly cause reactions. One category includes chemicals that are *highly toxic* at high levels of exposure, such as chlorine, ammonia and benzene. The second category is chemicals with *complex structures*, which appear more prone to cause reactions than other chemicals, for instance, complex hydrocarbons, such as organic solvents or many fragrances. Thirdly, and most important, are chemicals *that release vapour* or are more volatile so that they are readily inhaled or absorbed into the system.

It is worth emphasising that natural chemicals can be as troublesome as synthetic chemicals. Some natural chemicals (especially those that are volatile, give off fumes and have complex structures) can be very troublesome. These include natural plant oils and fragrances, such as menthol, lavender oil, oil of wintergreen, oil from orange or lemon peel; resins such as natural turpentine or rosin; terpenes such as grass sap; and other natural vegetable and plant products such as latex, acetic acid (vinegar), Balsam of Peru (a flavouring and perfuming agent), pyrethrum and derris (used as pesticides in organic gardening). >PLANTS AND TREES for a full discussion.

In What Situations Do Chemicals Cause Reactions?

So where are all these types of chemicals found? Answer: in very many places in everyday life. Before coming to that, however, you need to understand a few more concepts about how, and in what circumstances, chemicals can cause trouble. Even if you are sensitive or allergic to particular chemicals found commonly in everyday life, you can function quite well and use things that contain chemicals to which you are sensitive, provided you take certain precautions.

Chemicals are most likely to cause you reactions when they are found in *higher concentrations*. If you use chemicals extensively at work, say as a hairdresser; in building and decorating; or if you work in a place where chemical vapours can accumulate (say, in a shop selling paper or new clothes with chemical finishes, or in an office with poor ventilation, new building materials, office machines, and lots of paper), you may have problems with these, but not elsewhere.

Where you have lower exposures, it is when chemicals give off vapour or fumes that they are most troublesome. This happens most commonly when things are new, or when they heat up or become hot. It also happens obviously when exhaust or combustion fumes are given off when things such as engines, fires, cigarettes or stoves burn.

To give an example of how this may affect you, the chemicals used in many plastics and foams used in the interiors of cars are known to cause sensitivity. Most chemically sensitive people, however, are perfectly able to travel in a car that is not new on most days of the year without feeling unduly ill, even if they are sensitive to those particular chemicals. Brand new cars, however, give off high levels of fumes as the chemicals air off, and chemically sensitive people are often made ill by a new car, until it has aired off for some months, sometimes even for a couple of years. Problems can arise again on a hot day in an aired-off car that is normally fine; the heat causes the plastics and foams to start releasing fumes again and people may react where usually they have no problems.

There are numerous other examples of this kind of situation – of chemicals only being a problem when things are new, or subject to heat. An unread newspaper or magazine can cause problems, while one already read and left to air will not. A newly painted room may make you ill at first, but not as time goes on. A new item of clothing that has been washed a few times will be virtually free of fabric finishes and cause no reactions, but if it is worn straight after purchase it may cause trouble. A new pair of shoes left to air will soon lose fumes and any chemical vapours. Some people cannot tolerate synthetic fabrics if they wear them or use them for bedding – when the fibres get warm and give off fumes – but can live with them very happily in carpets, curtains or furnishings where the fumes are much less intense.

If you are exceptionally sensitive, you may continue to react even to very tiny levels of fumes once things are aired off, and you may have to avoid some chemicals totally, but this is extremely rare. For most people, taking care with specific situations means they can live happily with substances that upset them.

If you investigate for yourself what chemicals are found in anything you use, it is also worth remembering that chemicals are usually only troublesome when they are given off as vapour or released into the atmosphere. If a chemical has been used in the manufacture or finishing of a product, it may not be released as free vapour at all and it will not bother you. Formaldehyde, for instance, is commonly a troublesome chemical when it is released as free formaldehyde. It is used in the manufacture of many products, but in some circumstances is not released after manufacture as free formaldehyde and should pose no problems. Formaldehyde resins are used in the making of plywood, for instance, but, if manufacture has been correct, no free formaldehyde is given off at all, and plywood should not give problems. Formaldehyde resins are also used in the manufacture of chipboard but, in this case, free formaldehyde continues to be released after manufacture is complete, and chipboard is known to cause some people persistent reactions.

Another example is that some people are extremely sensitive to chlorine if they inhale its fumes as free chlorine (for instance, from liquid bleach, from tapwater, or at swimming pools) but find they have absolutely no problems using products which have been bleached with chlorine during manufacture (such as white fabrics, paper, toilet paper, or disposable nappies). (Some exceptionally sensitive people still do react, but that is highly unusual.)

Some materials that do not give off vapours are problem free, even though they are chemically related to materials that do cause sensitivity. Perspex, for instance, and cellophane – both synthetic materials – do not give off vapour and do not cause reactions at all. By contrast, plastic film and soft polythene do give off vapours, especially when new or hot, and they commonly cause reactions. Hard plastics, such as those used in radios, buckets, guttering and bowls, do not generally cause problems once aired-off. (For one exception, see below.)

So if you find out, or are told, that chemicals to which you know you react have been used in the manufacture of something you want to use, it helps to ask yourself:

- Is the chemical present in high concentrations in the item I want to use?
- Does it give off vapours?
- Do I need to use it when new, when vapours are fresh, or can I wash or rinse it before use?
- How long will it take to air off?
- Will I use it in a situation where it will heat up, and give off vapours?

A final factor in judging where chemicals are likely to cause reactions is that of 'chemical load' or overload of the system. The load effect is also known as the 'cocktail effect'. People with chemical sensitivity often appear to react to a wide range of chemicals and their tolerance to specific chemicals can vary. Sometimes they will react to a given chemical and at other times they can tolerate up to a certain amount. One explanation for this may lie with the body's mechanisms for detoxifying chemicals. From studies of toxic exposures, it has been shown that exposure to two or more chemicals can be much more harmful than exposure to one alone, the reason being that if the same enzyme is required to break down the chemicals, there can be an inadequate supply of the enzyme, and of the catalyst or cofactors needed to help that and other chemical processes in the body. The chemically sensitive person's ability to cope with chemicals in their environment may, therefore, depend on their overall 'load' of chemicals (and hence demands on their enzyme systems). This is perhaps the reason why a tiny extra amount of chemical load can often be enough to take a chemically sensitive person over their tolerance level and cause reactions.

The load effect is important when thinking about what chemicals might cause you to react. Some chemicals are more troublesome than others and consistently cause problems, but your overall load of chemicals may aggravate the situation by overloading your system.

This is why, when talking about avoidance of chemicals below, it is often good to try to reduce your overall load of chemicals, as well as to avoid chemicals to which you know you are specifically sensitive. Reducing overall load can actually improve your tolerance of specific substances.

In addition, some people cross-react to chemicals, that is their bodies recognise substances that are chemically related and react to them.

This can add to the load effect. If you think you cross-react to chemicals, >CROSS-REACTION for more information.

Where Are Troublesome Chemicals Found?

If you are chemically sensitive, it is important to know where your specific troublemakers are found so that you can try and avoid them. Often you start out like a detective, when you first learn that you are chemically sensitive, trying to track down the contents of every product or item that you use, to find those you can tolerate.

The process soon becomes overwhelming. Take a look at Table 5, which gives information about chemicals that commonly cause allergy and sensitivity – formaldehyde, chlorine, ammonia and rosin. Formaldehyde, also called formalin, has many, many uses. It is used as a preservative in cosmetics, cleaning products and pharmaceuticals; as a coating, it confers wet strength and grease resistance, so it is used extensively in paper production and as a fabric finish. It is used as an adhesive resin in all kinds of manufacture, and as a protective treatment on some building materials. It gasses off from some types of plastic foams, melamine sheeting, from computer plastics and some car interiors. In short, you find it almost everywhere in modern life. However, not *every* kind of cosmetic or cleaning product, nor *every* type of product named, contains formaldehyde, but how would you know, and what if you are also sensitive to other chemicals that may or may not be contained in things that also contain formaldehyde?

Chlorine, ammonia and rosin are also other common troublemakers. Each of these chemicals is potentially found where other potentially aggressive chemicals are also found – in household cleaners, cosmetics, toiletries, paper, fabric finishes and pharmaceuticals. Moreover, these chemicals are not necessarily found in all products in any category – not *all* soaps contain rosin, not *all* toothpastes contain ammonia – but soon you realise that you begin to feel quietly (or not so quietly) desperate about working out where chemicals are and what to use – let alone detecting what you react to.

A much more helpful and workable approach is to turn things around and to look at areas of your life where you come into contact with chemicals and to work out what the major potential troublemakers are in each. The list on pages 82–3 gives you the main areas of most people's lives and a short list of the chemicals that occur in each and could cause problems to the chemically sensitive.

If you want to know how to track down much more precise information about specific products or chemicals, and discover exactly where

Table 5: **Locating Common Chemical Troublemakers**

WHERE IS FORMALDEHYDE FOUND?

Tobacco smoke
Vehicle exhausts
Cavity wall insulation
Paper coatings and finishes
Printing inks
Newsprint
Textile and fabric finishes
Chipboard, blockboard and other
    building boards
Glass fibre insulation
Resin adhesive
Melamine
Foam rubber fillings and fascia
Photographic chemicals
Tanned leather
Insecticides and moth-proofing
Fungicides
Propellant in spray aerosols
Preservative in cosmetics, toiletries,
    personal hygiene products, phar-
    maceuticals and cleaning prod-
    ucts of all kinds:
        disinfectants
        cleaning liquids
        antiseptics
        toothpastes
        shampoo
        soaps
        cosmetics
        hair treatments

WHERE IS CHLORINE FOUND?

Liquid bleaches
Powder bleaches
Household cleaners
Disinfectants
Sterilisers and hand rinses
Tapwater
Swimming pool water
Bleached fabrics
Bleached paper
Fungicides
Mould inhibitors

WHERE IS AMMONIA FOUND?

Household cleaners
Disinfectants
Deodorants
Toothpastes
Preservative in some latex products
Permanent wave solution
Hair bleaches

WHERE IS ROSIN FOUND?

Adhesives
Chewing-gum
Grease removers
Cosmetics
Paper coatings and finishes
Soaps
Grip aids and resins
Varnishes and lacquers
Waxes and polishes
Fabric finishes
Pharmaceutical ointments and
    plasters

they are found, read **How to Find Out About Chemicals**, page 84.

If you want to explore any of these areas of life in particular detail before you read any further here, look at the individual sections in the rest of the book. For example, for more specific information on chemicals in school-life, >CHILDCARE. If you want to investigate specific chemicals further, >the INDEX.

Chemicals in Life

AREA OF LIFE	*Chemicals*
COSMETICS, TOILETRIES, SKINCARE PERSONAL HYGIENE FIRST AID AND HOME MEDICINE DRUGS AND PHARMACEUTICALS	Fragrances Preservatives Solvents Active ingredients Flavourings Formaldehyde Parabens Balsam of Peru Ammonia Lanolin Paraphenylenediamine (PPDA)
PAPER AND BOOKS	Formaldehyde Rosin Chlorine Coatings Finishes Inks Photographic chemicals
WRITINGS AND PLAY MATERIALS	Adhesives Solvents Paints
COMPUTERS AND TELEVISION	Plastic fumes
GARDENING	Pesticides Insecticides Fungicides Bonfire smoke
TAPWATER	Chlorine Contaminants
CHEMICALS IN FOOD	Pesticide residues Additives
CAR INTERIORS	Vehicle exhausts Fabrics, foam and plastics

AREA OF LIFE	*Chemicals*
INDOOR POLLUTION	Gas fumes
	Paraffin fumes
	Tobacco smoke
	Solid fuel fumes
	Wood fire fumes
FURNITURE AND FLOORING	Synthetic fibres and materials
	Carpet underlay
	Adhesives
	Fabric finishes
	Stain-resistance treatments
	Fire-resistance treatments
	Foam rubber
BEDDING	Synthetic fibres and materials
BUILDING AND DECORATING MATERIALS	Solvents
	Formaldehyde
	Fungicides
	Insecticides
	Pesticides
	Adhesives
	Chipboard
	Cavity wall insulation
	Rot and woodworm treatments
AIR POLLUTION	Vehicle exhausts
	Industrial discharges
	Sulphur dioxide
PUBLIC BUILDINGS	Disinfectants
	Cleaning products
	Building and decorating materials
	Tobacco smoke
	Paper and books
	Writing and play materials
	Office products
	Computer fumes
	Furniture and flooring
	Other people's toiletries

How to Find Out About Chemicals

Books

If you want to find out for yourself what chemicals are, and where they are found, the following books are useful:

C for Chemicals by Michael Birkin and Brian Price (1989) concentrates on issues of toxicity and the impact of chemicals on the environment, rather than on sensitivity and allergy, but it is very informative on the nature of common chemicals and where they are found. It is factual, accessible and readable.

Contact Dermatitis by Alexander A. Fisher (Editor, 1986) is a massive tome, a medical reference work for doctors, but it is a useful source-book for the lay-person, whether or not you have contact dermatitis. It is clear, readable and a sound source of information on where many chemicals are to be found, often giving brand and product names. It has an American bias, but is helpful for the UK. Any public library can order it for you.

For a basic dictionary of chemical terms, use *The Penguin Dictionary of Chemistry* by D. W. A. Sharp (Editor, 1983).

Two other books that are useful for information on where chemicals are found in everyday life are: *Chemical Victims* by Dr Richard Mackarness (1980) and *Chemical Children* by Dr Peter Mansfield and Dr Jean Monro (1987).

Manufacturers

If you contact manufacturers directly to find out the contents of any product you want to buy, they are usually very helpful if you explain your reasons, and will often supply full contents lists. Write to them directly or telephone. For building and decorating materials, ask for Technical Data Sheets, which are usually accessible to the lay-person.

National Eczema Society (NES)

The NES has a computerised database with the chemical contents of many common products. This has been compiled with the collaboration of many product manufacturers and has good, although not complete, coverage.

The database covers:

- Emollients
- Steroids
- Foods
- Skincare products
- Cosmetics
- Laundry products

You can search the database, check the ingredients of products you are using, and obtain the names of products with ingredients you may tolerate better. The service is available to any member of the public, not just to NES members, and no fee is charged, although donations are appreciated.

Contact: The National Eczema Society
                Tavistock House East
                Tavistock Square
                London WC1H 9SR
                Tel: 071–388 4097

How to Detect Sensitivity to Chemicals

Allergic contact dermatitis can be identified by patch testing with chemicals, and the specific chemical causes pinpointed (>DETECTING YOUR ALLERGIES for a full description of tests). Patch testing is not wholly reliable, however, and will not give results if you have irritant, rather than allergic, dermatitis. Nor will it help you if you have symptoms other than dermatitis, or if you are chemically sensitive, not allergic. Your GP can refer you for patch testing.

Sublingual challenge tests (>DETECTING YOUR ALLERGIES for description) will identify chemical sensitivity and its specific causes, but it is not widely practised across the UK and is rarely available on the National Health Service. The British Society for Allergy and Environmental Medicine (address in MEDICAL HELP) will give you names of doctors who do these tests. Your GP can refer you for these.

To investigate for yourself, analyse the pattern of your symptoms using the questionnaire opposite. If you answer 'yes' to several or all of the questions, then you may well be chemically sensitive. It may then be worth considering a chemical avoidance and reintroduction programme (see page 87) for a while to see whether your symptoms improve at all.

Further indicators of chemical sensitivity include the following factors, which are not really specific symptoms, but general characteristics often displayed by chemically sensitive people. *Rapid onset of symptoms* on exposure is a common characteristic of sensitivity. Chemically sensitive people often have an *abnormal sense of smell* – either almost totally absent or unusually heightened, and it can swing between the two extremes. They often display *passions or strong likings for particular smells* or chemicals – for instance, shoe polish, glues, nail varnish, air fresheners – and this is frequently an indicator of specific sensitivity. They often have 'shiners', big black rings under their eyes, although this is also often typical of people with nasal allergies.

People with chemical sensitivity commonly *do not tolerate alcohol* well; sometimes they have an addictive relationship with it – not alcoholism, but a craving or desire for a drink at regular intervals. They

When Do You Feel Worse?

	YES	NO
When doing DIY	—	—
After a long journey	—	—
In tobacco smoke	—	—
Using cleaning products	—	—
Handling new paper	—	—
When wearing aftershave or perfume	—	—
Using glues, office products or play materials	—	—
When a gas or paraffin appliance is on	—	—
In clothes shops, furniture shops or chemists	—	—
When the television is on	—	—
In a hospital or doctor's surgery	—	—
Filling a car with petrol or diesel	—	—
At a bus or train station	—	—
Using a computer	—	—
Reading a newspaper or new magazine	—	—
Wearing new clothes	—	—
In a modern office building	—	—

also often display *unexplained mood swings*, or tempers; these can often be linked to sudden exposures to chemicals when entering a vaporous environment such as a hospital, a chemist's shop or a petrol station, or using a toiletry or cleaning product. People who live with someone who is chemically sensitive say they can often identify a chemical trigger by a sudden change in the person's mood or behaviour. Such unexplained irritability is a prime indicator of chemical sensitivity.

To identify specific causes, you can use the Sniff Test or the Patch Test (see page 88). It is not wise to do these using strong chemicals, such as building and decorating materials, strong cleaning products, or any other chemical that you would not usually use directly on yourself, or wear. Many such chemicals will cause irritation even to people who are not chemically sensitive if inhaled or applied directly to the skin. Use the Sniff Test for polishes, mild cleaners, mild chemicals, fabrics, paper, fibres or toiletries and cosmetics. Use the Patch Test only for any chemical you would normally use on your skin.

For stronger chemicals, such as building and decorating materials, or strong cleaning products, you can use the Tile Test. Details of how to do this are given in BUILDING AND DECORATING MATERIALS. For fibres, fabrics and bedding, you can also use the Pillow Test. Details of how to do this are given in FIBRES. You can use the Iron Test for fabric finishes on clothing or fabrics (>CLOTHING and FABRICS for details).

The most reliable way to establish what causes your reactions is to *avoid chemicals*, removing them from your environment as far as you can, and then reintroducing them carefully, after a period of time, monitoring your symptoms on reintroduction. Leave them out or avoid them as much as you can for two or three weeks. You may experience withdrawal symptoms if you are very sensitive (>SYMPTOMS).

How to Avoid Chemicals

Before you start

If you smoke, or if you drink alcohol every day, you should stop and avoid them totally for a period of at least two or three weeks, to see if symptoms clear. There is no point in systematically avoiding other chemicals if you continue daily ingestion of smoke and alcohol. If you do not smoke, but live with a smoker or work in a smoky atmosphere, it may be difficult to get clear results unless you can escape from tobacco smoke for a while. Arrange this if you possibly can. See the box on page 90 for advice on clearing out tobacco residues.

If you already know that you are chemically sensitive, and want

The Sniff Test

Sniff any product gently before buying to see if it upsets you. You can sniff fabrics, clothing or footwear as well as cosmetics and other products. If you find the smell distasteful or it gives you strong symptoms, do not buy it. If you find the smell peculiarly alluring, even addictive, this is also an indication of sensitivity.

To test a product you already have at home, remove the lid and place the container in a glass jar. Alternatively, soak a small piece of cotton lint with a chemical you want to test, and place it in a glass jar. Seal the glass jar and leave it for a few days. You get the best results if you can totally avoid the product you want to test during the period of waiting. Open the jar carefully and sniff gently. If symptoms develop, do not use the product.

Take great care if you have a history of anaphylactic shock or life-threatening asthma attack. >EMERGENCY INFORMATION *for precautions to take.*

The Patch Test

To do a simple patch test at home, take a tiny dab of chemical and place it on the skin behind your ear or on your forearm. Try to use an area that you have never tested on before, and which is not inflamed if you have sensitive skin. If you have nowhere left in these places, get someone to help and use the skin in the centre of your upper back, between your shoulder blades. Mark in pen beside the spot where the product has been applied, then wait for 24–48 hours. If the area has reddened and is raised or swollen, it is wise not to use the chemical.

Patch tests can give false positive results, particularly if you have very irritable or sensitive skin. False negatives sometimes result as well, so a negative result does not mean that you tolerate the chemical. Patch-testing is not foolproof, therefore, and not totally reliable. However, it can be a help and at least some indication of whether or not you are sensitive to something.

advice on basic long-term avoidance measures, see page 98.

If you are just starting out and want advice on how to carry out an *elimination programme*, primarily to test out what does or doesn't upset you, read on from here.

Elimination Programme

You have a choice of four ways in which to eliminate chemicals from your environment in order to test what you are sensitive to:

- totally avoid one or a small number of specific chemicals
- eliminate chemicals in one area of your life (e.g. clothing or cosmetics)
- create an oasis in one room
- have a radical clear-out

Selective strategies

The first two strategies are usually where people start, as they are much less disruptive and can, if you pick on the obvious candidates first time, bring quick results.

If you choose the first option, of avoiding specific chemicals, use the information under **How to Find Out About Chemicals** on page 84, as well as the main Index, which will guide you into other sections useful to you.

If you choose the second strategy, to pick off selected areas of your life, use the various relevant sections in this book to help you in your avoidance.

The drawbacks of the selective approaches is that you sometimes get confusing results. The first strategy can turn out to be very difficult for the reasons given on page 80, that it is almost impossible to eliminate a specific chemical. The second strategy often fails because you are only eliminating certain chemicals partially – you may not get benefits or clear results until you go much further. You may think that you are not sensitive to a particular chemical when in fact you are, and your symptoms would clear if you were more thorough about elimination.

Creating An Oasis

Creating an oasis in one room of your house is often a better method of working out whether you are actually chemically sensitive than either of the selective routes above. It sounds like more work at the outset, but in the long term, it often turns out to be more economical of effort if you are indeed chemically sensitive. It has the added benefit that it lowers your load of chemicals and can help you be generally better while you are testing. It is less radical than the total clear-out strategy described on page 91.

To use your oasis as a basis for testing and elimination, follow the instructions in the box on page 92.

Clearing Out Tobacco Smoke

Residues from tobacco smoke impregnate many surfaces in places where people smoke regularly, and can give persistent problems for some time after, even if smoking has been banned. These may trouble you if you have just given up smoking, or recently banned it from your home, or if you have just moved to a house where smokers lived before. It helps to clear out and remove the residues as far as you can.

Wash and clean anything you can. Wash curtains, rugs, soft toys, pets' bedding, all clothing – anything you see. Steam-clean carpets, upholstered furniture, cushions, anything large. (>CLEAN-ING PRODUCTS for advice on detergents if you want to use them.) Wipe down toys, storage jars and kitchen utensils – anything that has been exposed. Wash down all surfaces thoroughly – walls, windows, furniture, skirtings, bare floors, doors, ceilings. Wash inside the vacuum cleaner. Even clean inside cupboards if smoking has been heavy.

TIP

Washing surfaces with a Borax solution can help neutralise fumes. Put 1 dessertspoonful of Borax in a bowl of warm water and wipe down. Domestic Borax is available from chemists.

If you dry-clean things to remove tobacco fumes, air them well in a shed or spare room, or on a washing line, before using again.

Put things to air. Washing and cleaning may not be enough, so air everything as much as you can – put furniture outside, or in a shed or spare room with plenty of ventilation. Remember to air duvets, cushions and soft furnishings. Put books and paper outside in the wind and sun to air. Open up windows as much as you can and let the air through. Do this for as long as it takes.

TIP

Do not forget to clean and air cars. Scrub out used car ashtrays and open them to air off.

If these measures do not go far enough, *redecorate* to cover up walls and building surfaces. Use low-hazard materials (>BUILDING AND DECORATING MATERIALS) and ventilate well afterwards.

You may also eventually have to *replace things* – furniture, furnishings, carpets and curtains, even lampshades and bedding, if residues still give you trouble. (See the relevant sections for suggestions for replacements.)

TIP

If you cannot manage to do the whole home, do just one room thoroughly to give you somewhere free of tobacco residues.

If you get stuck halfway through any of the above strategies, and get confusing results, either start from scratch and follow the radical clean-out programme (below), or go to page 98 and follow the long-term avoidance measures.

Radical Clear-out

The fourth strategy for eliminating chemicals is a radical clear-out. It is only worth doing this if you are seriously affected by chemicals and, even then, most people come to it only after a period of selective elimination. It can be disruptive and can cause a lot of tension with family and housemates, so you have to weigh up whether it is worth it to you to do it. Sometimes, however, it is the only way actually to know what you react to, or what you can use without trouble.

The basic approach of this strategy is to clear potential troublemakers out of your environment, especially your home, for as long as you can. If your symptoms improve or clear, this will confirm that chemicals are responsible. Then, to work out what you can tolerate, you reintroduce things you would like to use again systematically – one at a time (preferably one every few days and not more than one a day) – and see if you can tolerate them.

This strategy will achieve what is known as 'unmasking' of chemical sensitivity. If you are surrounded constantly by a chemical or chemicals to which you react, you will have permanent symptoms; you may not even identify them as symptoms if you are used to things like constant gut pain, headaches, cystitis, sweating and irritability. When

Creating an Oasis

The idea of creating an oasis is to give you one room which is as clean of chemicals as you can manage, where you can go to clear out of chemicals whenever possible; a room which can be a resource for you if ever you have high exposures to chemicals that you cannot avoid. It is not a refuge; it is a source of strength and renewed energy.

If you use an oasis as a means of testing whether you are chemically sensitive, set up the oasis and use only a minimum of common chemicals when you have to – outside the oasis if possible as well as inside. Wait for a week, and then reintroduce any chemicals you want to test, either using them outside the oasis, or bringing them in if you need to.

Having an oasis is also a way of handling tension within a household when other members want, or are obliged, to do things that upset the chemically sensitive member. If there is a rule that one room is a no-go area for certain activities, but that they are permitted elsewhere or outside the home, it helps defuse squabbles and emotional competition, especially between children.

The bedroom is usually the best place for an oasis, partly because most people spend so much of their lives there, and partly because it is usually recognised as a place for privacy and individual expression. If you share the room with a partner, or if a chemically sensitive child shares with a sibling, there may have to be a compromise on how far you go. If you have enough space in your home, you can also create an oasis living-room or playroom, in addition to the bedroom, but for most people, this is not feasible.

How To Do It

Start from zero. Put in the room only what you actually need to have. For most people, at first, this is a bed and a light. Start from that base, and then add to it. For testing and elimination purposes, move anything not essential out temporarily. Reintroduce them one by one to see if they cause a reaction. Only put in what you really want to have and things that are important to you for decoration and pleasure. Have the minimum of furniture and objects. If you put things in that are made of materials that can upset you, make sure they are not new and are well aired off. If you have a radio and clock, make sure they are aired off. If you have veneered chipboard furniture, for instance, it will probably not be a problem once it is a few years old and has gassed out the fumes. Keep pictures to a minimum, and make sure they do not smell. If you have toys, air them off and wash them well (>CHILD-CARE).

Keep things elsewhere if you can. Do you need to have all your clothes in your bedroom, for instance? Could you not keep them in cupboards or drawers elsewhere, in a passage or in the bathroom? Do you need a bookcase or toy shelf actually in the room? Keep toiletries and cosmetics in the bathroom cupboard or in another room. Do make-up in the bathroom or elsewhere. If you do keep things in the room or by the bed, keep them covered up in drawers or behind a cupboard door. Put things away when they are not in use. Put books and magazines in a drawer overnight and keep their number to a minimum.

TIP

If you have an air filter, run it in the oasis if you are out during the day to keep it really clear of fumes (>AIR FILTERS for choice).

Once you know what you react to, if you find that things already in your bedroom (such as the bed, carpet, curtains, bedding, furniture, or even building and decorating materials) upset you even when aired off, it may help to go further and replace them. For advice on choices, >BEDDING, BUILDING AND DECORATING MATERIALS, FABRICS, and FURNITURE.

Ban things that upset you from your oasis. Make your own rules about what comes into it. If you do not want perfumes, after-shave or hairspray in your oasis, or tobacco smoke, then people may have to stay outside, or change clothes or shower before entering. If you do not want polish or detergents, keep them out. Negotiate with family and housemates, but stick to your conditions if they are important to you. Be prepared to have to retreat to your oasis when other people do what they want to, elsewhere

you unmask through avoidance, you clear away these masking, background symptoms and you will recognise them when they recur on exposure. You learn, in effect, what it is like to feel well again.

The strategy of reintroducing everyday chemicals you want to use will also help you to decide what you can tolerate. To get through life,

you may well *have* to use some things that upset you, but if you use
them seldom, or do it in an environment basically clear of chemicals,
they become manageable. You are starting from close to a zero-base and
you have some degree of control over the load of chemicals in your life.

To carry out a radical clean-out elimination programme, follow the
instructions given below. Use this for testing, work out what you can
tolerate, then go on to the next part of this section for advice on long-
term measures for avoidance.

What do I do?

Clear chemicals as far as you can out of your immediate environment,
especially at home, for as long a period as you are able – for at least a
week and for up to two or three weeks if you can. It can take up to a
few weeks sometimes for fumes to disperse and symptoms to clear, so
give it time.

Remember that you may get withdrawal symptoms and may feel
worse or different at first, especially if you are very sensitive to something. (>SYMPTOMS for a full description of withdrawal symptoms). A
teaspoon of sodium bicarbonate in a glass of water (not more than
three times a day) will help relieve these. Paracetamol, in preference to
aspirin, will relieve any pain.

If you can start the programme with a few days spent mainly at
home, it works best. You can, of course, still go out and about, but it
helps to be mainly where you have control over things. So start it over
a weekend or public holiday; for a child, during school holidays or at
half-term; or take time off work. Pretend to yourself that you have
gone to a health farm, if you like.

The programme also works better if you get good co-operation from
the people you live with, work with or from school or nursery. If they
can co-operate – just a bit, if not totally – and try to limit their use of
things like fragrances, toiletries, cleaning products, DIY materials,
glues, paints, etc., it helps a lot. If there have been, or still are, smokers
in your home, you would be best to clear out smoke residues before
you go much further. (>box on page 90). If you are going to have to
cope while still living with smokers, then it is still worth doing the
programme, although results may be a bit clouded.

Create an oasis

If you have not already done so, create an oasis in your bedroom or in
another little-used room in the house where you can go to clear out.
(>box on page 92).

Stop using chemicals

Stop using chemicals that you commonly use on yourself, or around the home. For best results, get a box or bag and go around your home, putting in it anything you find – such as toothpaste, soap, deodorant, shaving gels, the contents of your bathroom cupboard or shelves, talc, all perfumes and aftershaves, bubble baths, hair gels, sprays, mousses, cosmetics, baby wipes and lotions. Include all cleaning products – soap powder and liquid, fabric softeners, bleaches, disinfectants, toilet cleaner, bath cleaner, oven cleaner, washing-up liquid, polishes, shoe polish, everything. Remember to include air fresheners and toilet fresheners; remove any that are stuck to surfaces. Collect up any DIY products, gardening chemicals, and glues, sticky tapes, felt-pens or similar stationery products. Take anything you see. You will probably be amazed at how much there is.

Put the box or bag in a shed or outside the house where the fumes will not reach you. Open the windows and doors and air the place right through for a short while – a few hours or longer, if you can. Keep it well ventilated.

Use only basic personal hygiene and cleaning products as listed below for the length of the programme. Persuade people who live with you to use the same things if you possibly can, to reduce your exposure still further. The same things can also be used on babies and children.

- For *tooth powder*, use sodium bicarbonate or table salt
- For *soap*, use Simple Soap or Kay's Vegetable Oil Soap
- For *shampoo*, use Simple Shampoo or Crimpers Shampoo
- For *shaving gel*, use Simple shaving gel or soap as above

For full details of sources and instructions for use, or if you need to use other things, such as contact lens solution or deodorant, >PERSONAL HYGIENE.

For names of products that chemically sensitive people tolerate well for laundry, dish-washing, general cleaning and toilet cleaners, >CLEANING PRODUCTS. Use the products recommended there for the elimination period, or:

- For *laundry*, use Borax, or sodium bicarbonate or washing soda
- For *dish-washing*, use washing soda
- For *general cleaning*, use washing soda
- For *toilets*, use Borax

>CLEANING PRODUCTS for full instructions for use.

Only use drugs and medicines during the programme that you absolutely have to have. Consult a doctor about whether you can leave

out or change any medication before starting the programme. If you
use emollients or ointments for eczema or dermatitis, try to do without
them completely during the test period – you may actually be sensitive to them. Do not use home medicines. If you need something
urgently, follow the advice in FIRST AID AND HOME MEDICINE. If you
cannot do without a painkiller, use Paracetamol rather than aspirin or
other compounds.

Avoid doing tasks that use strong chemicals if you can, such as DIY,
car maintenance, or using glues and solvent-based writing materials.
Do not use garden sprays or chemicals. Avoid solvent-based felt-tip
pens and white correction fluid.

Reduce your exposure

Reduce your exposure to chemicals and fumes as much as you can
during the test period. Stay out of places where chemicals are heavily
used, such as hospitals, doctors' surgeries, hairdressers' or barbers',
and swimming baths. Some shops are full of chemical fumes –
chemists', perfumeries, newsagents', shoe shops, DIY shops, television
shops, clothes shops – so do not spend too long in any of these. Keep
out of dry-cleaners' and away from agricultural spraying. Drive or
travel as little as you can. If you walk through traffic, try to stay away
from busy roads and junctions.

Ban smoking in your home and elsewhere around you if you can.
Avoid pubs, or public places where people smoke. If you go out to a
cinema, concert or evening event, other people's toiletries may bother
you – perfumes, cologne and hairsprays, in particular – so limit how
much you go out during the elimination programme.

Do what you can at work. If you work with chemicals, say in a
shop, at a hairdressers', at a garage, in a dry-cleaners' or in a factory,
there may be little you can do, but try. In offices, computers, photocopiers, paper stores, and new furniture are potent sources of fumes.
You may have no choice but to stay close to them, but keep away as
much as you can. Make sure the office is well ventilated and take frequent breaks in the fresh air.

At home, it helps if you can avoid using gas and paraffin cookers
and fires that give off strong fumes. Use alternative heaters; perhaps
borrow a microwave for cooking if you can. If you have to use a gas
cooker, keep its use to a minimum, and ventilate well. (Gas central
heating, and gas Agas, offer little problem unless you are extremely
sensitive, so continue using these unless you notice they are causing
you to react.)

Keep television watching to a minimum; only have your set on if
you are actually watching something. Fumes from televisions do not

bother some people at all, but they can give others real trouble. Take care with computers in the same way.

Put newspapers, brochures, magazines and any other paper away, in a drawer or cupboard for preference, unless they are actually being read or used. These can be potent sources of fumes. Stop using paper handkerchieves and kitchen paper towels.

Avoid buying anything new during the test period. If you do, leave it in a spare room or outside the home to air.

Once you have done these things, you should have eliminated most of the major hazards in your immediate environment. If you find anything around you that particularly bothers you (such as a piece of furniture, or plastic equipment), then put it in a spare room, outside the home, or cover it up with a sheet or cloth for the period of testing.

Follow this programme for at least a week, and up to three weeks, if you can sustain it.

After this time, you can reintroduce things you want to use, or increase your exposure to everyday chemicals and see what you are able to tolerate. Do this one thing at a time, preferably only once every few days, and no more than one a day. Monitor your symptoms as you proceed. See how things go, and gradually find out exactly what you can and cannot tolerate.

If you want to go further

If you want to go beyond this and reduce your exposure to chemicals even further, then there is more that you can do. You can avoid contaminants in water and food, avoid using plastics and you can avoid synthetic fibres and fabrics. You can also, if you are prepared to do it, stay indoors totally for the elimination programme and place conditions on what the people who live with you, or come into your home, use and wear. This is really hard-line and does not make you popular, but it can sometimes bring results.

To avoid contaminants in water, use a jug filter for water for drinking, cooking, food preparation, and for washing as far as you can. Alternatively, use bottled water – Malvern, Evian and Buxton are good choices (in glass bottles, if possible). For full advice, >WATER AND WATER FILTERS.

To avoid contaminants in food, eat fresh, unprocessed food – organic, if possible. >FOOD AND DRINK for full advice.

To reduce your use of plastics, stop using plastic containers, wraps and bags for food – use glass or ceramic containers, if possible. Cellophane poses no problems. Do not use plastic carrier bags – old ones are usually little problem, but avoid new ones particularly.

To avoid synthetic fibres and fabrics, wear pure cotton clothes, for preference. Make sure these are well washed if they are new. Avoid pure synthetics where possible – polycotton blends are usually better tolerated than synthetics if you have no pure cotton clothes at all. For bedding, use a pure cotton pillowcase, well washed before use, and lay a well-washed pure cotton cloth or sheet over the top of the duvet or blankets if you cannot borrow or replace a synthetic duvet or blankets with others of a different material.

If you are allergic to cotton, >BEDDING and CLOTHING for advice.

Basic Avoidance Measures

If you have just been diagnosed as chemically sensitive, or have just come through one of the elimination programmes just described, you are probably feeling very unnerved by what you have discovered, wondering how you will cope.

Take heart, it is not as bad as it seems. It is perfectly possible to live with even very severe sensitivity and to function quite happily in everyday life, if you take precautions and follow some basic guidelines. You are not sentenced to a prison cut off from ordinary life. There will inevitably be things in your life that have to change, and you may well have to give up some things that you cherish, but you will not have to become a hermit, remote from the world.

There are no really effective treatments for chemical sensitivity and allergy. Neutralisation therapy can work for some people (>MEDICAL HELP), and some people find that complementary therapies help (>COMPLEMENTARY THERAPY). Taking high doses of vitamins and minerals can also help (>MEDICAL HELP). The only thing that is consistently of any benefit is avoiding chemicals and eliminating them from your environment as far as you can.

Your basic precautions for coping with chemicals are to:

- Manage your load
- Air things when new
- Take care when things get warm
- Avoid fumes
- Think twice before using chemicals

Manage Your Load

What you choose to avoid depends very largely on what sort of life you lead, and what things make you particularly ill. You will probably have to work out your own strategy for balancing what you have to do in life, and what you can tolerate.

Remember the load effect (see page 79). Managing your load of chemicals is an important element in keeping yourself well and on an even keel. If you overload yourself with chemicals that make demands on your system, you may find that you are more prone to react to the chemicals that particularly upset you, or that you feel generally less well. Reduce your load as far as you can. Most people find that they reach an acceptable compromise by:

• reducing generally the level of chemical exposure in their lives
• avoiding their own particular troublemakers

No one person's metabolism is the same as another's – chemical sensitivity is very idiosyncratic; while *you* might be able to tolerate mild amounts of certain chemicals, other people with chemical sensitivity might not tolerate those particular ones at all (and vice versa).

Work out for yourself what you want to use and what you can tolerate. If your system can tolerate plastic bags and cosmetics, for instance, and it is important to you to use them, then go ahead. But listen to your body. If, for instance, you really do get very ill when the gas fire is on, or when you read a newspaper, do not fool yourself, and be prepared to stop doing things, or to cut down on them. Manage your load and you may find that you can do many things in moderation.

Clearing chemicals out of your home can give you a springboard for coping with life. If you do this, it can give you the tolerance to deal with the load of chemicals you meet outside your home. Treat it as a resource where you can go to clean out, rather than a refuge to hide from the world.

If you do not have the energy or money to sort out all or most of your home, or if you have a difficult domestic situation and friction with family or housemates, a good option is to create an oasis in your own bedroom, the place where you clean out (see page 92).

Air Things When New

Take special care when things are new. Air or wash whatever you can. If you air things off or wash them before you use them, you may have no problem at all. If you buy new furniture or furnishings – such as curtains, beds, cushions or rugs – always leave them in a spare room, or get the supplier to air them for you before delivery. Even if they are of materials that you can tolerate reasonably, airing will help. Let new shoes or bags air before using them to get rid of fumes. Wash new clothes before wearing, especially if they are pure cotton, polycotton or viscose, as they may have fabric finishes (>CLOTHING).

Air a newspaper, magazine or book before reading it. Keep newspapers and magazines in a drawer when not in use; their fumes can be very bothersome. Use an old plastic bag rather than a new one. Put new paper, stationery or sticky tape into a drawer or box to air before you use it. Air a new plastic appliance – a radio or audio equipment – before you bring it into the living-room for constant use. Air and wash new toys before use.

Take Care When Things Get Warm

Chemicals that normally would not bother you can give off fumes when they get hot. You may suddenly notice fumes from asphalt surfaces, from car tyres, or from car interiors on hot days. Open up cars and air them before driving off in hot weather. You may be able to tolerate synthetic materials unless you wear them or sleep on them – thereby making them warm enough to give off fumes. You may be able to use plastic bags, boxes, or plastic wrap, unless you use them on warm food. Decorating and furnishing materials, such as paints and plastics, may not bother you unless they get heated, so take care with paint on radiators, around windows and doors, and with lagging and insulating materials (>BUILDING AND DECORATING MATERIALS), and with fabric or plastic lampshades that get heated. Televisions, computers and audio equipment can give off fumes when hot, so you may have to moderate their use and ventilate well when they are on.

TIP

Avoid using a foam padded ironing board cover, or one with a metallic cover. Use a pure cotton cover, and pad with a pure cotton sheet or blanket.

Avoid Chemical Fumes

Avoid doing DIY, car maintenance, using garden chemicals or other tasks yourself unless it is imperative. Avoid newly decorated or treated buildings if you can. Do not use newly dry-cleaned clothes or bedding – hang them up to air for a few days before use (or else avoid dry-cleaning totally). Buy washable clothes whenever possible.

TIP

If you go to the hairdresser or barber, make an appointment to go when the place is not busy – first thing on Monday or Tuesday is a good time to go.

Avoid using gas and paraffin ovens and fires if you possibly can. If you are very sensitive to fumes, replace them with other forms of cooking and heating (gas central heating and Agas are usually less

TIP

Some plants actually absorb formaldehyde from the atmosphere. They have been used by NASA on spacecraft, and are often recommended for use in office buildings where there have been persistent health problems. Try keeping any of these in your home, workplace or school to reduce formaldehyde levels.

Chrysthanthemum	Spathiphylum
Coconut palm	Spider plant
Dracaena	Weeping fig
Gerbera	

>MOULDS for information on how to keep indoor plants if you are allergic to moulds.

Plants for Clean Air can supply these plants for home and office use.

Plants for Clean Air
Unit 2
69 St Mark's Road
London W10 6JG
Tel: 081–964 1110

trouble). If you retain gas appliances, get them and inlet pipes serviced and checked to be sure that they are operating properly.

Take care with barbecues, bonfires and solid fuel appliances. Some people find these no problem, but others are badly upset by them. Do not burn food – charring and burning give off chemical fumes known to upset people. Watch the toast!

Avoid tobacco smoke as much as you can. If you or your house-mates have been smokers, but have now stopped, or if you move into a house where smokers lived before, it helps to try and clear out the residues of tobacco fumes which impregnate carpets, furniture, curtains, even walls (see page 90).

Most hard plastic – used for radios, audio equipment, televisions and computers – does not give problems with fumes, once aired off, unless it gets hot. Some audio equipment is made of a type of hard plastic that can give off persistent fumes, however. It is usually distinguished by a sweet, aromatic smell – stronger than other types of audio equipment – and often has a black/greyish, metallic finish. Sniff equipment carefully before buying to try and avoid this problem.

TIP

If you have any plastic items which bother you with persistent fumes, covering them with a cloth when not in use helps keep down fumes to manageable levels.

Wash new plastic items in a solution of 1 dessertspoonful Borax in a bowl of warm water. This helps neutralise fumes.

Avoid situations where any spraying is being done – spray polish, agricultural spraying, gardening, hairdressing.

TIP

If you live near crop fields, or other places where spraying is done, ask the people responsible to warn you so that you can arrange to keep doors and windows shut, or to be away at those times.

The location of your home may expose you to heavy levels of fumes from vehicles or industry. You are best to live away from heavy traffic if you can, and upwind of local industry. Upper storeys of buildings are usually affected less by vehicle pollution; living in upper storeys of a high rise building may help you cope in a city centre. The eastern side of the UK is generally less favourable for people sensitive to industrial fumes than the western side; the prevailing westerly winds carry pollution eastwards across the country.

Chemical pollution can be aggravated by low, damp, cloudy weather that holds down fumes and discharges. You may be better to restrict going outdoors on such days if you can manage it, or to take extra care if you cannot avoid going out.

TIP

Changing wind direction may affect you if you are sensitive to pollution. Your symptoms may improve on certain days if the wind veers and carries pollution away.

Fumes from a built-in garage can seep into a house. Try and avoid a house with an integrated garage. If in flats with a basement garage, live as high above it as you can.

Chemical sensitivity can also be exacerbated when pollens and moulds are high in the atmosphere, even if you are not actually allergic to these things themselves. Chemical molecules adhere to the surface of the larger molecules of pollens and moulds, and are inhaled in greater concentrations and absorbed at higher levels into the bloodstream. You may therefore feel worse at high pollen and mould seasons (>POLLENS and MOULDS).

TIP

If you are extremely sensitive, it can help to change your clothes and wash your hair or shower after contact with fumes – say, after coming in from work, after an evening out, or after travelling. Hang clothes to air in a spare room or shed.

Fumes from other people – their toiletries, aftershave, perfume, traces of tobacco smoke, soap powder – may upset you if you are exceptionally sensitive. For people with whom you live, it helps if they only wear or use things that you can tolerate. It can also help if family and housemates change clothes or shower if they have lingering fumes about them, when they come into the house – say, after an evening in a pub or at a party, or after a long drive, or even after work.

If you are badly affected, ask visitors to your house not to wear aftershave, perfume or hairspray, and ban smoking. Keep a cloth or headscarf handy, for people to wrap or lay over hair or clothes that really upset you. Some chemically sensitive people even keep a pure cotton gown or apron for visitors to wear. This dampens down fumes very effectively. These are sold by mail order from Sander and Kay:

> Sander and Kay
> 101–113 Scrubs Lane
> London NW10 6QU
> Tel: 081–969 3553

If people sitting next to you at work, school or at leisure activities are using products that bother you, see if you can persuade them to use others – giving them to them to try, if necessary. If they will not, ask to be moved.

TIP

Using an air filter can help cope with chemical fumes (>AIR FIL-TERS for full advice).

Wearing a face mask and covering your hands can help protect you when you have to use chemicals, or are exposed to fumes that upset you (>FACE MASKS and HAND PROTECTION).

For advice on coping with fumes on public transport; with traffic as a pedestrian; choosing and buying a car; car maintenance and driving, >TRAVEL.

TIP

A dose of alkali salts can help relieve, or even stop, a severe reaction to chemicals. A simple version of this is to take 1 teaspoon of sodium bicarbonate in a glass of water. Do not take this more than three times a day for adults, and only once a day for children. For alternative alkali salts and more information, >FIRST AID AND HOME MEDICINE.

TIP

Before trying any new product, use the Sniff Test (page 88) or the Patch Test (page 88) to see if the product upsets you.

Rather than buying a product before patch-testing, ask the shop assistant to apply a sample for you from a product or apply a patch from samples on display.

You can also write to manufacturers or suppliers to ask for samples to test.

Think Twice Before Using Chemicals

Stop to think before you use any chemical, apply it to yourself, or swallow it. Do you really need to use it, or is there a less aggressive alternative? Use the relevant sections of the *Guide* to help you find what to use without problems.

TIP

Take care with toiletry fumes in changing areas at swimming pools and sports centres. Watch out for sprays, etc. Either go when the place is not busy, or go ready-changed and leave fast. Wait outside change areas for friends and companions.

Take care if buying anything secondhand as fumes from cleaning products, tobacco smoke, toiletries and soap powder can still cling. Air things well, and wash them if possible before use.

Put things away when you are not actually using them. Use a spare room or outhouse to put anything that gives off even slight fumes. Put paper and books in drawers or cupboards. This helps cut the general level of fumes.

Fumes from your neighbours' activities – lighting fires, car maintenance, creosoting fences, barbecues – may affect you. Try and reach agreement that they let you know in advance what they intend, or that they do things while you are out or away.

Try to limit the drugs, medication and home medicines that you take to the absolutely essential. Take your doctor's advice before stopping or reducing any prescribed medicines. >MEDICAL HELP for a fuller discussion; >FIRST AID AND HOME MEDICINE for well-tolerated alternatives.

___TIP___

If you have any doubts about a product you intend to buy, check with manufacturers for any information you feel you need (see page 84).

What Next?

This section has given general advice about living with chemical sensitivity. Much of the rest of the *Guide* deals with specific advice on chemical avoidance. In many sections, you will find much more detailed information on where chemicals are found, on detection and tips for avoidance. There is also a lot more advice on what to do if you are very highly sensitive and unable to use even usually well-tolerated substances. The easiest (and cheapest) sections to start with are:

- CLEANING PRODUCTS
- COSMETICS, TOILETRIES AND SKINCARE
- FIRST AID AND HOME MEDICINE
- PERSONAL HYGIENE

The more tricky (and often more costly) areas are:

- BEDDING
- FURNITURE
- BUILDING AND DECORATING MATERIALS
- SEX AND CONTRACEPTION
- CLOTHING
- TRAVEL
- FABRICS
- WATER AND WATER FILTERS
- FOOD AND DRINK

Choose for yourself where to start. If you have difficulty finding the information you need, refer to the Index.

For special advice on avoidance for babies and children, >BABYCARE and CHILDCARE.

For more information on dealing with natural chemicals from plants, >PLANTS AND TREES.

For information on cross-reaction to chemicals, >CROSS-REACTION.

For advice on taking drugs, using medication, and anaesthetics, >MEDICAL HELP.

For advice on dental treatment, >MEDICAL HELP.

Fibres

This section covers natural and synthetic fibres. The fibres discussed are:

- Coir
- Cotton
- Horsehair
- Jute, Sisal and Hemp
- Kapok
- Linen

- Ramie
- Silk
- Synthetics and Blends
- Viscose and Rayon
- Wool

For feathers and down, >MISCELLANEOUS ALLERGENS.
For leather, >MISCELLANEOUS ALLERGENS.
For animal fur and pelts, >PETS AND OTHER ANIMALS.
For latex, >MISCELLANEOUS ALLERGENS.

This section covers:

- How to detect allergy or sensitivity to fibres
- Where fibres are found

At the end, it refers you on to other sections of the *Guide* for detailed advice on avoidance and substitutes.

If You Are Just Starting Out

You might find it useful to read other sections before you start to investigate fibres. Fibres often appear to be the first suspect if you react, say, to your bedding, clothing or furniture, but they are frequently not the prime cause of reactions.

The most common cause of reactions to bedding, for instance, is house dust mites rather than the material of your bedding (>BEDDING for more details). If you react to your clothing, the cause may be chemical treatments and finishes, such as resins or dyes, for instance, rather than the fibre itself (>CLOTHING). If you react to a piece of furniture, the cause can often be house dust mites or chemical treatments (>FURNITURE and FABRICS).

Your laundry agents may also be the cause of apparent reactions to fibres (>CLEANING PRODUCTS). Finally, tiny traces of mould spores cling invisibly to even slightly damp fabrics or bedding. If you know you are extremely allergic to moulds, these may be the cause of reactions to fibres (>MOULDS).

How to Detect Allergy and Sensitivity to Fibres

Wool and synthetic fibres are the most common causes of allergy and sensitivity to fibres. Cotton, silk and linen are much less likely to cause reactions. Fibres most commonly cause breathing, nasal and skin symptoms, though other allergic symptoms, such as headaches, joint pain and gut pain, are also recorded. Synthetic fibres and polycotton mixes can cause chemical sensitivity as well as allergy, and other symptoms such as mental symptoms are possible (>SYMPTOMS for more information).

Standard skin and laboratory tests for allergy are quite reliable at detecting allergy to inhaled fibre particles such as wool and cotton (>DETECTING YOUR ALLERGIES). There are no reliable tests other than avoidance and reintroduction for chemical sensitivity to synthetic fibres.

Allergic and sensitivity reactions to fibres are caused by *inhaling* particles or vapours as well as by *touching* the fibres directly. Other people's clothes, or fibres from furniture or furnishings, or fibres at work, may therefore affect you if you are very sensitive, since particles and fumes will circulate in the air and you will breathe them in. If you get symptoms when you fold laundry, sort clothes or make beds, then inhaling fibres may be the cause, although moulds and house dust mites are possible culprits as well.

If you only get symptoms when you wear, sleep on, or come close to specific fibres, then you will have a clear guide to the source of the trouble. If there is a label, consult it to see what the fabric composition is, and think whether you can see any pattern to your reactions.

There is a relatively cheap and easy way to test at home for allergy or sensitivity to specific fibres – the Pillow Test (overleaf). Washing the cloth with sodium bicarbornate and drying thoroughly before use will minimise the possibility of sensitivity to laundry agents, chemical treatments or moulds interfering with the test.

You will get clearer results from the test if you are able to avoid totally the fibre you are planning to test for at least a day, preferably several days, before you do the test. You can then confirm the Pillow Test by avoiding totally (or as far as is practicable) the fibre that you

The Pillow Test

This test is a shortcut to testing fibres without major expenditure. This should help you tell whether it is the fibre itself causing reactions.

Choose an item made of the fibre you want to test:

COTTON: a T-shirt, pillowcase, cotton towel or cotton blanket.

LINEN: a pure linen tea-towel.

SILK: a silk scarf.

SYNTHETICS AND BLENDS: a garment of your choice.

VISCOSE AND RAYON: a garment.

WOOL: a rug, scarf or sweater.

Wash the item several times, placing 1 dessertspoonful of sodium bicarbonate in the washing machine or bowl. Dry thoroughly and make sure it is bone dry.

Remove the pillow from your bed. Fold the item into a pillow and sleep on it. If you have obvious symptoms, then you can be reasonably confident that you react to the fibre tested.

If you have strong symptoms early on in the Pillow Test, then *stop*. Do not persist if you get an early result.

Take great care if you have a history of anaphylactic shock, or of life-threatening asthma attack (>EMERGENCY INFORMATION for precautions to take).

suspect for a period of a week, and then reintroducing it by wearing or using it again. Monitor any symptoms for the period of avoidance and on reintroduction.

TIP

You may not need to replace totally anything you use or wear. It may be sufficient to place a cloth of a material you tolerate over your pillow or over the upper part of your bed clothes, or wear underclothes of a fibre you tolerate next to your skin or around your neck. Try this before replacing anything.

Where Fibres Are Found

Coir

Coir is a fibre made from the outer husk of the coconut. It is used to make doormats (the bristly type), floor matting and ropes. It is also used as a filling in mattresses and can be used in upholstery. It gives off few particles and rarely causes reactions. Unless you have significant exposure to handling it, say at work, it is an uncommon cause of allergy.

Cotton

As pure cotton, and in blends with synthetics, cotton is very widely used. Allergy to cotton is very rare, despite its wide exposure. It is a cellulose fibre, not a protein fibre like wool, and is hence less likely to provoke an allergic reaction. However, if a reaction does occur, it is the cotton flock – the small particles given off from the fibre – which causes reactions when inhaled. Some people allergic to cotton find they can tolerate it if they avoid very fibrous cotton, such as towelling, knitted cotton or cotton wadding. (For more advice on avoidance, >CLOTHING).

When people react to cotton fabrics, it is often found that they are sensitive to resins applied to the fabric to give easy-care properties, rather than to the cotton itself. If you follow the guidelines for testing cotton in the Pillow Test (see left), resins should not interfere with the test. They are not applied to cotton towels or blankets; and they are rarely or lightly applied to T-shirts and pillowcases. They are also usually washed out after several washes, so using a well-washed cloth for testing should prevent problems for even those highly sensitive to resins. (>CLOTHING for full advice on fabric treatments and finishes.)

TIP

Always wash clothes or fabrics well before using. It may prevent any problem with chemical treatments unless you are highly sensitive.

Fabric resins are applied to furnishing fabrics as well as to clothing fabrics. In addition, pure cotton furnishing fabrics are often treated with fire-retardant chemicals to meet with fire regulations, and some have stain-protection chemicals applied as well. These chemicals may be responsible for apparent reactions to cotton (>FABRICS and FURNI-TURE).

Horsehair

This is hair taken from the mane and tail of horses. It used to be a common material in upholstery and furniture-making but is now much less used. If you are allergic to horses (>PETS AND OTHER ANIMALS), you may be sensitive to horsehair used in furniture. Generally, older furniture is more likely to contain it than modern furniture. For most people, however, exposure to horsehair is low and allergy uncommon.

Jute, Sisal and Hemp

These fibres come from three plants and are commonly used in rope-making. Hemp has been recorded to cause allergy among workers handling it in production. Otherwise, sensitivity is not common.

Kapok

Kapok is a fibre that surrounds the seeds of a tropical tree. It looks and feels rather like a pink-coloured cotton wool. It is used for filling cushions and soft toys. Children are sometimes allergic to kapok in soft toys that they cuddle closely, although sensitivity to house dust mites and other types of filling material is more common. (For a source of supply, >page 278).

Linen

Also known as flax, linen is a cellulose fibre in common domestic use for tea-towels. It can also be used for clothing (often in a blend with cotton), tablecloths and napkins, and for sheets. It is an expensive fabric, which creases easily and so exposure to it, apart from tea-towels, is low. Allergy to linen is rare.

Starches and resins are sometimes applied to linen, and these can cause sensitivity reactions. However, linen without finishes, as in tea-towels, rarely causes allergic reactions. Despite its creasing, it is hard-wearing and can be a useful fabric for people with multiple allergies.

Ramie

Ramie is a yarn made from a plant with fibrous leaves. It is used in clothing, especially knitted garments, often in blends with cotton or linen. It is uncommon and most people never wear it, so allergy is not reported.

Silk

Like linen, silk is an expensive and often impractical fabric in daily life. Silk has few everyday uses, apart from clothing, ties and accessories. It is a protein fibre, like wool, and is known to cause allergy, but because so few people have any significant exposure to it in everyday life, allergy to silk is uncommon.

Resins are not used on silk at all, since they accentuate the fibre's natural tendency to break and abrade. Silk is therefore a very useful fibre for the chemically sensitive. Starches and sizes are sometimes applied, but these usually wash out.

Synthetics and blends

Pure synthetics and synthetic blends commonly cause allergy and chemical sensitivity. Moreover, using synthetics can cause irritation, even if you are not actually allergic or sensitive to the fibres themselves; many people with sensitive skin, for instance, find that wearing or sleeping on synthetics makes their skin worse. This is because the materials do not allow sweat to escape and dry as well as natural materials do. Sweat on the skin increases its permeability to allergens, as well as causing friction and irritation. If you avoid synthetics (even if you are not specifically allergic or sensitive to them), it can be of general benefit and help you relieve other reactions.

Synthetic materials and blends are found everywhere and in every application, from carpets to clothes to insulating materials. Many different chemicals are used, and it may be that you are sensitive to one type of chemical and not to another. Although it is generally better, if you are chemically sensitive, to reduce your load of potential troublemakers as far as you can (>CHEMICALS for reasons), you may find that you can use or wear some fabrics or fibres and not others.

To help you work out if there are synthetics that suit you, the three main types of synthetic fibre in general use are:

Fibre	Brand Name
Polyamide	Nylon
Polyester	Terylene, Crimplene, Dacron
Acrylics	Acrilan, Courtelle, Orlon, Dralon

Lycra is a brand name for polyurethane elastomer.

Some people who react to pure cotton find they can tolerate it in a blend with a synthetic fibre (polycotton or polyester cotton). Similarly, some people who react to pure synthetics can also tolerate polycotton blends. Fabric resins are applied to polycotton blends, although, again, they wash out readily.

Synthetic materials are often used in fastenings, trimmings, elastic and in thread, even on garments or items of cotton or other natural fibres. If you are very sensitive, these may be enough to cause reactions. (>CLOTHING for further information and advice.)

TIP

Wearing synthetic fibres or using synthetic bedding may give you problems, while using it in furnishings may not. This is because the fibres warm up as you wear or sleep on them and give off fumes. You may not need to avoid synthetics except in clothing and bedding.

Dyes on synthetic fibres can sometimes cause allergy and sensitivity and you may mistake this for sensitivity to the fibre. Dyes do not generally cause reactions but Disperse azo dyes are known to be troublesome. These are rarely used on cotton, rayon or wool, but usually on synthetics. Dyes in nylon stockings and tights (even flesh-coloured) are a known area of sensitivity. (See **Socks, Stockings and Hosiery** in CLOTHING for further advice.)

Viscose and Rayon

These are man-made fibres, processed from natural wood fibres or cellulose. Viscose is now more common than rayon, and viscose fabric is very common in clothing. Viscose is also used in cotton blend wadding in tampons, and often in cotton wool pads and bandages. (Sanitary towels are made of wood pulp, not of viscose.)

Resins are used in significant amounts on viscose fabric and appear to wash out less well than from other fabrics; people sensitive to resins often report continuing problems with viscose. Glycerol, a mild solvent, is used on the viscose/cotton wadding in some brands of tampons and can cause sensitivity. Chlorine bleaches are also used in many brands (>PERSONAL HYGIENE for advice on avoidance).

Wool

Wool is a very common cause of allergic reactions, leading to breathing, nasal and skin symptoms, and headaches and joint pains. It can also irritate the skin, even if you are not actually allergic to wool itself. Some people who are sensitive to lanolin also find that wool triggers reactions, since the fat is present in the fibre.

Wool is found widely in most uses, including clothing, bedding, carpets, rugs and furniture. Cashmere, angora, mohair yarns and sheepskin products can also upset you and are best avoided if you are sensitive to wool.

Some people who are allergic to wool find they can tolerate very fine and smooth woollen garments, such as Botany wool knitted garments, woven gabardines or men's suiting. These give off less particles to inhale and are less irritant to the skin.

Easy-care resins are rarely applied to wool fabrics for clothing and furniture. Fire-retardant chemicals are never applied to wool used for furnishing since it meets fire safety standards without any treatment being necessary. Stain-protection chemicals are often applied to wool or wool blend carpets, however, and to wool fabric used for upholstery (>FABRICS and FURNITURE for more information).

How to Avoid and Eliminate Fibres

Full advice on how to avoid and eliminate fibres, or how to find substitutes, is given in further sections of the *Guide*. The sections that are of prime importance are: BEDDING, CLOTHING, FABRICS and FURNITURE.

The following sections may also be of interest to you: BABYCARE, CHILDCARE, FIRST AID AND HOME MEDICINE, HAND PROTECTION and PERSONAL HYGIENE.

Food and Drink

This section tackles a vast subject – allergy and intolerance to food and drink – and cannot deal with every aspect of living with food sensitivity. It concentrates therefore on four main topics:

- what food sensitivity is
- how to work out what you react to
- how to organise and live with special diets
- sources of unusual foods

NOTE: Drinks, with the exception of simple water, are derived from foods – from fruits in juices, from fruits, grains and vegetables in alcoholic drinks, and from natural and synthesised chemicals, such as cola, tea, coffee and flavourings. The terms 'food', and 'food sensitivity', 'allergy' or 'intolerance' always include drinks in this section, unless otherwise specified. For more information on water, >WATER AND WATER FILTERS.

The topic of food sensitivity – of allergy or intolerance to food and drink – is probably the most difficult area of this book. Not only is the subject the most controversial and the one which arouses most hostility from sceptics, but it is also the most demanding area to manage if you are trying to discover what upsets you. Futhermore, food sensitivity is one of the most difficult types of allergy or sensitivity to live with. Avoiding certain foods can affect your family life profoundly, particularly if children are involved. It impinges on your social life and your worklife, and engages you frequently on complicated endeavours of organisation and planning.

Working out a diet that suits you can often be a quite straightforward process if you go about it in an orderly fashion. The vast majority of people find that they can solve their problems by avoiding just one or a tiny number of foods – even if it takes them some time to work out which ones.

However, a small handful of people have much more severe problems, discovering that they are sensitive to a wide range of foods. Often such people do not suspect wide-ranging sensitivity before embarking, and only discover it in the process of eliminating and testing foods.

It is *best to do any exclusion dieting under medical supervision*, because the process of identifying food allergy and intolerance can occasionally be complicated, because some (rare) individuals can become quite ill in the process of sorting out their diet, and because specialist advice on nutritional balance is often necessary. This is especially important if you are working out a diet for a baby or child.

Some doctors, however, are unsympathetic or even hostile to the idea of reactions to food. Many GPs will not consider giving you any help in the process, let alone refer you to someone else who can help. If you meet this reaction from your doctor, remember that it is worth persisting in asking for a referral to a specialist. Your doctor may eventually agree, if only because he or she believes it will exclude food allergy or intolerance as a possible cause of your symptoms. You have also the right to change your doctor without giving a reason and, if you meet with real hostility, it may be necessary to do this. For how to find doctors who specialise in the field, >MEDICAL HELP.

If, despite all your efforts, you cannot get satisfactory help from a doctor, you may decide to carry through a limited exclusion diet by yourself. If you do so, *go gently*. You should only exclude foods selectively, rather than go for a comprehensive exclusion diet (see below for full advice), and take your time, rather than to try to identify problem foods quickly. *Never go on a fast or a one- or two-food-diet without supervision.*

If you suspect food allergy or intolerance, and want advice on how to work out what you react to, go straight to page 121 for advice on how to detect food sensitivity. If you have been testing foods for some time, and feel confused by your results, there is advice on how to sort things out on page 131. If you know you are sensitive to foods and want advice on how to deal with it, >page 154. For specific advice on managing a rotation diet, >page 148. For sources of unusual foods by mail order, >page 166.

If you are caring for a baby or child, read this section first, and then go to BABYCARE and CHILDCARE. In these sections, there is specialised advice on how to apply this section's advice on detection and dietary management to babies and children, plus advice on feeding and weaning babies, handling young children on special diets, and dealing with school. Hyperactivity (or hyperkinesis) in children is dealt with in CHILDCARE.

For full advice on treatments for food sensitivity, >MEDICAL HELP and COMPLEMENTARY THERAPY.

For a short summary of what food allergy and intolerance are, read on from here.

What is Food Sensitivity?

Food sensitivity manifests itself in people who react adversely to food and drink that they consume. You can be 'allergic to', or 'intolerant' of a substance. The distinction between allergy and intolerance is important; allergy and the various forms of intolerance have different patterns of symptoms, and they are detected by different tests and diets, so detection and diagnosis are very much affected by this distinction.

Allergy and intolerance also respond to different types of treatment, and, perhaps most importantly, to differing ways of managing your diet. It is often possible, for instance, if you are intolerant of a food, to keep it in your diet, provided you do not eat too much of it too often. However, if you are severely allergic to something, you may be unable ever to eat even tiny amounts of it. It can therefore be crucial to know whether you have food allergy or intolerance, especially if you have a very restricted diet and need to take care with its nutritional balance.

Unfortunately, there is no quick nor totally conclusive way of telling whether you have food allergy or intolerance. Skin and laboratory tests for allergy – for the involvement of the immune system – can be inconclusive and misleading, although very helpful if they show positive results that correspond to your pattern of symptoms and history of illness. (>DETECTING YOUR ALLERGIES for full details of tests.)

Exclusion dieting – leaving out foods and reintroducing them in systematic fashion – is the most reliable method of sorting out what you react to and whether you have allergy or intolerance. Such dieting takes time and patience and can be confusing if you turn out to be sensitive to several foods, but it is really the only way to be sure.

A detailed discussion of what food allergy is, and of the different types of food intolerance, is to be found in DEFINING ALLERGY, and a full description of the symptoms of each is set out in SYMPTOMS. The main points of definition are as follows:

Food Allergy

Food allergy is probably less common than most people believe, since many cases of reactions to food are food intolerance rather than true allergy. Allergy to foods will show positive results to skin and blood tests. You are likely to react whenever you eat a food to which you are allergic, even if you have not eaten it for a very long time. You are more likely to have an immediate reaction, even to a small or tiny amount of food, although reactions can be delayed. You may be able to recollect a specific date or occasion when you first reacted to a food.

The symptoms of allergy to food are those of the classic allergic diseases – asthma, eczema, hay fever, rhinitis, urticaria, anaphylaxsis. Nausea, vomiting, diarrhoea, gut pain, gut spasm, oedema, joint pain, severe headaches and other late or remote allergic reactions are also symptoms which can be linked to food allergy.

Almost any food can cause allergy, but the common ones are cow's milk and its products, eggs, wheat, yeast, citrus fruits, nuts, and beans and pulses. Proteins are more prone to cause allergy than other foods.

Allergy to foods can respond to treatment with anti-histamine drugs, and to sodium cromoglycate (Nalcrom) (>MEDICAL HELP). Severe allergy to foods may not be helped by these, and in these cases, total avoidance of the offending food is the best remedy.

Even if your symptoms are mild, if you have food allergy, you will usually be advised to avoid the food totally. Unlike food intolerance, reducing the amount you eat or leaving the food out of your diet will not make you able to tolerate it again.

Food Intolerance

Food intolerance is an umbrella term covering a number of adverse reactions to foods, including some in which the specific causes have been identified, such as false food allergy; reactions to histamine, caffeine and other chemicals in food; and enzyme defects. For information on whether these might cause your symptoms, >page 121.

The main type of food intolerance of concern to this section is one in which the mechanisms and causes are not known, but in which the involvement of the immune system is unproven. No single set of symptoms characterises the disorder but the main ones include:

Headache	Vomiting
Migraine	Nausea
Fatigue	Stomach ulcers
Hyperactivity in children	Duodenal ulcers
Recurrent mouth ulcers	Diarrhoea
Aching muscles	Irritable bowel syndrome
Joint pain	Constipation
Rheumatoid arthritis	Wind, bloating
	Crohn's disease
	Oedema (water retention)

(From *The Complete Guide to Food Allergy and Intolerance* by Dr Jonathan Brostoff and Linda Gamlin.)

The onset of this type of intolerance can be very hard to identify. Often people report that symptoms are mild at first, but then steadily get worse, almost imperceptibly, until they realise that they feel generally unwell, often tired and exhausted, as well as having specific problems. Symptoms can also disappear for a while, and then come and go. New symptoms can develop over time, as well, which complicates diagnosis. Many systems of the body can be affected and different individuals are affected in various ways, according to their own constitution and metabolism.

Reactions are usually slower than those of true food allergy, and more likely to be delayed. You are more likely to be sensitive to foods that you eat regularly, probably at each meal; and this regular intake appears to help 'mask' symptoms and lead to the general, background feelings of malaise, lack of energy and being unwell that typify food intolerance. Another characteristic feature of food intolerance is that people are often able to tolerate a food in small amounts, only reacting if they eat a lot of it, or if they eat it very frequently.

Leaving out foods of which you are intolerant often leads to withdrawal symptoms, so you feel worse initially (>SYMPTOMS for details), and then better after a few days. Reintroduction of an offending food can sometimes provoke intense, severe reactions – often different from the kind of general masked symptoms of which the person had been complaining. The severity of these reactions can diminish in time, however, if the food is left out for a long while, or if it is eaten only at regular intervals of a few days, or in small amounts. It appears that the body has a capacity, in food intolerance of this kind, to cope with a certain amount of the food, so you may be able to keep it within your diet, provided that you do not exceed your body's tolerance of it.

People who have sorted out their diets often report that all kinds of vague symptoms that they did not consider linked to food sensitivity (such as earache, vaginal discharge, cystitis, insomnia, irritability, tension and tiredness) clear up as well as their principal symptoms.

Food intolerance of this kind is also found associated with other diseases, such as rheumatoid arthritis, irritable bowel syndrome, candidiasis and Crohn's disease. Some people with these conditions improve following changes to their diet, although the specific reasons for the links between their disease and food intolerance are not known.

There are no medical tests to detect this kind of intolerance. The only method of detection is exclusion dieting, leaving out foods and reintroducing them systematically, while monitoring symptoms. Almost any food can cause intolerance but the most common culprits are also those which often cause allergy (see page 119). Why this should be so is not understood.

Some people seem to be intolerant to specific groups of foods. Some people do not tolerate proteins (for instance, meat and poultry) but have no problem with other types of food. Other people find, by contrast, that they do not tolerate fruit and vegetables well, but tolerate proteins or grains better.

Most people with food intolerance are sensitive to only one, or a tiny number of foods, and find that their problems can be resolved by avoiding those foods. Sometimes it can be something as simple as leaving out tea, coffee, chocolate, monosodium glutamate, alcohol or sugar. People with multiple food sensitivities often find that totally excluding their main troublemakers helps their overall tolerance level and they react less severely to foods that sometimes upset them. The 'load factor' that applies to chemical sensitivity (>CHEMICALS) appears to operate with food intolerance as well.

The only treatment for this type of food intolerance is *managing your diet* with the aim of reducing or totally avoiding the foods upset you. Advice on managing diets is given below. Some people are also helped by high doses of vitamins and minerals, especially if they are also chemically sensitive. Again, why this should be so is not known. Some people respond to neutralisation – a form of desensitisation. (For more advice, >MEDICAL HELP.)

How to Detect Sensitivity to Food and Drink

Skin and laboratory tests for allergy to foods are not always conclusive or reliable. They need to be considered in the context of a detailed history of symptoms (>DETECTING YOUR ALLERGIES for more information). Exclusion dieting, followed by challenge testing – eating a food to see if you react – is the most reliable method of testing for both food allergy and all types of food intolerance.

One specific form of food intolerance, which reproduces the symptoms of allergy and responds to treatment with anti-histamines, is called 'false food allergy' (described in DEFINING ALLERGY). It can be detected by modified laboratory tests for allergy. Certain foods are known to cause false food allergy (i.e. peanuts, beans, pulses, wheat, egg white, shellfish, pork, fish, chocolate, tomatoes and strawberries) and other foods are suspected of causing it (i.e. buckwheat, mango, mustard, papaya, raw pineapple, sunflower seeds). If you have classic allergic symptoms caused by any of these foods, respond to anti-histamine treatment, but have negative results to tests for allergy, false food allergy may be the cause.

Food intolerance caused by specific chemicals found naturally in certain foods can only be confirmed by exclusion dieting. Some foods contain chemicals that have effects directly on the body, such as histamine, other vasoactive amines and caffeine. Histamine is found naturally in fermented foods, cheeses, well-ripened foods such as salamis and sausages, and fish of the mackerel family that has been kept too warm. Other vasoactive amines are found in cheeses, fermented and pickled foods, yeast extract, chocolate, bananas, avocados, wine and citrus fruits. Caffeine is found in tea, coffee, chocolate, cola drinks and some painkillers. For a full description of this kind of intolerance, >DEFINING ALLERGY and SYMPTOMS.

Exclusion dieting will also help identify known enzyme defects that can cause food intolerance and specific symptoms, or coeliac disease, a form of wheat and gluten intolerance. A specialist doctor will be able to identify such defects readily from your pattern of symptoms.

Hyperactivity in children has been linked to enzyme defects and food intolerance. (>CHILDCARE for full advice on detection).

TIP

People with food sensitivity often exhibit some identifiable traits of character or behaviour. While not precisely symptoms, these are strong indicators of sensitivity. >the box opposite for details.

How to Carry Out an Exclusion Diet

There are a number of ways in which you can carry out an exclusion diet – that is, a diet in which you leave out foods that you suspect and then reintroduce them to monitor symptoms. Whichever way you go about it, it is important that you *do it thoroughly*. If you leave a food out of your diet (even if it is only one food), you have to leave it out totally during the testing period to be confident of your results. You may not get clear results if you cheat a bit, or eat 'just a little' of something. Only you and your conscience need know what you actually do eat, but *be honest with yourself* and be prepared to redo the exclusion period if you succumb to temptation.

Be aware also that *it can take time* to get clear results. You need to leave a food out, wait for a while and then try it again. Even to test one food, it can take up to a few weeks to be absolutely sure about it, and if you are sensitive to a number of foods it can take longer. So be

Am I Food Sensitive?

The following characteristics are often typical of people who are sensitive to foods. Some of them are also common to people who are sensitive to chemicals (>CHEMICALS). If you see anything of yourself in one or more of these traits, then suspect food sensitivity.

I Have Food Addictions or Obsessions

People sensitive to a food or drink often have an addictive or obsessive relationship with it. Certain foods are extraordinarily important to them. Sometimes they eat or drink an excessive amount of a food, but more often they need to consume it constantly, craving it and often feeling better when they first eat or drink it again. If you wake up in the morning and do not feel well until you have consumed a particular drink or food, this is a prime indicator of food sensitivity. Feeling awful in the morning, to the point of feeling sick or even vomiting, is often a symptom of withdrawal from a food.

A child who craves constant biscuits/milk/cheese/juice/anything else may well be sensitive to that food. An addictive relationship with alcohol is sometimes caused by the foods (e.g. grapes, grains, hops, yeast) from which the drink is made, or the yeast in the alcohol.

I Have Unsatisfied Hunger or Thirst

Another indicator of food sensitivity is excessive hunger or thirst that is not satisfied by eating or drinking. Still feeling hungry after a big meal is often linked to sensitivity to a food. Excessive and constant thirst, often accompanied by constant need to urinate, is also a sign – particularly noticeable in young children. It sometimes accompanies puffiness and weight swings (see below). In adults, excessive sweating also often accompanies heavy thirst.

I Have a Puffy Face

Puffiness, particularly noticeable around the face, is a trait of food sensitivity. Fingers, ankles and other joints also suffer as well. Fluid retention can result from reactions to foods and this puffiness is a sign.

I Have Big 'Shiners' Under My Eyes

Big black rings – so-called 'shiners' – are another indicator, although they can also be a sign of nasal allergies. A constant sniff, a runny nose, and persistent sinusitis, are often linked to shiners.

I Can Never Lose Weight

Failure to lose weight on a weight reduction or slimming diet is a common sign of food sensitivity, possibly due to fluid retention.

I Lose and Gain Weight Sharply

Some people with food sensitivity have very erratic weight patterns, with sudden sharp losses and swings in their weight. Some people are capable of gaining or losing several pounds overnight, or during a day. The reason for this is probably fluid gain or loss.

I Have Erratic Mood Swings

Sudden variability of temper and mood – highs and lows, and sudden anger or irritability – is a strong indicator of food sensitivity, although it is also linked to chemical sensitivity. People who become very animated or excitable after a meal, drink or snack (or children who become hyperactive), are often found to be sensitive to a food they have eaten. Sudden vagueness and distance, sudden swings into depression or moroseness also result.

My Symptoms Come and Go

Variability of symptoms is often a sign of food intolerance, rather than allergy. Capricious symptoms that often worsen for no apparent reason, or disappear, are a feature of the disorder.

I Feel Constantly Rotten and Exhausted

Feeling generally awful and always tired is a common sign of food intolerance. It often accompanies multiple food sensitivity although it can be caused by one food alone.

patient and do not be in too much of a hurry – it is better to get good results eventually, than to get confusing results straightaway.

If you are testing for an adult, do not worry overmuch about nutritional balance for the period of exclusion dieting, unless you continue with it for a period of more than a few weeks, or unless you are already in poor health. Providing you are eating a variety of different foods and are in generally good health, leaving out a few foods that are important to general nutrition will not do you permanent harm. *Seek advice from a doctor if you are worried.*

If you are pregnant, breastfeeding, or thinking of conceiving within the next year, you should not go on an exclusion diet unless a doctor advises.

Working out a diet for a baby or young child should *always* be done with a doctor's advice.

Single-Food Exclusion Diet

The way that most people start an exclusion diet is by leaving a single food out of their diet totally. If you have an obvious suspect in mind – one that you think makes you ill, or one with which you have an addictive relationship, or which you particularly crave (>box on page 123) – start with that one.

The benefits of the single-food approach are that you are not excluding many foods at once, so that if there is absolutely no change, or if you feel substantially better straightaway, you know that you have a clear result from this food. If you have really no idea which food to choose first, but want to follow a single-food diet, there is advice on page 130 on how to keep a Foods Diary and to choose where to start.

If you go the single-food-exclusion route, choose your food and leave it out of your diet *totally* for a minimum of four days, and preferably for a week. This gives your system time to clear the food. If you are sensitive to that particular food, you may feel worse at first and get withdrawal symptoms, including cravings for that food. (>SYMPTOMS for a description of withdrawal symptoms.) As your system clears the food, you should start to feel better and, by the fourth day, you should feel significantly improved if that food is the source of your problems.

If you feel a lot better, you may decide to leave the food out permanently, provided you can find ready substitutes in your diet. If you get inconclusive results from exclusion, or if you want to confirm whether the food actually does make you ill, test-eat the food following the protocol in the box on page 126. If the first food you exclude and test gets no result, then proceed on to another candidate and test that systematically, using the same total exclusion and reintroduction procedures.

There *are* drawbacks to the single-food approach, however. The first is that it is very difficult *totally* to exclude the common allergens, such as cow's milk, eggs, wheat, yeast and corn, from your diet, unless you leave out virtually all processed foods. Cow's milk products, for instance, are found not just in milk, yogurt, cheese and butter, but also in all sorts of processed foods like biscuits, pies, white sauces, even in

How to Test a Food after Exclusion

Before Starting

If you are extremely sensitive to a food, have a history of anaphylactic reactions to food, or of life-threatening asthma attack, your doctor will advise whether it is safe for you to test foods or not, but you should always take emergency precautions before testing (>EMERGENCY INFORMATION) and not test unsupervised. If you have no such history, such precautions would not be essential.

If you have had immediate allergic reactions to a food, or are nervous about testing, one useful test you can carry out prior to actually eating the food is the Cheek Test. Smear a small amount of the food or its juice on the skin of your cheek and leave for half an hour. If you develop symptoms in that time, do not test-eat the food without further consulting a doctor. This is a useful test to do for babies and young children.

How to Monitor Symptoms

Before starting to eat, note down how you feel, and whether you have any specific symptoms already so that you will notice any change.

Eat the food you want to test, as a single food (see below for full advice). If you have a history of allergic reaction, you may only need to eat a little and your doctor may advise you not to eat too much. If you have no clear history of allergy, you may need to eat a lot of the chosen food: you may only react if you eat a large amount and it is better to get a clear result on the first round of testing. (You can experiment later to see if you can tolerate smaller amounts.)

Next, *wait and see if symptoms develop*. Note down any adverse changes (physical or mental) that you notice, and the time when they occur. Most people find that, if they are going to react, symptoms start to develop within the first four hours after eating. Delayed reactions can occur, especially with proteins and grains, and you can develop symptoms up to eight hours later or even the next day.

Do not take food or drink other than water for at least four hours after testing so that you do not confuse the results. Some people like to test foods in the late afternoon or evening, so that they can be at home resting and are able to monitor symptoms for several hours after eating.

TIP

If you get very hungry when testing or on an exclusion diet, a drink of hot boiled water helps quell hunger cravings and get you through to the next meal or snack.

If you feel worse the next day or get withdrawal symptoms (>SYMPTOMS for description), these will confirm any symptoms that you noted on eating the food.

If you have no reactions to a food first time round, it can be a good idea to wait a week (or a minimum of four days) before eating it again, and then repeat the test to be absolutely sure of negative reaction.

Pulse and Weight Checks

If you want to be more rigorous about testing foods, you can take your pulse and weigh yourself before and after eating. Some people, not all, have significant pulse changes on eating a food. Take your resting pulse rate before eating as follows: Rest for 10 minutes, then place your finger on your pulse at neck or wrist and count the beats for 15 seconds. Multiply the number of beats by four, to give your pulse rate per minute. Take your resting pulse rate again at 20, 40, and 60 minutes after eating. A rise or fall of more than 10 beats per minute after eating a food is an indication of a reaction. It must be a *resting* pulse rate – rest for 10 minutes before taking the pulse, otherwise it will rise and fall naturally as you move around.

To check your weight, weigh yourself morning and evening on the day that you test. If you put on more than 0.5 kg (1 lb) during the day, that is a sign of a reaction.

TIP

A further indicator of a reaction is to take a sample of handwriting an hour after eating. Many people find that the quality of their script degrades significantly, beyond their control, after a food reaction. It is a useful check on children testing and can be done without them knowing it is part of the test.

How Often to Test?

If you are testing foods on a single-food exclusion diet, or on a special low-allergen diet, under medical supervision, you will be advised as to how often you can test new foods. It is best not to test too often, and most people are recommended to test one food a week, or not more than one every four days. If you are on a total exclusion diet, you will be given specific advice as to what and how often you can test.

If you are on a permanent diet, such as a rotation diet, it is a good idea to use this testing protocol if ever you want to introduce a new food into the diet. If you want to test water, or anything else you swallow or ingest, such as toothpaste or medicines, use the same test procedure as above.

Testing Foods Singly

When you test a food, the best way to do it is to *eat it singly, on its own*, without any accompanying foods. You should not use any cooking oil or fat, flavouring, sugar, sweeteners, or herbs or spices on it. You can use salt, but it is best to use sea salt or Pure Salt BP (available from chemists or Green Farm Foodwatch – see page 168 for address). Either grill, bake or boil foods which need cooking. If you cook in water, use filtered water or bottled Evian, Buxton or Malvern. Alternatively, cooking in a microwave can be a useful way of cooking meat, poultry, fish, vegetables or eggs, since no fat and little water are required.

It *is* possible to test a food without eating it as a single food. You can combine it with others, but if you do so, you must be sure that you do not react to the foods with which it is combined. You can sometimes get confusing results, as well, since combining can affect some people's ability to tolerate a food (see page 134). So only combine foods when testing if it is really important to you.

Eat common foods in the following ways:

BEET SUGAR	Silver Spoon white sugar *or* plain boiled beetroot
CANE SUGAR	Tate and Lyle white sugar *or* golden syrup
CHOCOLATE	Cocoa made with water, no sugar
COFFEE	Black coffee, no sugar, not instant
CORN	Sweetcorn

TIP

Remember that a food must be just that one food. Roast potatoes are cooked in cooking fat or oil, as are chips and crisps. Fish fingers are not just cod or haddock, but breadcrumbs, batter, flavouring and colouring. Eat just the food and nothing but the food!

Pure orange juice in cartons or bottles is not always 100 per cent orange. Manufacturers are permitted to add tiny amounts of sweeteners, even if the juice is labelled unsweetened. Malic acid from apples is used as a sweetener in some brands. Do not use processed orange juice for testing, to be certain.

COW'S MILK	A glass of cow's milk (test butter, yogurt and cheese separately; they can give different results)
EGGS	Soft- or hard-boiled *or* scrambled in microwave (no fat)
EGG WHITE	Whipped into meringue and baked (no sugar)
EGG YOLK	Scrambled in microwave (no fat)
FRUIT	Fresh or stewed in water Avoid dried fruit if mould sensitive Avoid canned fruits Avoid juices unless freshly squeezed
OATS	Porridge oats made with water
OILS	*Either* sip a tablespoon of oil *or* Corn: eat sweetcorn Groundnut: eat unprocessed peanuts (from wholefood shops) Olive: eat olives Sesame: eat sesame seeds Sunflower: eat sunflower seeds Soya: >below
POTATOES	Plain baked, boiled or jacket
RICE	Plain boiled rice Ricecakes (from wholefood shops) Rice noodles (from wholefood shops) Kallo Rice puffs without honey (from wholefood shops)

RYE	Original Ryvita crispbread
SOYA	Plain boiled soya beans
	Make own soya milk (recipe below)
	Tofu
	Unsweetened soya milk
TEA	Black tea, no sugar, not instant
WHEAT	Allinsons Wholemeal Crispbread
	Matzos (Jewish crackers)
	Shredded Wheat (no milk or sugar)
	Weetabix (no milk or sugar)
	Pasta (check no egg included)
YEAST	Fresh yeast (from wholefood shops)
	Brewers' Yeast Tablets

To Make Your Own Soya Milk

50 g (2 oz) soya flour
600 ml (1 pint) water (preferably bottled or filtered)

Soak the soya flour in the water in a heatproof bowl for 2 hours. Place the bowl in a large pan of boiling water and cook for 20 minutes. Cool, then strain through a fine sieve. Stir before using.

pills, home medicines and margarine. *You have to leave the food out totally to get results.* For guidance on where common foods are found so that you can avoid them totally, >the boxes on pages 136–43. If you get inconclusive results after testing one of the most common foods, look at the relevant box and check that you have excluded it totally. Retest a food, if necessary, before turning to another food. If you still get inconclusive results after testing several foods, see page 131. If you are in fact sensitive to more than one food, you may get only partial improvement in your symptoms on single-food exclusion and it can take a long time for you then to work through other suspects individually. If you suspect multiple sensitivity, you may be better starting off on a more stringent diet (>page 147).

A single-food exclusion diet is also not always helpful if you have no obvious suspects and really do not know where to start. If this applies to you, and you do want to try this approach, rather than a more radical diet from the outset, keeping a Foods Diary for a week to 10 days will help identify possible candidates to test. Note down every time you eat, drink or ingest something (whether it is food, drink, drugs, home medicine or even toothpaste). Note down any change in symptoms, whenever they occur, and see if you can detect any pattern at all.

Watch out for delayed reactions – if you feel worse at night or the morning after eating a particular food, this may be a sign of intolerance, especially with grains and proteins, which the body takes longer to break down. Watch out also for withdrawal or cravings. If you feel unwell until you can consume a drink or particular food in the morning, or until you eat something specific at a snack or meal, then suspect that food or foods.

If you really cannot see an obvious suspect, then pick one of the most common causes of allergy and intolerance, such as wheat, eggs, corn, yeast or cow's milk, and leave that out totally. Alternatively, you could choose a food that is not such an extensive part of basic diet and hence easier to leave out – such as tea, coffee, chocolate or oranges – and start there.

If You Get Confusing Results

If you get confusing results while you are testing foods on an exclusion diet, or if you get confused on a permanent avoidance diet, investigate any of the following.

Are You Leaving Out a Food Totally?

Even a tiny trace of a food to which you are sensitive can be enough to make you react. >the boxes on pages 136–43 for advice on totally avoiding corn, cow's milk, eggs, soya, wheat and yeast. Avoid *all* processed foods if you want to be absolutely sure that you are leaving out any food totally. Remember oils, herbs and spices are foods as well – leave these off any food you are testing.

Are you consuming anything else that might contain the offending food, even if you are not actually eating it as a single food? Avoid home medicines (including homeopathic) and drugs, if at all possible – they may contain the food in tabletting, syrups or flavouring. You may have to stop using toothpaste, mouthwashes and other such products. Avoid licking stamps, envelopes or other gummed surfaces – these are often gummed with glues derived from wheat, corn or potato. Avoid taking vitamins and minerals unless it is essential and you know exactly what is in the formulation. Think of anything else you might lick or chew – chewing-gum, paper, anything at all?

You May Be Suffering Withdrawal Symptoms or Delayed Reactions

You can get delayed reactions to a food, and withdrawal symptoms after eating it. If these occur within the next day, or two days, after eating a food, they can be hard to tell apart, although withdrawal symptoms have certain characteristics (>SYMPTOMS for full details). If you feel well on eating a food, and do not feel ill until several hours after a meal, this is most likely a delayed reaction. If you feel ill the next day, it can be either delayed or withdrawal reaction. Either way, it is the food you ate the day before that is upsetting you.

If you get unexplained reactions, keep a note of the foods you ate the day before and see if there is any pattern. Proteins and grains are particularly prone to cause delayed reactions.

Delayed reactions can occur up to several days after eating a food. This is more common in cases of dermatitis. To track this down, you may have to eat suspect foods only once every two weeks and see what happens. Long delayed reactions of this kind are very rare in children, who usually react within a few hours of eating a food.

Reactions May Be Due to Overload

People sometimes react unexpectedly to a food that they normally tolerate, if they are under a great deal of load or stress.

If you have multiple sensitivity – are allergic or sensitive to many other things – sometimes the overall load seems to affect your system. Your tolerance drops unexpectedly and you start reacting to many things at once. High pollen season or high mould season (>POLLENS and MOULDS) often seems to bring on food sensitivity in people who are fine at other times of the year. Exposure to places with high levels of chemical fumes can bring on food reactions, often temporarily. Eating too much of foods to which you react, but which you tolerate normally at low levels of consumption, can tip you over into reacting more often. Watch out for triggers of this kind. Test foods again when your system is less under stress.

The process of exclusion dieting sometimes brings on temporary intolerances as well, which disappear once a permanent diet is established. Some people seem to go into a downward spiral, starting to react to many things which normally they tolerate. If you react to a lot of things suddenly on an exclusion diet, it does not mean the situation is permanent – it is sometimes just the body's response to the process of testing. *Test foods less often and less intensively* – spread out testing to wider intervals if you can possibly do so, to give your system a rest. A rotation diet (see page 148) following testing will help to settle things down.

Women are prone to react more to foods at times when their hormones are fluctuating – at ovulation in mid-cycle, or at pre-menstrual times. See if your food reactions correspond to your menstrual cycle. If your cycle is erratic, look back at when reactions occurred and see if there is any pattern. Hormonal surges at the menopause, or during and after pregnancy, childbirth and breastfeeding, can bring on temporary food sensitivity.

A virus, especially a gastric upset, can induce food sensitivity temporarily. Gastric upsets, in particular, disturb the natural balance of the gut and can exacerbate mild intolerance and allergy or bring on new intolerances. Take extra care after a gastric upset, if necessary going back to a strict diet for a while. Viruses, such as colds or flu, can also knock the system temporarily. Take extra care when you have a virus and afterwards; avoid food testing then, if possible.

Taking drugs, or having an operation, can also affect food sensitivity. Antibiotics, particularly, often affect the system.

Babies often develop temporary food intolerance when teething. Take extra care with diet at those times.

Overgrowth of Candida – candidiasis – can cause unexplained food reactions (>page 146).

Finally, but not least important, emotional stress and worries can bring on, and exacerbate, food sensitivity. A sudden shock, a car accident, prolonged family or money worries, stresses at work – any kind of stress can affect your tolerance of food. Sometimes the effects can be delayed – the response to a bereavement, for instance, can take years to work through, and it is only in hindsight that you can see the connection. If you have stress or worries, even half-hidden, acknowledging their presence will help deal with food sensitivity.

Are You Eating Too Much of a Food?

You may be able to tolerate a food if you eat just a little of it. Eat smaller portions and see if things improve. If you are on a rotation diet (>page 148), put the food on a longer rotation – eat it once a month for a while, then once a week and see if things improve. Try eating a food only once in a day, especially if on a rotation. Eat it just at one meal or snack and see if that makes it tolerable.

Are You Cross-Reacting to Closely Related Foods?

You may get unexpected reactions through cross-reaction to foods

which are closely related to other foods to which you are sensitive
Read the section on CROSS-REACTION to learn more. Some foods are
related in ways you would not expect – for instance, peanuts to beans,
peas and pulses; potatoes to tomatoes, aubergines and peppers; carrots
to parsley and parsnips; avocado to bay leaves and cinnamon. Obtain
a full list of food families, if necessary (>FURTHER READING), for understanding these relationships may make sense of the pattern of your
reactions.

Are You Eating a Food in Combination?

Some people can only tolerate a food if they eat it completely on its
own, without any other food with it (including herbs, spices and oils
for cooking). Try eating a food singly, to see if it helps. Leave a three-
or four-hour gap before you eat anything else.

Alternatively, you might respond to eating foods on the Hay
System, which is of benefit to some people with food intolerance. This
is a way of eating, the main principles of which are to eat fruit before
meals, and not to mix acid and alkali foods at the same meal. >FUR-
THER READING for a list of books that are helpful.

Are You Bingeing on Substitutes?

Having left out a food or foods that upset you, are you going over-
board on their substitutes? If you overload on substitutes (such as
oats, soya or goat's milk), you can become sensitive to them, even if
they were fine at first. Go easy, eat substitutes in moderation and keep
your diet varied and unrepetitive to protect against new intolerances
or allergies.

Are You Eating Pure Foods?

Some people do not tolerate certain food additives well – this is well-
recognised in some cases of hyperactivity in children (>CHILDCARE).
Avoid processed food generally to avoid additives.

Some people who are chemically sensitive react to traces of chemicals in foods and drink. To see if this applies to you, try eating an
organic or additive-free version of a food to see if you tolerate it better
(>pages 168–169 for sources). You can be sensitive to foods or drugs
ingested by an animal you consume (>pages 154–169 for advice on
avoidance).

Drink pure water and eat foods free of water from processing
(>WATER AND WATER FILTERS).

Do not use plastic wrapping or containers on foods. Use ceramic,
glass or marble kitchen utensils.

Some people are sensitive to tiny traces of invisible moulds on foods, even fresh or organic foods. (>MOULDS for full advice on how to avoid these problems.)

If All Else Fails

If you are still confused about food testing or diet, either go back to a strict diet if you were once on one, or go back to page 126 and test foods systematically from the start.

If you still cannot sort things out, >MULTIPLE SENSITIVITY and DETECTING YOUR ALLERGIES.

Special Exclusion Diets

If single-food dieting has been inconclusive or confusing, or if you appear to have multiple food sensitivity, the next step recommended by doctors is often a special exclusion diet. It is a halfway stage between single food testing and a total exclusion diet (which is described below).

There are two basic kinds of special diet. The first type is a so-called low-allergen diet in which all the major foods that commonly cause allergy or intolerance are omitted. The second type is a much more specific type of diet, in which a specific range of foods is suspected of causing allergy or intolerance. These only are omitted, often leaving some common allergens in the diet. Specific diets of this kind include gluten-free, anti-candida, mould-free and low-salicylate diets. More of these below.

Before a doctor chooses which diet to put you on, you will usually be asked to keep a Foods Diary, noting down absolutely everything you eat, swallow or ingest, and monitoring the timing and nature of symptoms. The doctor will then choose the specific range of foods according to your particular pattern of symptoms and food habits.

The principles of low-allergen diets are to leave out all foods commonly causing allergy and intolerance, to leave out processed and manufactured foods, and to eat foods which are as free of additives and chemicals as possible. The best known of the so-called low-allergen diets is the Stone-Age Diet pioneered by Dr Richard Mackarness. A typical comprehensive low-allergen diet is given on page 144.

It is usually recommended that you follow this type of diet for five days to a week, giving time for your symptoms to clear. You may, as with the single-food diet above, find you feel worse at first and have withdrawal symptoms. However, if you have excluded the foods that upset you, you should begin to feel much better after five days. You

Avoiding Corn

As well as being a food in itself, corn (or maize) is used very commonly as a sweetener, and as a starch in food processing.
To avoid corn you have to stop eating the following foods:

Sweetcorn	Maize
Corn on the Cob	Maizemeal
Cornflakes	Polenta
Popcorn	Corn Snacks
Buttercorn	

Do not use the following *in cooking*:

Corn Oil
Maize Oil
Cornflour
Baking Powder

Avoid any processed foods containing corn or maize. Read labels. Avoid any foods containing the following, which are derived from corn:

Corn Meal
Corn Starch
Corn Syrup

The following ingredients are usually derived from corn, although they can be from other sources. *Avoid any food containing these* to be absolutely sure:

Dextrimaltose	Fructose
Dextin	Glucose
Dextrose	Glucose Syrup

Avoid the following glucose products that are usually corn-based:

Glucose drinks (e.g. Lucozade)
Glucose tablets (e.g. Dextrosol)

Avoid the following ingredients, which are derived either from corn or wheat:

Cereal Starch
Edible Starch
Modified Starch
Starch

If a product contains *vegetable oil* of unspecified nature, it can often be corn oil. Avoid this. Similarly, if a product contains *sweet-*

ening or *syrup* of unspecified nature, it may well be corn. Avoid these.

To avoid all the above ingredients means *avoiding most processed foods*, especially sweetened ones such as snack foods, cakes, confectionery, biscuits and puddings. Children's sweets are a common source. Pies, sauces, prepared savoury dishes, sauce mixes, custard powder, gravy mixes and stock cubes also often contain corn in the form of starch and oil. Corned beef and some brands of instant coffee also contain corn, although this is not always clear from the labels. If in doubt, leave a product out of your diet.

Corn is often, with other cereals, a base material for *beers*, *lagers* and *spirits*. Avoid these while excluding corn.

Corn is used in tabletting and coating many drugs, and in syrups for medicines. *Take your doctor's advice* about avoiding prescribed medicine. Stop taking any home medicines. Vitamin C (ascorbic acid) is sometimes derived from corn.

Corn is sometimes used as a glue on envelopes and other similar uses. Avoid licking envelopes and stamps.

Corn starch is sometimes used to stiffen and seal paper and waxed cups and cartons. Avoid using these for food use. It is sometimes used as a starch on cotton clothes, for instance on some denim clothes, but washes out readily, and should not cause problems on contact after clothes have been washed several times.

can then reintroduce foods into your diet, using the protocol described on page 126.

The benefits of a special exclusion diet of this kind are primarily for people who have had confused results from leaving out single foods, or who can identify no obvious candidates for single-food exclusion, or who have other multiple allergies or sensitivity with competing symptoms. It is a less rigorous approach than a total exclusion diet, and more balanced nutritionally, but more rapid and effective than single-food dieting.

Two major drawbacks of a special exclusion diet are that it is expensive and inconvenient. You have to rely on being able to eat mainly at home, or carry packed foods with you. It is also eccentric and makes you conspicuous. You often feel ravenous and empty, although these can be withdrawal symptoms. A final drawback is that, if you really have very severe problems with multiple sensitivity, it will not be adequate to sort them out straightaway. Only a total exclusion diet on a rotation basis will do that.

Avoiding Cow's Milk

To avoid cow's milk, you have to *stop eating dairy products* made from it:

Milk	Soured cream	Evaporated milk
Butter	Fromage frais	Condensed milk
Yogurt	Buttermilk	UHT milk
Cream	Ghee	
Cheese	Milk powder	

(For advice on baby formula feeds, >BABYCARE.)

You need to *avoid using any of the above in cooking* and avoid using butter as a cooking fat (e.g. in scrambled eggs and omelettes). Remember to avoid using milk products in:

Mashed potatoes	Waffles	Cakes
Sauces and gravy	Yorkshire puddings	Biscuits
Butter	Breaded coatings	Custards
Pancakes	Puddings	Any other baking

Avoid any processed foods containing milk products. Read labels. Avoid any foods containing the following which are components of cow's milk:

Whey and whey powder	Lactose
Casein	Lactalbumin
Caseinates	

Avoid the following processed foods that contain milk and its products:

Battered products (e.g. fish)	Anything containing cheese
Pancakes	Custards
Waffles	Egg custards
Yorkshire puddings	Rice puddings
Ice cream	Milk sauces
Sorbets	Cheese sauces
Anything made of or containing milk chocolate	

In addition, many types of the following foods contain milk products. *Avoid these* unless you have checked the labels, or you know from the manufacturer exactly what has gone into them. Many types of bread contain milk products. You will find them not just in bread, but also in breaded products such as fish, and in bread-

crumbs in stuffing. A local baker or wholefood shop may be able
to supply bread without milk components.

Bread	Pies
Breadcrumbs	Dumplings
Breaded products (e.g. fish,	Cakes and baked goods
chicken legs)	Soups
Margarine	Sauces
Biscuits	Canned food in sauces (e.g.
Puddings	baked beans)
Powdered beverages	

The following brands of margarine do not contain milk components: Granose, Tomor, Vitaquell, Vitasieg, found in wholefood
shops. Look also for Jewish *pareve* or *parve* bread or margarine.
Prepared to kosher laws, they will contain no trace of cow's milk.

Lactose, a sugar derived from cow's milk, is used commonly in
tabletting drugs and home medicine remedies. *Take your doctor's
advice* about avoiding this in prescribed drugs. *Stop taking any
home medicines*, including homeopathic remedies, which are
sometimes tabletted in lactose. (>COMPLEMENTARY THERAPY for
advice on alternative ways to take homeopathic remedies.)

TIP

>pages 157–159 for advice on substitutes for cow's milk.

Some people who are sensitive to cow's milk generally can
tolerate it in heat-treated forms. >page 158 for full advice on
things to try.

If you are specifically lactose intolerant, >page 159 for cow's
milk products which are well tolerated by people with your
condition.

Some types of Feta cheese, usually made with sheep's milk,
are made with cow's milk. Check before buying.

Some brands of sheep's yogurt include tiny traces of cow's
milk. Check before buying.

Avoiding Eggs

To avoid eggs, you have to *stop eating eggs cooked by themselves* (e.g. scrambled, poached, fried, etc). You have to *stop using* them in *cooking* as follows:

Batter

Pancakes

Waffles

Yorkshire puddings

Puddings

Biscuits

Cakes

Glazing on bakery

Custard

Egg custard

Meringues

Macaroons

Quiches and flans

Soufflés

Sauces (e.g. mayonnaise, hollandaise)

Avoid any processed foods containing eggs or egg products. Read labels and avoid any food containing *egg yolk, egg white* or *ovalbumin*.

Lecithin is sometimes derived from eggs and sometimes from soya. Avoid products containing this (e.g. ice cream and margarine) to be absolutely sure. Eggs are often used for glazing baked products, such as pies, buns or sausage rolls. These are best avoided.

Avoid the following processed foods which contain eggs:

Quiches and flans

Battered products (e.g. fish)

Pancakes

Waffles

Yorkshire pudding

Breaded products
(e.g. fish, chicken legs)

Sorbets

Scotch eggs

Custard

Egg custard

Confectioners' custard

Meringues

Macaroons

Mayonnaise

Hollandaise sauce

Tartare sauce

Egg noodles

In addition, some of the following processed products often contain eggs, although not always. If you are not sure of their contents from their labels, leave them out.

Bread

Biscuits

Cakes

Confectionery

Soups

Sauces

Puddings

Baking powder

Pasta

Avoiding Soya

To avoid eating soya, you have to *stop eating*:

Soya milk	Soya oil
Soya beans	TVP
Tofu	Soya sauce
Soya flour	Miso

(For advice on baby soya milks, >BABYCARE.)

Soya, in its various forms, is found commonly as an ingredient in processed foods (e.g. pies, bakery, prepared dishes). Read labels to see if any of the above products are mentioned. If a product contains *vegetable oil* of unspecified nature, it can often be soya oil. Avoid this. If it contains *vegetable protein*, this is invariably soya, and should be avoided.

Lecithin is sometimes derived from soya and sometimes from eggs; products containing this (e.g. ice cream and margarine) are best avoided to be absolutely sure.

Many breads now contain *soya flour* as well as wheat flour. You will not know this if you buy unlabelled bread from a local baker or wholefood shop. Check with them as to what ingredients they use. *Avoid bread* if you are not sure whether it contains soya or not.

TIP

If you are chemically sensitive, you may react to the water used to make up processed soya milks rather than soya itself (>WATER AND WATER FILTERS for more information). For information on how to test soya as a single food, or to make your own soya milk, >page 130.

Avoiding Wheat

To avoid wheat, you have to stop eating foods made entirely or mainly from it:

Breakfast wheat cereals	Wheat bran
Bread	Wheat germ
Pasta	Cracked wheat (bulgur)

Most of the following foods are commonly made with wheat; unless you know for sure they are made totally without wheat, *you must avoid them*:

Biscuits	Breadcrumb stuffing
Crackers	Batter
Pastry	Battered foods (e.g. fish)
Pies	Pancakes
Sausage rolls	Waffles
Cakes and bakery	Yorkshire pudding
Puddings	Dumplings
Breaded food (e.g. fish, chicken legs)	Suet puddings
Gravies and mixes	Pretzels
Sauces and mixes	Snack foods
Stock cubes	Croûtons
Casserole sauces	Melba toast
Soups	Baking powder

Wheat is commonly used as a cereal filler and thickener in processed foods. Read labels and *avoid foods containing the following* which are usually wheat:

Cereal binder	Cereal protein
Cereal filler	Flour

Avoid the following ingredients which are derived either from wheat or corn:

Cereal starch	Modified starch
Edible starch	Starch

To *avoid wheat as an ingredient* in processed foods, you may have to avoid the following which often contain it. If not absolutely sure, avoid the food.

Sausages	Pastes
Frankfurters	Spreads
Luncheon meats	Powdered beverages
Pâtés	

Wheat is often, with other cereals, a base material for *beers*, *lagers* and *spirits*. Avoid these while excluding wheat.

Wheat is used in tabletting some drugs and home medicines. *Take advice from your doctor* about avoiding prescribed medicines. Stop taking any home medicines.

Wheat is sometimes used as a glue on envelopes and similar uses. Avoid licking envelopes and stamps.

Communion wafers are made of wheat. It is best to avoid swallowing or licking these if you can. Your minister or priest will be able to advise you on what to do. Holding the wafer in your mouth without touching it, or touching it without licking it, is often a satisfactory solution.

Avoiding Yeast

To avoid yeast, you have to *stop eating* the following foods:

Bread	Vitamins based on yeast
Breaded food (e.g. fish, chicken legs)	Oxo cubes
	Stock cubes
Breadcrumbs	Bovril
Yeast bakery (e.g. crumpets, muffins, doughnuts, croissants)	Vinegar
	Pickles
Alcohol of all kinds	Sauerkraut
Ginger ale, ginger beer	
Yeast spreads (e.g. Marmite)	
Brewers' yeast	

Yeast is often contained as an ingredient in all kinds of processed foods, biscuits and baked goods. Read labels and *avoid any foods containing the following*:

Hydrolysed protein
Hydrolysed vegetable protein
Leavening

If you are highly sensitive to yeast, it may also benefit you to leave out other mould- and fungi-containing foods (including cheese, mushrooms and malts). (>MOULDS for a comprehensive mould-free diet.) You may also respond to an anti-Candida programme (>page 146).

A Typical Low-Allergen Diet

The following diet is typical of the kind sometimes recommended if you get confusing results from single-food testing, or if you are suspected of multiple food sensitivity. Often called a low-allergen diet, it is helpful in identifying both food allergy and intolerance. It excludes all foods that commonly cause sensitivity, plus all manufactured and processed foods and drinks.

Permitted Foods

All fresh meat, poultry and game (except chicken and smoked, salted or pickled foods)

All fresh vegetables

All fresh fruit, except citrus. Do *not* eat:

Orange	Citron
Grapefruit	Tangelo
Lemon	Pomelo
Satsuma	Ugli
Tangerine	Kumquat
Clementine	Lime

Buckwheat, Sago, Tapioca, Quinoa

Olive oil

Sea salt or Pure Salt BP

Black pepper, white pepper

Herbs

Spices

To drink: Water (preferably filtered or bottled Buxton, Evian, or Malvern)

Some versions of the diet also permit the following foods, unless you already know that you are sensitive to them.

Free-range chicken

All fresh fish (not smoked, salted, pickled or canned)

All nuts and seeds

All beans and pulses (not canned, nor manufactured, processed e.g. not baked beans or soya milk)

Vegetable, fruit and nut oils (not corn oil, or rice oil)

Honey

It is preferable to eat organic foods and field-fed meat and free-range poultry, if you can possibly manage it (>pages 166–7 for sources).

Foods to Avoid

All eggs

Milk (cow, goat, sheep) and its products (butter, yogurt, cream, cheese)

Grains and cereals (wheat, oats, rice, corn, barley, millet) and all their products (e.g. bread, cakes, biscuits, crackers, crispbreads, pies, pastry, oils, malt, pasta, bakery etc)

All sugars (cane, beet, maple, fructose) and their products (treacle, syrup, molasses)

Citrus fruits (see list above)

Salted, smoked and pickled meat, poultry and fish (e.g. bacon, ham, kippers)

Coffee, tea, cocoa, chocolate and beverages

Alcohol

Vinegar

Yeast and yeast extract

All manufactured and processed foods

Do *not* eat:
- Canned food and drink
- Fruit juices, drinks and squashes
- Dried fruit
- Sweets and chocolate
- Chewing-gum
- Margarine
- Jams, marmalades and spreads
- Pickles
- Sauces and mustard
- Bread and baked foods
- Snack foods, nuts and crisps
- Cooked meats, sausages and pies
- Pastes and spreads
- Prepared dishes, cook-chill foods

Organising the Diet

You can eat as much of the permitted foods as you want and at any time of day. You follow the diet for five to seven days to see if symptoms clear, and then start to reintroduce foods to test them.

Most people find that they get very hungry on this diet and need to eat large amounts of the permitted foods to keep going. Root vegetables, such as potatoes, sweet potato, carrot, swedes, parsnip or turnip can be very useful to fill you up, as can buckwheat. If you are able to eat nuts, seeds and beans and pulses, these are also filling. You may also have to eat unconventional meals – a grilled chop for breakfast, say, or a baked potato as a mid-morning meal to keep you going.

If you get unusual symptoms or confusing results while on the diet, >page 131. When you come to reintroduce foods, >the box on page 126.

If you get confusing results on a special exclusion diet, your doctor may advise you to go on to a total exclusion diet. For details of this, see opposite.

If your doctor suspects specific types of intolerance or allergy, you may be put on a very specific type of exclusion diet, such as a gluten-free diet for coeliac sufferers. If you are highly allergic to moulds, you may cross-react to moulds in foods and a mould-free diet will be proposed. Details of this diet are given in MOULDS. If you are sensitive to aspirin, you may react to foods that contain salicylates, the active ingredient chemicals. Details of this diet are given in CROSS-REACTION.

If you suffer from overgrowth of Candida – candidiasis (>SYMPTOMS) – you may be put on an anti-Candida diet. Although candidiasis is not itself a form of food intolerance, it appears to exacerbate the condition of people with food intolerance and allergy. One treatment for candidiasis is through diet. This is not specifically a treatment for food intolerance or allergy, but works rather by depriving the Candida organism of the nutrients it needs to survive in the human body. Candida thrives on sugars – both pure sugars and those produced during digestion from the breakdown of fruit sugars, carbohydrates and yeasts. An anti-Candida diet excludes any foods that feed the Candida fungus. (If you are, coincidentally, also allergic to, or intolerant of, those foods, or allergic to Candida, you get a double or treble bonus of clearing those symptoms as well as the candidiasis.) A full anti-Candida programme, including diets, is given in *The Complete Guide to Food Allergy and Intolerance* by Dr Jonathan Brostoff and Linda Gamlin (>FURTHER READING).

If You Are Vegetarian

If you are vegetarian, you will have realised by now that it is difficult to undertake an exclusion diet and to stick to a vegetarian regime. Some of the most common problem foods – eggs, cow's milk, cheese, grains, nuts, beans, soya, pulses – are the building blocks of a vegetarian diet. Many vegetarians have, in food sensitivity terms, a high-risk and repetitive diet with a heavy load of potential troublemakers.

You may have to renounce your vegetarian diet for at least the period of exclusion dieting. Use unusual cereals such as sago, tapioca and buckwheat. Use pulses and nuts sparingly and only eat types that you rarely eat. Introduce fish if your principles permit, but take care as fish can be allergenic.

If You Have an Ethnic or Religious Diet

If you eat a particular diet because of your religion or because of your ethnic background, add to the list of the potentially most allergenic foods any foods that you eat a great deal as part of the diet. Do not forget spices, or flavourings such as monosodium glutamate.

Total Exclusion Diet

The principle of a total exclusion diet is that you either fast, or eat just one or two specific foods, for a period of up to five days, then reintroduce and test foods. The fast or two-food period will clear your system of foods that you eat commonly, and should unmask background symptoms. *You can become very weak and ill on a diet of this kind. You can do it at home, but should never do it without a doctor's knowledge and supervision.*

The best-known version of a two-food diet, the lamb and pear diet, is often prescribed for up to five days. You eat nothing but lamb (baked or grilled, with no oil or cooking fat) and pears, and drink nothing but water, preferably filtered or bottled. You can eat as much of these two foods as you want or need – for breakfast, lunch, tea or dinner – but nothing else at all.

Lamb and pears are chosen for the diet because, it is argued, they rarely cause reactions. The diet originated in the United States where lamb and pears are not common items in the diet, and hence are uncommon causes of allergy and intolerance. In the UK, however, they are much more frequently eaten and do cause reactions, although relatively rarely. Some doctors in the UK therefore prefer to use other, less often eaten foods, such as turkey and peaches, or rabbit and raspberry.

After the fast, or two-food diet, you start reintroducing and testing foods. Reintroduction is usually done on a stricter basis than for single-food testing or a special exclusion diet. It is usually recommended that you eat foods singly (not combined with any other foods), that you leave four hours or more in between testing foods, and that you organise foods on a rotation, so as to avoid problems with cross-reaction between related foods. (For more information on testing foods and organising a rotation diet, >pages 126 and below.) A doctor will usually give you a diet sheet to follow, based on your own history and preferences, which will help you with the complexity of planning. Depending on how many foods you test (and how many you react to), it can take between two and four weeks to devise a permanent diet.

The drawbacks of this type of exclusion diet are fairly obvious. It is time-consuming and almost impossible to combine with an active life. The foods you eat can be costly. You can be very weak and hungry while carrying it through, apart from any reactions you might get to foods you test. If you have a lot of food sensitivities, it can take a long time to devise a manageable diet.

On the other hand, if you are as highly sensitive as that, this is the only way to work out a tolerable diet, and it can turn up some sur-prises. People often find that they are not sensitive to foods that they had assumed to be a problem, and that, conversely, something unex-pected turns up to be a real villain. Often just one or two foods turn out to be the root causes of symptoms and that can be an enormous relief. It really does sort out what is going on and if you can stick it out, it is an invaluable process.

There are two in-patient units in the UK where you can go through this type of diet with constant medical supervision. For details, >MED-ICAL HELP.

Rotation Diet

What is a Rotation Diet?

The principle of a rotation diet is to manage your diet formally, so that you only eat certain foods at given intervals. *Its purpose is both to pre-vent and to cure.* It helps prevent you developing new intolerances or allergies by keeping your diet varied and unrepetitive. It can help cure mild allergy or intolerance by reducing the load of a food in your diet, while still allowing you to eat it in moderation.

A rotation diet is usually planned on a four-day basis. You are allowed to eat a particular food on one day in the rotation, and not again until that day comes around once more. The foods that you tol-erate are allocated to each of the days of the rotation and you stick to that system. So on Day One you have a list of foods from which you can choose what you will eat that day; on Day Two, you have your Day Two list, and so on.

A four-day basis is chosen because four days gives the body time to clear the food from the system, and most people are able to tolerate foods well at four-day intervals. You usually start out on a four-day rotation, keep to it strictly and then modify it to suit your own system, or way of life.

Organising a Rotation Diet

Table 6 shows an example of a typical rotation diet for someone with mild sensitivity who can eat a wide range of foods, and can tolerate some commonly troublesome foods, such as cow's milk, eggs and wheat, if eaten on a rotation.

This diet treats all fish, all eggs, all birds and all nuts, as if each category is one food. Some people react to all fish, irrespective of the species or type, and a strict diet will confine all fish to one day – similarly with eggs, birds and nuts. A less strict diet allows you to eat different types of fish, nuts, birds and eggs on each day of the rotation and greatly expands your choice. (Peanuts are legumes, not nuts, and can be eaten separately from other nuts.)

This diet is also constructed to take account of 'food families'. Some people cross-react to foods that are closely related. On a rotation diet, foods that are closely related have to be eaten on the same day, or else can be eaten at a two-day interval. In one example in the diet in Table 6, you can see that cow's milk is eaten on Day One, while goat's and sheep's milk, which are closely related to it, can be eaten on Day Three. In addition, cow's milk is related to beef and to lamb. Beef has been allocated to the same day as cow's milk, and lamb has been allocated two days away, on the same day as sheep's milk.

A doctor or dietitian will usually draw up a rotation diet for you and help you with any changes you eventually want to make, so that it is planned correctly. If you want to know more about how to make changes yourself, >below and also **CROSS-REACTION**.

The diet in Table 6 is based around a core of fairly ordinary foods. If you find you cannot tolerate foods like these, even on a rotation, it is usual to substitute more unusual foods such as game, rare fish, exotic fruit and rare grains.

Some people prefer to move, once they are established on a rotation diet which they tolerate, to a seven-day rotation based on the days of the week. This has the advantage of simplicity in planning, but it can be monotonous, and even exasperating always to eat certain foods on certain days of the week. It is also not feasible if you have very few foods that you tolerate, or if you cross-react to related foods, and need

Table 6: **A Typical Rotation Diet**

DAY	ONE	TWO	THREE	FOUR
PROTEINS	Beef	Pork	Lamb	Birds
	Rabbit	Eggs	Fish	Turkey
		Venison		Chicken
				Duck
MILKS	Cow's milk		Goat's milk	
	Cheese		and cheese	
	Butter		Sheep's milk	
	Yogurt		and cheese	
GRAINS AND	Wheat	Tapioca	Rice	Buckwheat
STARCHES	Oats		Corn	Sago
	Rye		Millet	
FRUIT	Apple	Banana	Pear	Dates
	Berries	Melon	Apricot	Kiwi
	Grapes		Peach	All Citrus
				Rhubarb
VEGETABLES	Carrot	Sweet Potato	Sweetcorn	Potato
PULSES AND	Avocado	Green Beans	Cabbage	Tomato
BEANS	Parsnip	Peas	Broccoli	Lettuce
	Onion	Courgettes	Sprouts	
	Garlic	Cucumber	Watercress	
	Olive	Soya		
	Spinach	Lentils		
	Mushroom			
NUTS AND SEEDS	Nuts	Peanuts	Sesame	Sunflower
OILS	Olive Oil	Groundnut	Corn	Sunflower
	Grapeseed Oil	Soya	Sesame	Palm Oil
	Nut Oils			
SUGARS	Beet Sugar	Honey	Cane Sugar	Maple Sugar
				and Syrup
BEVERAGES	Chocolate	Tea	Coffee	Dandelion
				Coffee
HERBS AND SPICES	Bay Leaf	Nutmeg	Allspice	Tarragon
	Cinnamon	Rosemary	Clove	Mint
	Chives	Oregano	Coriander	Sage
	Parsley	Basil	Cumin	Thyme
	Ginger		Dill	
MISCELLANEOUS	Yeast			
	Alcohol			
	Vinegar			

to organise your diet to allow for food families, which requires an even number of days in the rotation.

A longer rotation, however, suits some people better, not just for reasons of practicality. They find they cannot tolerate foods on a four-day rotation, but are able to do so on a longer rotation, say once a week, or even once a month. A compromise solution that often works well is to keep a basic four-day rotation as the core of the diet, and to include other foods occasionally, as often as you find you are able to tolerate them.

If you tolerate foods reasonably well after a while, you can move to a two-day diet, eating foods in rotation every other day. This is pretty close to normality and easier to live with.

If you are extremely sensitive and have very few foods, you may have to reduce your rotation to less than four days, although this has the risk that you build up sensitivity again and find that you start to react to the foods that previously were fine. If this happens, lengthen out the rotation as far as you can, eating foods that you have not eaten for a while, and give the foods you have been eating intensively a rest for a short time.

It is best to start strictly with a rotation diet and then, once you feel well enough, experiment with what you can tolerate, and work out your own compromise. If you feel worse, you can always go back to the strict rotation, get things straight and then try again. It takes time but, provided you are not eating things that upset you badly, you can generally work out something acceptable.

TIP

Remember that everyone is different. What suits you may not suit someone else with food sensitivity. Work out your rotation for yourself and do not worry if it is not the same as anybody else's.

People often get worried about their nutritional balance when on a rotation diet. The individual days of a rotation often look to be lacking in important nutrients. A doctor or dietitian will have taken this into account, however, and what they look for is an adequate supply of nutrients over several days of the diet, rather than on specific days, or at individual meals. If there is inadequate supply of an important nutrient, they will propose a supplement. They will advise you if there are specific foods that you should always eat on the allocated day. A well-constructed rotation diet will also give you a good balance of protein, carbohydrate and fat, so that you feel nourished and full.

Modifying a Rotation Diet

If you want to modify your diet after you have been on it for a while, or change the days of allocation because you are bored with the combinations of foods, there are a few tricks which help in planning.

Step one

Most people find that the core of their diet, around which the rest is organised, are the proteins, milks, and grains and starches. Start with these, using the headings of the chart in Table 6 if you like, and allocate the proteins, milks and grains that you tolerate to the number of days that you want for your rotation.

Observe the food families unless you know that you have no tendency to cross-react >FURTHER READING for sources of lists of food families. Allocate related foods either all to the same day, or keep them at least two days apart.

Step two

The next step for most people is to allocate other carbohydrate-rich and filling foods to balance up days on which there is not adequate proteins, grains or milk. Foods which are important here are potato, sweet potato, parsnip, swede, turnip, soya, lentils, nuts and seeds, mushrooms, avocado, and vegetable grains such as buckwheat, sago and tapioca, if these are not already allocated. Follow the food families.

Step three

After that, there remain the rest of the vegetables, fruits, and the culinary necessities such as oils, sugars, herbs and spices, plus beverages, alcohol, yeast and vinegar. The allocation of these will be driven in part by taste preferences, but the food families will probably play a large role in where things need to go, plus the question of preferred food combinations.

It is a good idea, for instance, to allocate wheat and yeast on the same day so that you have the option of eating bread. Most people then allocate cow's milk to that day as well, plus beet or cane sugar, so that they can use butter on toast, scones or bread, or can bake wheat cakes, biscuits or puddings. However, once cow's milk is allocated, it usually brings with it beef or lamb because they are related, and chocolate too, if you tolerate it, so that you can eat milk chocolate. Yeast brings with it cheese, mushrooms, yeast spread and vinegar, because they contain yeasts or moulds related to it. Alcohol, if you can tolerate it, must also accompany yeast, and it usually needs to go with grapes (for wine, port or sherry), apples (for cider), or grass family grains (base material for many spirits). Beet sugar is related to spinach and needs to be allocated in relation to that. Cane sugar is related to corn and the grass family. For how to tell beet sugar from cane sugar by brand and product, >page 161.

So, pretty soon, after just a few decisions, major parts of your rotation will be set. Now allocate the rest of your foods to balance up the diet. Consult a food families list (>FURTHER READING) to check that you have allocated foods correctly. Some of the key foods to double-check since they have unexpected or multiple relations are:

Apple	Lettuce
Berries	Peanuts
Cabbage	Pear
Carrot	Peas, beans, pulses
Chicken	Potato
Cucumber	Sunflower
Dates	Tomato

Foods that are particularly useful in planning a rotation are those that have relatively few or unimportant relations. They can be very useful for adjusting the balance of a rotation once the main food families and food groups are fixed. These include:

Avocado	Olive
Banana	Pineapple
Buckwheat	Pork
Coffee	Rabbit
Duck	Sesame
Fig	Sweet Potato
Ginger	Tapioca
Kiwi	Tea
Maple Sugar and Syrup	Turkey
Nutmeg	Venison

Allocate herbs and spices last since they, like oils, are largely dictated by food families of other important food groups. Herb teas can follow where culinary herbs are allocated.

>page 164 for more practical tips on running a rotation diet.

How to Deal with Food Allergy and Intolerance

How you deal with any food allergy or intolerance you have depends on how severe your reactions are, and how many foods you react to.

Basic Avoidance Measures

Avoid foods

The best course of action wherever possible is to avoid the foods to which you are sensitive. If you have had very severe reactions to a food on exclusion dieting, you should leave it out of your diet totally, and will probably need no encouragement to do so. >the boxes on avoiding cow's milk, corn, eggs, soya, wheat and yeast (pages 136–43), for advice on total avoidance of these foods.

Use substitutes in your diet where possible (>page 157 for tips and ideas for substitutes for common foods). A doctor can advise you on nutrition and on any need for vitamin and mineral supplements. You can also ask for a referral to a dietitian which can be very helpful, especially if you are managing a baby or child's diet.

Manage your diet

If you are sensitive to many foods, or even to a small number of basic foods, it can be virtually impossible to avoid everything to which you react. If you have come through exclusion dieting and found this to be the case, *do not despair*. Except for some very rare individuals, it is quite possible to manage your diet and live with multiple sensitivity. Food intolerance and mild allergies respond to dietary management – eating foods seldom and in small quantities will help you to keep them in your diet and maintain some kind of balance.

With food intolerance and mild allergy, the severity of reactions often declines markedly if you do not eat a food constantly or in large quantities. The body seems able to build up a certain level of tolerance. Therefore, a doctor may recommend that you keep a food to which you are sensitive in your diet, but eat it in moderation.

You may also be recommended to leave a food out for a long time – say, a few months or even a year – and then try it again, even if you had severe reactions to it on testing. (Doctors are only likely to recommend this where you have food intolerance rather than allergy.) The reason for trying this is that many people find that they regain tolerance for a food to which they been sensitive after leaving it out for a long time. You can then include the food in your diet, but again eating it in moderation and at intervals.

A rotation diet (as described on pages 148–53) will also help to maintain the body's level of tolerance to foods, and to prevent you developing new sensitivities.

When you first start on managing your diet, it is best to start by being very strict, avoiding troublesome foods and sticking to the guidelines of the diet you have been advised to follow. After a while, many people find that, as their wellbeing improves, their overall tolerance of foods improves as well and they can be less strict or even eat foods that previously upset them. Many people prescribed a rotation diet find after a while that they do not have to continue to rotate foods and that they can return to a more or less ordinary diet, avoiding only certain foods to which they are very highly sensitive.

Special diets are therefore not necessarily a life sentence. Follow them strictly at first and then ease off, to see how you go. You can always go back to the strict diet to get yourself well again if you find your symptoms creeping back. Find out for yourself what you can tolerate – eat a little of a problem food occasionally and see what amount of it you might be able to bear. Watch out for masked symptoms (feeling generally rotten, and having background symptoms again), which can return when you eat a problem food regularly.

You may have to get used to being very organised about your meals – taking food with you to work or school, speaking to restaurants or hosts in advance to make sure they cater for you. It pays to be assertive – most people are very helpful, provided they have enough information on what you need.

Some of the biggest problems that arise in managing a permanent special diet stem from organising them alongside normal family meals. If one or two foods have to be avoided, it is not usually much of a problem to accommodate within ordinary household catering; but if more foods are involved, or if more than one household member has a special diet, then it can become a nightmare of planning and juggling.

One solution that people sometimes adopt is to put the whole household on to the special diet, or something close to it. It is often easier to organise and plan this way, but it has some drawbacks. It often causes stupendous rows, it can be very costly (depending on the foods you have to eat), and it can have one unforeseen consequence – it occasionally reveals that other family members have food allergies and intolerances too, unmasked by the special diet, and they start to get sharp reactions typical of an exclusion diet. It is not a good idea to put anyone through that process without good reason, without supervision or without foresight.

You may well have hidden food sensitivity in your family, given that allergy and food intolerance often run in families, and that mild symptoms often go undetected and unreported. It is better either to leave it alone, or to sort it out systematically, rather than find it out by accident when one family member starts following another's special diet. So keep the special diet just for the person for whom it is designed.

For advice on how to cope with a baby or young child on a special diet, >BABYCARE and CHILDCARE. For more advice on practical organisation and planning, >page 164.

Some people with multiple food sensitivity find that 'neutralisation therapy' – a form of desensitisation – can help them eat foods to which they react. For some people, it works very well. For others, it is less successful and still usually needs to be combined with a rotation diet (>MEDICAL HELP for full information). High doses of vitamins and minerals can also be of benefit (>MEDICAL HELP).

For short-term help, say a special-occasion meal, taking the drug Nalcrom can enable you to eat things to which you usually react (>MEDICAL HELP).

TIP

If you are very short of money on a special diet, then use cheap, filling foods that you tolerate as much as possible. Use potato, sweet potato and unusual grains, such as buckwheat, if you can, and beans and pulses for cheap protein. Fish can also be good value if you tolerate it.

Severe reactions to a food can be relieved by a dose of alkali salts (>FIRST AID AND HOME MEDICINE).

It is common for people with a tendency to multiple food allergy and intolerance to develop new sensitivities, especially when run down and already reacting severely to other foods or other allergens. These are often temporary intolerances and disappear with managing your diet, but they can be demoralising and confusing. You may suddenly find you react to something you thought relatively safe. Be warned that reactions like this sometimes occur during exclusion dieting. For other causes of temporary reactions, see pages 131–4. The way to cope with them is, again, to manage your diet. In particular, it is a good idea not to binge on or eat any food in excess, as this seems to pre-dispose to sensitivity. If you leave a food out, for instance, do not binge to compensate on its substitute or on other foods. Eating a varied diet in moderation is the best policy to keep new food sensitivities at bay. It is often very difficult on a vegetarian diet to eat a sufficiently varied range of foods (>page 146 for more advice).

You are also much less likely to react to foods that you have eaten seldom, infrequently or never. This is why, if you have even just a few food sensitivities, you are often advised to eat unusual foods and to make your diet as wide and as varied as you can. This helps the body to maintain its level of tolerance.

Some people cross-react to foods which are closely related. A rotation diet is usually planned to avoid problems of this kind. For more information, >pages 148–53 and CROSS-REACTION.

If you get confusing symptoms while on a diet that has been fine for a time, >page 131.

Further Measures

There are many other practical things you can do to help you live with food sensitivity. These include:

- finding substitutes
- eating and cooking food in different ways
- organising and planning diets
- finding pure foods
- handling and preparing foods

Finding substitutes

People differ widely in how they like to deal with having to avoid common foods such as cow's milk, wheat or bread, coffee or tea. Some people like to try and find as near a substitute as they can to the food they omit, so that their diet appears as normal as possible. Others find it frustrating and disappointing to eat things that taste different from the real thing, and prefer simply not to try to create substitutes.

Be careful not to binge or overload if you use substitutes that are closely related to things to which you are sensitive, in case you become sensitive to those as well. If you have to leave cow's milk out of your diet, you can try goat's milk or sheep's milk as a substitute, but take care not to overload since they are related to cow's milk. Goat's milk, in particular, is very closely related to cow's milk and it is common for people to become sensitive to it. Put it in your diet, but rotate it – once every four days at first – and use it sparingly. Increase its use later if you tolerate it well.

Sheep's milk is generally much less troublesome than goat's milk or cow's milk, although this may be because it is more rare in the diet.

Rotate once every four days at first and keep it two days apart from goat's milk if you are on a four-day rotation. Mail order sources of sheep's and goat's milk powder and cheese are given on page 167. You can also buy yogurt and cheese culture so you can make your own.

Fresh bought goat's and sheep's milk and yogurts are often unpasteurised. Cook them before serving to babies and young children, pregnant women, the infirm or the elderly.

(>pages 138–9 for advice on finding cow's milk-free margarine and bread.)

You can also use soya milk and nut milks as a substitute for cow, goat or sheep milks. These are rich sources of calcium and particularly useful in casseroles and baked dishes. Be careful not to overuse these since both soya and nuts can cause reactions. Some people are sensitive to processed soya milk in cartons, but not if they make their own. The reason for this may possibly be minute contaminants, either from the water used or from the packaging. To make your own soya milk, see page 130.

You can make nut milks by liquidising 100 g (4 oz) nuts with 340 ml (½ pint) water. Hazelnut, almond, cashew and peanut are particularly delicious. You can use these as bases for puddings, to thicken soups or stews, or, sweetened, to drink.

Unless you are very highly allergic to cow's milk, you may be able to tolerate it in different forms. It is worth trying any of the following alternatives as they may enable you to keep a little cow's milk in your diet. Try a small amount once every four days at first.

Heating or cooking cow's milk and milk products modifies its proteins. Many people who cannot tolerate ordinary milk can tolerate it if it has been boiled, or if it is used in sauces, puddings, confectionery, milk chocolate, or baked products. Evaporated milk and UHT milk have been heat-treated – so try these to see if they are acceptable.

Baby formula milk, in which the proteins are heat modified, is often tolerated by babies and young children who do not tolerate cow's milk proteins in ordinary cow's milk. Try this for them, unless you know they are sensitive to formula, and also for adults (>also BABYCARE).

Ghee (clarified butter) is tolerated well by many people sensitive to cow's milk. You can buy it at Indian groceries and large supermarkets, or make it yourself. It can be used for cooking or spreading. To make ghee, melt butter over a gentle heat, allow to cool for a while, then pour into a glass jar, leaving the white residues (the proteins) in the pan. Keep in the fridge. Do not eat the white protein residues which will settle in the jar when the ghee is cold.

If you are lactose intolerant (intolerant of the sugar in cow's milk), rather than allergic to cow's milk proteins, you may be able to tolerate cow's milk products in which the lactose levels are low. Try any of the following to see:

Live yogurt	Camembert
Cheddar Cheese	Aged Gouda
Cheshire Cheese	Aged Edam
Cottage Cheese	Pasteurised processed cheese

If you have to leave out milks entirely, >page 160 for advice on foods rich in calcium. Get a doctor's advice on any need for supplements.

If you have to leave wheat out of your diet (and are not sensitive to other grains or gluten), oats, rice, millet, corn, barley and rye are cheap and easy substitutes. The information given on pages 148–53 (Rotation Diets) will help avoid any risk of cross-reaction. In place of wheat breakfast cereals, you can eat porridge oats, cornflakes or rice cereals. In place of wheat bread, you can make bread from oats or rye.

Rice is a good substitute for pasta, or you can buy noodles of rice and buckwheat. Use oatcakes, ricecakes and rye crispbreads as another substitute for bread or for savoury biscuits, but check that crispbreads are pure rye – some contain wheat or malt (Ryvita Original is one brand of pure rye crispbread). Other useful grains, which are not related to wheat or the other grasses, are buckwheat, sago, tapioca, quinoa. Breads can also be made with potato, chestnuts, soya and gram (chickpea) flours. (>FURTHER READING for useful cookbooks.)

As a substitute for baking powders, which usually contain wheat, use sodium bicarbonate or cream of tartar (made from grapes).

If you are sensitive to gluten, look for the gluten-free sign on foods. Many health food shops have extensive choices. If you are sensitive to eggs, some people react to egg white and not to egg yolk and vice versa. Test them separately (see page 126) to see if you can tolerate one or the other. A number of firms sell egg substitutes for baking, as well as sugars, chocolate substitutes and bakery mixes – for cakes, breads and biscuits – excluding foods commonly causing reactions. Sources are given on pages 166–9. One firm, The Custom Bake Company, will bake cakes and other products to your exact recipe by mail order. Wonderful for children's birthdays.

If you are sensitive to sugar, avoid using artifical sweeteners and saccharin as a substitute if you are chemically sensitive. The chemicals used can cause reactions. Some people react to sugars in any form (including honey and maple sugar and syrup) irrespective of the food from which it is derived. Other people can tolerate sugar derived from one food and not another. It is worth trying different types to see if you can tolerate them.

Sources of Calcium

Calcium is required by the body to form bones and teeth. It is especially important to growing children, and to pregnant and breastfeeding women. Most people on an ordinary diet get all their calcium needs from milk, cheese and yogurt. For children aged between one and nine, three-quarters of a pint of milk a day supplies their recommended intake of 500 milligrams. If you cut all milk (including goat and sheep's milk) out of your diet, you need to make sure you are eating enough calcium from alternative sources.

The recommended daily intake of calcium is as follows:

	Milligrams per day
Adult men and women	500
Pregnant and breastfeeding women	1200
Children: up to 1 year	600
1–8 years	500
9–14 years	700
15–17 years	600

Foods Rich in Calcium

Broccoli, watercress, soya, nuts, figs, sesame seeds, sunflower seeds, parsley and molasses are rich sources of calcium. Other good sources include most green leafy vegetables, beans and pulses, and carob powder.

White bread and other foods made of white flour are moderately good sources of calcium, but wholemeal bread is a poor source of calcium, containing phytic acid which interferes with calcium absorption. Spinach contains a high level of calcium but also contains oxalic acid which renders most of the calcium unabsorbable. The bones of fish in canned fish are high in calcium, but it is disputed whether calcium eaten in that form is absorbed by the body.

It is possible, even on a rotation diet, to keep up calcium levels by eating a variety of calcium-rich foods. In particular, it is useful to eat dried fruit, nuts and seeds as snacks, and to use garnishes of sesame seed, sunflower seed and parsley on salads and casseroles. Use tahini in salad dressing. You can use nut spreads and nut milks in soups and stews (>page 158 for instructions on making nut milks). Use carob, molasses, dried fruit, seeds and nuts in biscuits or cakes.

The portions below supply the following amount of calcium:

	Milligrams of Calcium	Per Cent Adult Daily Intake
125 g (4 oz) Cooked broccoli	180	36
50 g (2 oz) Watercress	130	26
50 g (2 oz) Soya beans (dry)	140	28
125 g (4 oz) Tofu (soya bean curd)	150	30
50 g (2 oz) Almonds, brazils, hazelnuts	170	34
50 g (2 oz) Walnuts	80	16
25 g (1 oz) Sesame seeds or tahini	135	27
25 g (1 oz) Sunflower seeds	135	27
50 g (2 oz) Figs	140	28
25 g (1 oz) Molasses	140	28
25 g (1 oz) Carob powder	90	18
25 g (1 oz) Parsley	90	18
125 g (4 oz) Raw cabbage	80	16
50 g (2 oz) Raw carrot	55	11
50 g (2 oz) Dried apricots	45	9

If the body has insufficient Vitamin D, calcium cannot be absorbed from the bloodstream. Vitamin D is formed naturally in the skin when exposed to sunlight and, if you encounter normal amounts of sunlight, you should have no deficiency at all. Fatty fish and fish liver oils are rich sources of Vitamin D, as are eggs, milk, butter, cheese and margarine (Vitamin D is added to the latter). Even if you have to leave any of these foods out of a special diet, you should have no problem with Vitamin D deficiency provided you are getting out of doors regularly.

Some sugars are derived from cane sugar. These include all brown sugars and demerara sugar, plus white sugar made by Tate & Lyle. Golden syrup, molasses and black treacle are also derived from cane. Silver Spoon white sugar is derived from beet sugar, not cane sugar. Treat this as a separate food from cane sugar. Most icing sugars are derived from beet sugar unless they specifically say otherwise.

As alternatives to cane or beet sugar, which are the most common sugars to which people react, you can try date syrup or maple sugar or syrup – available from Green Farm Foodwatch (>page 168) or health food shops. Some health food shops also sell pure corn syrup.

Honey and fructose are derived from various foods as a base. Treat these as separate foods from other sugars, and rotate them if you are on a rotation diet.

If you are sensitive to yeast, you can make bread with soda as a leavening agent (>FURTHER READING for cookbooks). Alternatively, some bakers and major supermarkets (e.g. Sainsbury's) sell soda bread.

Using unusual foods in your diet, especially in rotation, can help extend and vary your diet. You are less likely to react to a food if you have never or seldom eaten it. Use substitutes such as goat's and sheep's milk and cheese if you can, and unusual grains, such as buckwheat, sago or tapioca. Eat duck, venison, rabbit and turkey more frequently. A source for goat's meat by post is given on page 167.

Fish, if you tolerate it, can be a very useful, and relatively cheap, way to extend your rotation. There are a large number of families of fish, and you can have a wide diet by using this variety on a rotation (>CROSS-REACTION). Some people react to fish of any kind, however, so take care if you know you react consistently to all fish.

Pure nut butters can also be useful to extend your diet. You can buy almond, cashew and peanut butter without added oil.

Introduce herbs, spices and seeds into a rotation to give you variety and flavour. Treat each as a new food as you introduce it, and stick to the food families (>CROSS-REACTION).

You can use fruit oils or nut oils, such as grapeseed oil or hazelnut and walnut oils, for salad dressings. Do not use for baking or cooking as they produce unpleasant-tasting chemicals when cooked.

Trying foods in different forms

Try preparing food in different ways to see if you tolerate it better. Cooking food modifies its chemical structure. As an example, some people tolerate cooked food where they cannot eat it raw. Try baking or stewing fruit, for instance, if you cannot eat it raw. (Or, conversely, try food raw rather than cooked if it upsets you.) Prepare purées of gently cooked meat or vegetables – this can make foods easier to digest.

Do not burn or char foods when cooking. This can alter the chemical composition of foods and make you react to them. Burning meat when grilling or roasting produces the chemical acrolein which, even in tiny traces, can irritate. Do not burn toast.

If you have been eating whole grains in the form of wholewheat or brown rice, and cannot tolerate them, it is worth trying white wheat and white rice. These are sometimes better tolerated than whole grains, and may make you able to eat them.

Try different varieties of apples to see if you tolerate certain ones better. Some people find that they can tolerate one variety of apple and not another, so test Granny Smiths separately from Golden Delicious, and so on.

Some people tolerate processed and canned foods, such as canned fish or canned or dried fruit, better than their fresh equivalents. Some chemically sensitive people do not respond well to canned foods, however, so take care if you are sensitive to chemicals.

Some people find that they tolerate foods better if they add salt when eating. Other people find, conversely, that this makes things worse. Test this out to see. Use Pure Salt BP (available from Green Farm Foodwatch, address below) to avoid any additives in salt.

Some people are generally sensitive to alcohol, whatever the food or foods from which it is made. Other people can tolerate alcohol of different types, being able to tolerate the base foods. Ciders are based on apples. Wine, port, sherry and champagne are based on grapes. Most spirits are derived from various grains and cereals of the grass family (wheat, rye, oats, barley, corn, cane sugar) or from vegetables such as potato. Beers are brewed from grains and cereals, and hops; lagers are usually from grains and cereals only. Fruit wines and liqueurs are derived from various fruits.

Try buying poultry or meat from different shops or supermarkets to see if you can find one which suits you better than others. Some people find that one shop's produce makes them ill, while they tolerate another shop's quite well. This could be due to different feedstuffs or drugs used in production.

Some people tolerate fat on meat and poultry but not lean, and vice versa. Try cutting off fat, or only eating the fat on meats and poultry, and see if it helps.

Chew your food thoroughly. It can help break down foods and make them more digestible. It can be enough to make a difference. Take time to eat and digest food properly if you can. Do not eat on the run, and sit down for a short while to digest.

Try eating large meals at different times of the day to see if this helps at all. Some people find they cannot digest a large meal in the evening and have problems overnight, and are best having their main meal at lunch, or even breakfast. Other people are better if they have a large meal before sleeping. See what suits you. Grains and proteins, being slow to break down in the body, are especially affected by the timing of meals.

Some people find that they tolerate a food or drink if they eat it completely on its own but not if they combine it with any other foods. Eat foods and drinks singly, one food or drink for a meal, or else at a short interval apart, to see if this makes them tolerable.

The Hay System of food combining helps some people (see page 134).

Organising and planning diets

Organise and plan ahead as much as you can, even if it is not in your nature. Keeping a Foods Diary for the week ahead is a help for shopping and catering, especially if you have more than one household member on a special diet.

TIP

Do not go shopping for food when you are really hungry or withdrawing from a food. You are much more likely to buy forbidden things, break your diet or eat naughty snacks. Go shopping just after a big meal.

For running a rotation, if you tolerate frozen food well and you have a freezer, you can cook casseroles, sauces, purées or bakery in batches and freeze the surplus, labelled for each day of the rotation. This will help avoid food wastage, and save buying and cooking small amounts every few days. Use colour code labels for each day of the rotation. Frozen vegetables, although expensive, can save a lot of waste. Divide up fruit juice cartons and freeze them in portions for one day of the rotation.

Do not forget when working out a rotation diet to include things which can be eaten as snacks or fillers. These are particularly useful for babies and children. Use nuts, dried fruits, fresh fruit, seeds, ricecakes, rice puffs, rye crispbread, oatcakes.

TIP

If running a rotation diet for people taking packed lunches to work or school, try to work out lunch menus which look as normal as possible. It helps psychologically to cope with a special diet if you are not too conspicuous in public. Put herb teas or strange juices in thermoses. Mixed salads are useful, as are oatcakes, rye crispbread, ricecakes, and wholefood crisps (>pages 166–9).

Use colour codes if you are running a rotation diet. Use red jars and labels for Day One, and so on. Alternatively, keep separate shelves or cupboards for each day of the rotation and colour code them. Then you know that on a given day you can reach into that jar or that cupboard and eat anything in it. Particularly useful for hungry children just home from school.

Finding pure foods

Some people react to tiny traces of chemical contaminants and additives in foods. It is also known for people to be sensitive to water used in diluting drinks or processing foods. If you suspect water as a cause, >page 126 for information on testing foods, and WATER AND WATER FILTERS for advice on avoiding water in processed foods.

To avoid chemical contaminants in food, use processed foods as little as possible. Buy organic food wherever possible, cook your own food from fresh ingredients, and do not use canned foods. Avoid eating salted, smoked or pickled foods of any kind. Store food in glass jars wherever possible, and avoid using plastic boxes and film for food storage, especially when food is warm. Buy milk and other drinks in glass bottles rather than in waxed cartons or plastic bottles.

The rind of lemons and other citrus fruits are sometimes waxed to protect them in transit and against infestation. Do not grate rinds. Alternatively, use organic citrus fruit.

Cultivate your butcher. Small local butchers may be better able to obtain meat from field-fed stock, or free-range poultry, or will know more about the farms from which their products come. Some are also willing to make up batches of your own blend sausages (e.g. lamb and buckwheat, turkey and oats). For mail order sources of organic foods, pure meat, poultry and sausages, see below.

TIP

Dried fruit is often treated with sulphur dioxide as a preservative and with vegetable oils to keep it moist. See below for sources of untreated dried fruit.

Beware salad bars in restaurants, cafés and pubs. The salads are often sprayed with antioxidants to prevent deterioration.

Beware of chips. Frozen chips, and chips from fish and chip and fast food shops are sometimes treated with antioxidants.

For more information on food adulteration and additives, >FURTHER READING.

Handling and preparing foods

If you are extremely sensitive to a food or foods, you may react even to the smell or vapours of the foods, or to handling them. You may also be affected by other people eating them in your presence, or if you go into canteens, cafés or restaurants.

To protect your hands when preparing foods, wear gloves (>HAND PROTECTION). Use cooking methods that minimise cooking times and fumes. Ventilate well. Keep chopping boards separate if necessary to keep juices off your own food.

You may have to avoid public places where food fumes are found if you are badly affected. Members of your family or household may have to modify their diet and leave out things that upset you. Avoid situations that you know upset you.

Tiny traces of moulds adhere to cut or just prepared food, vegetables and fruit, and in refrigerators and freezers. These may upset you if you are highly sensitive to moulds (>MOULDS for full advice).

Sources of Supply

All the companies listed below provide a mail order service. Their addresses follow, on pages 168–9.

Bakery products and flours
The following firms supply bakery products and flours by post, including special mixes and food substitutes. Custom Bake will supply baked cakes and other products, using any ingredients you specify.

Cantassium
Custom Bake
Diet Care
General Designs

Green Farm Foodwatch
Nutricia
Suma

Organic foods

Church Farm
Countryside Wholefoods
Green Farm Foodwatch
Infinity Foods

Natural Foods (London area)
Naturally Yours
Organic Farmers and Growers
Suma

For other sources of organic foods, >FURTHER READING.

Organic fruit and vegetables

Church Farm
Countryside Wholefoods
Natural Foods (London area)

Organic Farmers and Growers
Red House Farm

Organic meat, conservation-grade and additive-free meat, poultry, sausages, ham, bacon

Church Farm
Greenway Organic Farms
Heal Farm
Longwood Farm
Murray Meats
Natural Foods (London area)

Organic Farmers and Growers
Pure Meat Company
Real Meat Company
Red House Farm

For sausages made to your recipe:

Church Farm
Heal Farm
Red House Farm

For goat's meat:

Murray Meats

Goat's cheese, goat's milk powder

Countryside Wholefoods
Green Farm Foodwatch
Market Pantry
Natural Foods (London area)

Paxton & Whitfield
Suma

Sheep's cheese, sheep's milk powder

Green Farm Foodwatch
Market Pantry
Natural Foods (London area)
Paxton & Whitfield

Suma
Sussex High Weald
Wells Stores

Yogurt culture, cheese culture, rennet

Smallholding Supplies
Suma

Addresses of Suppliers

Cantassium Company
Larkhill Natural Health
225 Putney Bridge Road
London SW15 2PY
Tel: 081–874 1130

Church Farm
Strixton
Wellingborough
Northamptonshire NN9 7PA
Tel: 0933 664378

Countryside Wholefoods
19 Forty Hill
Enfield
London EN2 9HT
Tel: 081–363 2933

Custom Bake Company
Ivestan
Crown Road
Marnhull
Dorset DT10 1LN
Tel: 0258 820743

Diet Care
34 Saxon Road
Hove
East Sussex BN3 4LF
Tel: 0273 417157

General Designs
PO Box 38E
Worcester Park
Surrey KT4 7LX
Tel: 081–337 9366

Green Farm Foodwatch
Burwash Common
East Sussex TN19 7LX
Tel: 0435 882482

Greenway Organic Farms
50 St Mary's Street
Edinburgh EH1 1XS
Tel: 031–557 8111

Heal Farm
Kings Nympton
Umberleigh
Devon EX37 9TB
Tel: 0769 572077

Infinity Foods
23 North Road
Brighton BN1 1YA
Tel: 0273 603563

Longwood Farm
Tuddenham St Mary
Bury St Edmunds
Suffolk IP28 6TB
Tel: 0638 717120

Market Pantry
Craven Court
High Street
Skipton
North Yorkshire BD23 1DG
Tel: 0756 700570

Murray Meats
Tordean Farm
Buckfastleigh
Devon TQ11 0LY
Tel: 0364 43305

Natural Foods Ltd
Unit 14
Hainault Road Industrial Estate
Hainault Road
London E11 1HD
Tel: 081–539 1034

Naturally Yours
The Horse and Gate
Witcham Toll
Sutton
Ely
Cambridgeshire CB6 2AB
Tel: 0353 778723

Nutricia Dietary
Products Ltd
494–496 Honeypot Lane
Stanmore
Middlesex HA7 1JH
Tel: 081–951 5155

Organic Farmers and Growers
Abacus House
Station Yard
Needham Market
Ipswich
Suffolk IP6 8AT
Tel: 0449 720838

Paxton & Whitfield
93 Jermyn Street
London SW1Y 6JE
Tel: 071–930 0250

The Pure Meat Company
Red Hill House
Saltney
Cheshire CH4 8BU
Tel: 0244 681333

Real Meat Company
East Hill Farm
Heytesbury
Warminster
Wiltshire BA12 0HR
Tel: 0985 40436

Red House Farm
F A & J Jones & Son
Red House Farm
North Scarle
Lincoln LN6 9HB
Tel: 052277 224

Smallholding Supplies
Pikes Farmhouse
East Pennard
Shepton Mallett
Somerset BA4 6RR
Tel: 0749 86688

Suma
Dean Clough
Halifax
West Yorkshire HX3 5AN
Tel: 0422 345513

(To buy from Suma you have to
be a registered co-operative
with at least five members.)

Sussex High Weald
Dairy Sheep
Putlands Farm
Duddleswell
Uckfield
East Sussex TN22 3BJ
Tel: 082571 2647

Wells Stores
29 Stert Street
Abingdon
Oxfordshire OX14 3JF
Tel: 0235 535978

House Dust Mites

House dust mites are tiny living creatures that co-habit in human environments. They are about a third of a millimetre in size and can just be seen with the naked eye, although they are indistinguishable from a speck of dust; their features and movements cannot be detected without magnification. They are one of the most common causes of allergy, resulting from inhaling minute debris from their body or of their droppings. Tests have shown that over 80 per cent of people with allergies show positive skin test results to house dust mites (although only a share of these may have positive clinical symptoms of allergy). (>DEFINING ALLERGY and DETECTING YOUR ALLERGIES)

The most common symptoms resulting from house dust mite allergy are nasal symptoms, including sneezing, runny nose, rhinitis (hay fever), as well as sinusitis, with related headaches and ear blockages. Breathing symptoms, such as wheezing, dry persistent cough, tightness of breath and asthma, also commonly result. Eczema and dermatitis are frequently caused by house dust mites. Some people sensitive to dust mites report joint pain, swelling of tissues, and muscle aches. (>SYMPTOMS for full description of likely symptoms.)

If you know you are allergic to house dust mites, and are looking for specific advice on how to deal with your allergy, >page 174.

If you want advice on how to help a child or baby with house dust mite allergy, read also pages 181–2.

If you need information on treatments to help you cope, >MEDICAL HELP and COMPLEMENTARY THERAPY.

If you want to know more about house dust mites and how to detect allergy to them, read on from here.

What are House Dust Mites? Where are They Found?

House dust mites live on the debris of human environments, and on other small living organisms. They do not cause harm directly to humans, apart from being a potential allergen. The species of mite particularly associated with allergy in the UK is called *Dermatophagoides pteronyssimus*. *Dermatophagoides* means 'skin-eating' and, in common with other mites, house dust mites feed especially on human skin scales. Humans shed on average up to one gram of skin scales a day – enough to feed many mites for months and these fall and collect around where humans live. House dust mites also feed on animal skin scales, and on micro-organisms such as moulds, bacteria and viruses.

Having house dust mites in your environment is not a sign of dirty or insanitary conditions, nor of slovenly or poor housekeeping. They need a particular ecology to survive and human environments provide the best conditions for them. House dust mites thrive where food supply is plentiful, and where the environment is moist, warm and dark. They like ideally a moisture level of 80 per cent relative humidity and a temperature of about 25°C (77°F). For humidity year round, the UK is ideal for them; and for temperature, many warm, dark places indoors such as unaired beds, duvets, chairs and carpets, are also well suited.

They are present all year round and hence are responsible for many cases of perennial rhinitis or other year-round symptoms. Their presence can increase when the weather is very damp and, like mould allergy (>MOULDS), allergy to house dust mites often gets worse in damp weather.

They can be found in very high densities where the environment is favourable to them. Up to thousands have been measured in one gram of surface dust. It is their droppings – their faecal pellets – that cause most problems with allergic reactions, although some people are allergic to debris of the mites themselves. The faecal pellets remain even when the mites themselves move on or die, so dust, bedding or pieces of furniture can continue to cause problems even if you kill the mites.

Mites (and their debris and faeces) are found particularly in beds and mattresses, and in house dust. They are also found in carpets and rugs, upholstered chairs, sofas and furniture, (especially old furniture), and they can cling to curtains and cushions. They often thrive in animal bedding, or where animals lie and sleep during the day. They frequently collect in corners or crevices, such as skirting-boards, where food for them, such as moulds, bacteria and viruses as well as human and animal skin scales, are found. They are found not just in home environments, but in any indoor environment such as offices and hotels – anywhere where there is human skin as food, and damp, dark places to live. Chairs and carpets at work can thus be sources of dust mite allergens.

It is when these environments are disturbed, and house dust mite allergens become airborne, that most allergic reactions happen. Vacuuming, cleaning or dusting are particularly hazardous, since they disperse mite allergens into the air. Tests have shown that levels of airborne allergens are higher during or just after vacuuming than before. Other types of housework (such as changing bed linen, turning mattresses, beating rugs or carpets, plumping up cushions and moving furniture around to clean) also throw house dust mite allergens into the air. Repair work, such as dismantling old skirtings or disturbing floorboards, can also stir up problems.

Another common trigger for reactions is when heating or fires are turned on, especially initially, when allergens are drawn into the air by convection currents and then circulated around the room. Warm air ducted central heating, convector heaters and fan heaters are particularly likely to trigger reactions this way. (These reactions can be caused by other airborne substances, such as moulds, animal allergens or fibres from carpets, or even by chemicals in the environment – >individual sections – but the most common cause is house dust mites.)

Beds, bedding and bedtime toys are also prime triggers for house dust mite reactions. Humans lose on average half a litre (just under a pint) of fluid overnight, so beds are invariably damp, unless thoroughly dried and aired. Not only do house dust mites love the damp, warm dark of mattresses, pillows, blankets or duvets, with their abundance of human skin scales, but they thrive in other places such as teddies, soft toys, padded headboards and bed-bases.

A damp environment encourages house dust mites. Living close to damp areas significantly increases mite populations: it has been shown that even living over an underground water course can correlate with increased incidence of house dust mite allergy. Rising or penetrating damp in the structure, using humidifiers, drying laundry indoors, having a lot of house plants, using heating such as gas fires or paraffin stoves which create water on burning, can all contribute to an increased population of house dust mites.

Poor ventilation, or failing to ventilate also contributes. Fixed windows, or keeping double glazing or windows tightly shut to conserve heat will stop through draughts, circulation of air and hence drying of the environment.

Certain environments do not favour house dust mites. They are killed by sunlight. The majority of mites live in the top 1–2 cm (¾ inch) of any surface, and sunlight can penetrate far enough to kill by light or drying many of the mites present, although it does not remove their faeces or debris. Washing at high temperatures (90°C/194°F plus) also kills mites, and, if thorough, can remove them and their faecal debris completely. A dry environment kills them. They do not survive at a relative humidity level below 55 per cent, and if you can create localised dry conditions, say by drying a pillow on a radiator or hot water tank, or by drying a bed with hot water bottles, or with an electric blanket, this will kill them, although again faeces and debris are not removed. House dust mites do not occur in any concentration in the Alps; the combination of low humidity and low temperatures is probably the reason for this.

Synthetic materials are often claimed to deter house dust mites and advice is often given to use synthetic bedding, to avoid problems with house dust mite allergy. Despite the prevalence of this advice, there is little evidence to substantiate it, and the experience of many people with allergies indicates the need for caution.

People who replace old bedding with new bedding (of any material) often get a great improvement if they are allergic to mites, but house dust mites will colonise new bedding, even if synthetic. Problems with mites can, and do, recur in synthetic bedding after a while, unless you take preventative measures to deter them (so the benefits can be due simply to the *newness* of the bedding, not to the change to synthetic material).

There is some evidence that synthetic carpets can reduce the level of airborne allergens (including house dust mites) because their increased level of static electricity attracts particles and holds them down. There are also some benefits to using synthetic bedding, compared to wool or feathers, in that it can be readily washed and dried. However, washing at low temperatures (40°C/105°F or less) does not kill mites. It simply rinses out the faecal pellets, but not always the mites themselves, who are tenacious and cling on to survive. You need a high temperature of wash to kill and eliminate mites. (This is possible with cotton bedding and some special anti-dust mite bedding.) See below and >BEDDING for a full discussion of how to choose bedding to meet your needs.

How to Detect Allergy to House Dust Mites

Skin tests for allergy are reasonably reliable at detecting allergy to house dust mite inhalants (>DETECTING YOUR ALLERGIES). You can ask your GP for a referral for such tests.

Another way to identify allergy to house dust mites is to analyse the pattern of your symptoms by answering the series of questions on page 174. If you answer 'yes' to several or all of these questions, then suspect allergy to house dust mites. Then try some of the avoidance measures outlined below. If these result in improvement of your symptoms, then house dust mites will be confirmed as a cause.

It is important to bear in mind that inhaling large amounts of dust is irritant for anyone, and can cause sneezing, coughing, itchy eyes or difficulty in breathing. If you need more help in working out whether your symptoms are irritation or allergy, >SYMPTOMS.

Are You Allergic to House Dust Mites?

DO YOU FEEL WORSE?

	Yes	No
When you first lie down in bed	—	—
On turning a mattress	—	—
When the heating comes on	—	—
Only in indoor environments	—	—
During or just after vacuuming	—	—
When making or changing beds	—	—
When dusting or sweeping	—	—
Overnight or first thing on waking	—	—
When shaking rugs or carpets	—	—
When sitting on old furniture	—	—
In places with carpets	—	—

How to Deal with House Dust Mite Allergy

Much of the advice commonly given to people with house dust mite allergy is unhelpful or impracticable in everyday life. The basic advice often given by doctors – to vacuum as much as possible to remove allergens and use plastic covers on mattresses – usually make things worse. Vacuuming actually increases the level of airborne allergens, and plastic covers trap damp and condensation in the mattress, making things worse when you come to change covers or air the mattress. At the other extreme, people often receive a long list of things which are very desirable to do, but which are totally overwhelming. You would need most of your life to carry them out, and no small amount of money. In practice, many people fail to carry through any of the measures, and are left feeling inadequate and guilty.

TIP

For some people, symptoms can last through the day, caused by heavy exposure from their bed, or other sources at home. The effects can last even when away from the source.

Some of the conditions that favour house dust mites also encourage moulds to grow invisibly in indoor environments. If you still feel unsure about how far house dust mites cause your symptoms, >MOULDS and see whether mould allergy might be the cause.

Reactions to house dust mites in bedding often manifest themselves in symptoms the following morning, rather than when you first lie down. If you feel worse when waking and then improve once you have left your bed, suspect house dust mites. >BEDDING also for guidance on sensitivity to fibres and choice of bedding.

Reactions to dusty old attics, storerooms, or to old dusty books are often caused more by moulds than by house dust mites. For advice on this, >MOULDS.

The advice that follows focuses on things that people have found to work without massive expenditure of energy or money, and without enormous upheaval. It focuses also on improving your home environment, especially your bed and bedroom. The reason for this is that, if you reduce your exposure to allergens for a significant portion of your life (especially in bed where you have intense exposure to house dust mites), your tolerance to them when you meet them somewhere else will generally be much better. You will not react so severely when you meet them elsewhere (in other people's homes, at work, or at school) if your home environment is reasonably clear.

How far you go to eliminate house dust mites depends ultimately on how badly affected you are, and on what investment of time and money you feel able to make. If you are not severely affected, it may be sufficient merely to improve your bedroom environment, take care with housework, and keep the home as well ventilated and as dry as possible. If you are severely affected, particularly if you have a highly allergic child, you may feel the need to make substantial changes.

Basic Avoidance Measures

The following are basic measures to avoid and eliminate house dust mites that people generally find to be very useful. Full advice is given below for the main measures, namely to:

- Use filters on your vacuum cleaner
- Damp dust and damp mop (explained below)
- Get someone else to do tasks that stir up dust
- Get rid of really old, dusty furniture and carpets
- Air and dry beds and bedding
- Keep the place as dry as you can

There are additional special measures which help babies and children (see page 181).

If you are not able to take precautions throughout your whole home, do not worry. Concentrate particularly on the bedroom first, and next on the main living room. Carry out the measures intensively at first to get things sorted out, but if you want to relax them later on, do so, say after a few weeks or a couple of months, and see how things go. If you manage to reduce mites significantly through intensive effort at first, then often it is enough to do just a little – particularly keeping beds and the home aired and dry – to keep them at bay.

If you have tried all these basic measures, and need more drastic action, see page 182 for more things worth doing. For full advice on the basic measures, read on.

Use Filters on Vacuum Cleaners

Conventional vacuum cleaners blow back a share of the dust they collect (including house dust mites and other allergens) into the room. It has been demonstrated that the level of airborne allergens actually increases during and after vacuuming. So, if you vacuum a great deal to remove house dust mite allergens, you actually stir things up.

If you only ever do one thing to combat house dust mites, then use filters on your vacuum cleaner. These take out over 99 per cent of allergens present in vacuum cleaner exhausts. Even if you are desperately short of money, do this. It has two benefits, immediate and long-term. The immediate benefit is that intensive vacuuming to remove old allergens from beds, carpets, wherever, is feasible without making the sufferer worse. This will not remove all traces of allergens at first – the real benefit of filters shows itself over the long term, as allergens are progressively removed. Users report that the level of allergens does steadily and perceptibly decline over time if they use filters.

For some people, this measure, combined with airing and drying as much as possible, has meant they have not been obliged to replace bedding, furniture or any other previous sources of allergens. After a period of intensive use, it is often enough to vacuum mattresses or carpets once a week or even less – an enormous bonus for many allergy sufferers.

To use filters, you can either buy special filtration vacuum cleaners or you can use fabric filters, which tape over vacuum cleaner exhausts. The filtration cleaners, although more expensive, are superior in performance, and much less troublesome to use. >VACUUM CLEANERS for detailed information.

TIP

Always change vacuum cleaner bags out of doors. Change them as often as recommended, so they do not overfill and discharge dust into the machine. Get someone else to change them if they affect you badly.

Use a carpet sweeper, or damp mopping (see below), for quick floor cleaning without creating too much dust.

If you get filters, or a filtration vacuum cleaner, have an intensive clean at first. Vacuum down curtains, upholstered furniture, duvets, pillows, blankets, bed-bases, headboards, cushions, rugs, soft toys – anything that might harbour dust mites. Repeat every so often, or spring clean once a year.

There are chemicals available that kill or denature house dust mites, but they have some drawbacks and do not always remove the need to vacuum (>page 184).

Steam cleaning a carpet can sometimes clear mites, but you need to dry the carpet well and fast to prevent damp conditions encouraging their return. For advice on cleaning materials, >CLEANING PRODUCTS.

Damp Dust and Damp Mop

Normal methods of dusting and sweeping simply disperse dust (and allergens) around the room. You can usually see it settling again on surfaces a short time after cleaning. To make dusting and sweeping possible, and to remove dust from the place, 'damp dust' and 'damp mop'.

To damp dust, take a duster or cloth, dip it in water, and wring it out so that it is only just damp. Then dust as usual, removing the dust as you go, and rinsing and wringing the cloth as often as you need. If you keep the cloth as dry as possible, it does not leave smears of dirt on surfaces.

To damp mop instead of sweeping, dampen a mop and wring out hard, as with the duster, above. Then mop the floor gently, rinsing and wringing frequently.

These measures, combined with vacuum filters, significantly reduce the level of airborne allergens.

Get Someone Else To Do Things

If you are the person responsible for the housework and you are highly allergic to house dust mites, then do whatever you can to get other people to do tasks that make you ill – be it turning mattresses, changing bedlinen, vacuuming or whatever.

If you live alone or if you have no luck with getting immediate family or housemates to help, then see if you can barter with a neighbour or friend to swap tasks that you can do for them if they do things for you that make you ill. Offer to do their ironing, do their shopping, do DIY, wash their car, babysit for them, or weed the garden, for instance, in return for them doing some of your jobs. Just ask – people are often glad to be needed, and don't feel guilty about not doing everything yourself. Nobody wants you to suffer.

TIP

If someone does tasks for you, stay out of the room while they are done. Allow the dust to settle before you go back in.

If you have to do household tasks which upset you, spread them out over the week or a few days. Do not do all your jobs on one day – you may be able to cope this way.

Get Rid of Dusty Objects

If you use vacuum filters and keep things dry and aired, you may not need to get rid of, or replace any major object. Vacuum thoroughly first, try the avoidance measures for beds and bedding (opposite), and see how you go. Sometimes, though, a piece of furniture, a carpet, or a mattress just sits there looking at you screaming that it really has to go – it is too dusty, too old and it cannot be retrieved. So get rid of what you have to and replace it. (>BEDDING and FURNITURE if you need guidance on choosing replacements.)

You can buy specially designed anti-dust mite covers for mattresses and pillows. These are cheap, relative to the cost of replacing old mattress and bedding, and can lessen the work required in airing and drying. These covers are reported by users to be very effective and worthwhile. Full details are given in BEDDING. If you are extremely chemically sensitive and do not tolerate synthetic fibres well, you may not be able to use them since they are made of synthetic blends. For most people, however, they are well tolerated and extremely useful.

Air and Dry Beds and Bedding

House dust mites hate light and dry air. Keep beds and bedding aired and dry as much as possible. You will deter mites and even kill them. You will not remove old allergens this way, but if you combine this with a bout of intensive vacuuming with filters, this will remove a high proportion of them. If you subsequently keep to an airing and drying regime, plus weekly vacuuming, you will keep mites at bay, if not totally absent.

Do not make beds in the morning. Turn back duvets or blankets to allow them and the mattress to dry. Prop pillows up to allow air to circulate. Open windows and let the bedroom ventilate – for a short time only if it is a damp day, but let the air pass through.

Make up beds in the late afternoon or early evening. One really worthwhile thing to do is to use hot water bottles for a few hours before bedtime to air and dry the beds. (Alternatively, use an electric blanket, if you tolerate one.) Wrap pillows over a hot water bottle to dry them. Get the bed really dry – house dust mites absolutely hate dryness. Do this even in summer to dry the bed.

The above measures will reduce and control the level of mites a great deal. If you want to go further and air bedding during the day, try any of the following.

Allow light to get to bedding as much as you can. In Continental Europe, people hang bedding out of windows to air in the early morning, and this works well if you can do it. Alternatively, lie pillows and other bedding just behind windows, to get the light. In summer, if you have energy and favourable weather, hang duvets and blankets outside to air. Lie pillows in the sun.

Another method of airing bedding during the day, particularly in

TIP

If you do not tolerate latex or synthetic rubber, use an old-fashioned ceramic bottle. Look in junk shops or your attic. They are still manufactured and sold direct by:

Pearsons of Chesterfield
Pottery Lane East
Whittington Moor
Chesterfield
Derbyshire S41 9BW
Tel: 0246 271111

winter or on damp days, is to put as much as you can in an airing cupboard, close to a hot water tank, or close to a boiler, or hang it over a towel rail or other heat source. Do just the pillows if you have limited space.

Again, you can do these things intensively for a while to get things under control, then ease off to see how things go. Some people need to keep doing them – other people do them just in winter, or on damp days – some people stop altogether after a while. Do what is right for you.

Keep the Place Dry

The final basic avoidance measure that is really useful is to keep your home as dry as you are able. Use heating to keep the place as warm and dry as you can afford – particularly avoiding damp in the bedroom, but remember to ventilate well, do not overinsulate to conserve energy, open windows or doors at least once a day and keep air circulating through the home.

Fix obvious damp spots or rising damp. Avoid using gas fires or paraffin stoves if you can; these generate water on burning and create damp in the environment. (Gas central heating creates no such problems with damp.) Dry laundry outside the home if possible, do not use humidifiers, and generally keep damp to a minimum.

If you want to take more thorough measures to create a dry environment, including using dehumidifiers, there is a full discussion on damp control in the section on controlling moulds (>MOULDS).

Avoidance Measures for Babies and Children

There are some things you can do specifically to help babies and young children who have house dust mite allergy, or to prevent it developing. Add these to any of the other measures you carry out.

Take Care with Soft Toys

Soft toys snuggled in bed are frequently a prime source of house dust mites for allergic children. To avoid such problems, buy washable toys and wash them frequently to remove the faecal pellets. Then hang outside to dry in the sun, vacuum them, or air and dry them, to remove the mites themselves. Buy a duplicate favourite toy if necessary, to substitute while washing is done.

TIP

Some parents report success in killing mites by freezing the soft toy after washing. (Poor Teddy!) Remember, if you do this, make sure the toy is thoroughly dry after defrosting.

Bunk Beds

It is better for an allergic child to sleep in the top bed rather than the bottom, if this is feasible. House dust mites are scattered from the top mattress as the inhabitant turns and moves during the night.

Childminders and Nurseries

If your child seems fine at home, but gets worse after going to a childminder's or nursery, the cause can be, amongst others, house dust mites – particularly in a warm, damp, carpeted environment. If this is worth taking action over, either look for a childcare place where the environment is more favourable – for instance, uncarpeted and well ventilated – or see if you can lend the childminder or nursery a filtered vacuum cleaner to see if things improve. Be tactful.

Take Care with Young Babies

If you have a history of any allergy in the family, it can help to take avoidance measures with young babies, to prevent them developing house dust mite allergy. Remember that very small babies spend much of their time with their noses stuffed into the

very surfaces that harbour dust mites – carpets, bedding and furniture. They have a much more intense exposure to house dust
mites than older children or adults have.

So do what you can with all the basic and other measures suggested to reduce the level of mites around a baby or young child.
In particular, use washable bedding, especially using cotton blankets (washable at high temperatures) rather than duvets. Keep
bedding and insulation around a baby to a minimum – avoiding
cot bumpers and pram 'nests' if possible, or washing and airing
them frequently. Air mattresses and keep them dry.

Pay particular attention to carpets and rugs where the baby
plays, crawls or rubs its nose a great deal. Vacuum with filters, or
wash if possible. Keep these mite-free if you can. Prevent pets
sleeping on beds or cots, or where a baby or young child plays a
great deal. Warmth, damp and animal skin scales encourage
mites to grow.

For more advice on general preventative measures for babies and
children, >BABYCARE and CHILDCARE.

Other Measures to Eliminate House Dust Mites

If you are extremely sensitive to house dust mites, there is much more
you can do to reduce or eliminate allergens.

If you have very little spare money, but really need to replace dusty
objects, start with your pillow first, and then bedding, such as duvets
and blankets. If money is not a constraint, one of the best things you
can do is to replace bedding, furniture or mattresses with new ones
free of house dust mites. If you start from scratch, free of mites, and
vacuum with filters, damp dust and keep things dry and aired, you
should prevent them recolonising. >BEDDING and FURNITURE for advice
on choices.

Another excellent thing to do is to take out fitted carpets. Many
people find this very difficult to do – not only are fitted carpets attractive, warm and comfortable, but they have often been a major expense
and chosen with care, with the expectation of long use. However,
people who have steeled themselves to do it say it is one of the best
things they have done – dust is considerably reduced and housework
drastically cut. So think about it seriously. Do just the bedroom if you
cannot bear to do it elsewhere.

There are alternatives to fitted carpets that can be attractive, warm and practical (as well as mite-free) – sanded and sealed wooden boards, linoleum or vinyl, cork, tiles: these are much quicker and easier to keep dust free. (Linoleum is very well tolerated by chemically sensitive people. >PLANTS AND TREES for more information.) Use scatter rugs, which can be vacuumed on both sides, hung on the line in sunlight to kill mites, or even washed.

Remove things that collect dust as far as you can – scatter cushions, dried flowers, other decorations or furnishings which can harbour dust or mites. Use curtains of light, washable fabric if you can: avoid velvets or flocky fabrics which trap dust. If you want warmth and insulation, use washable curtain linings – even hang two linings, or use a blind plus lined curtains to conserve energy. >FABRICS for fabric sources.

_TIP

Do not use venetian or other blinds or festoons which collect dust. If you have them, then vacuum or wipe down regularly.

Choose furniture that does not collect dust. Avoid flocky fabrics on upholstered furniture. Use furniture without upholstery as far as possible, particularly beds. Avoid padded headboards and solid divan or bed-bases. A simple, slatted bed-frame in wood or metal allows ventilation and drying of a mattress and does not itself harbour mites. For choices and sources, >FABRICS and FURNITURE.

Put away as many dust-collecting objects as possible. (>MOULDS for advice on controlling dusts from books and paper.) Keep clothes in drawers or wardrobes if you can, or hang a light curtain over open shelves to stop dust accumulating. Avoid fussy lightshades or ornaments which collect dust.

In the long term, if you live in a very damp location, and it is not possible to keep your home as dry as you like, you may have to move. If looking for a new home, check out the dampness of the location – is it near a river, canal or even over an underground waterway?

_TIP

Some people find using a dehumidifier very helpful in keeping down damp and controlling mite levels. (>MOULDS for full information.)

Air filters can also be very helpful, although they will not solve mite problems if you take no other measures. (>AIR FILTERS for a full discussion.)

Remember to clean out cars – house dust mites thrive in cars as well. Vacuum seats with filtered vacuum cleaner as often as possible.

Be careful of buying secondhand furniture or of carpets in a new house. Take extra care at first.

If going on holiday or on a visit, take your bedding with you if you want to be extra careful about mites. Avoid damp locations if you can.

Always air things you use seldom – like sleeping bags or camping blankets – before putting them away, to control mites. Air them before use as well.

Anti-Dust Mite Chemicals

There are treatments available which either kill or denature house dust mites. If you use a treatment that *kills* house dust mites, you still have to remove the mite dropping allergens which remain potent unless you get rid of them in other ways. You have to follow up these treatments with rigorous filter vacuuming to remove the allergens. So they save you no work and you are no better off unless you vacuum. Acarosan, one such treatment, is sold at chemists, in department stores, and by mail order from ServiceMaster (address on page 186).

Treatments that *denature* the mites work by physically changing the structure of the dust mite's droppings, so that they become unrecognisable to the immune system and do not then trigger an allergic reaction. Suppliers of these treatments also recommend following up treatment with filter vacuuming, although it is not so critically important. Users of these sprays report improvement in symptoms without vacuuming, although they need to re-apply the spray often. These sprays are supplied by Allerayde, The Healthy House and Medivac.

Other treatments available include a paint containing mite-killing chemicals (from Gem Services), treatment with gas which freezes the mites to death (Cadogan Medical), and a chemical which loosens the mite's grip on surfaces (Allerite by Vax). These too require rigorous follow-up filter vacuuming to remove mites and are of no benefit unless you do this.

Drawbacks and Benefits

Apart from the need for follow-up vacuuming, the major disadvantage of chemical products is the need to re-apply (recommended between fortnightly and every six months, depending on make, except for the anti-mite paint) and the consequent cost. The cost of re-applying the treatments runs at somewhere between £100–£200 a year, depending on how extensively you do it, and on which chemical you use. You could pay for an increase in your heating bills to keep things dry, several vacuum filters or a large share of an allergy vacuum cleaner with the same amount of money.

You can treat soft toys with sprays, but being often an awkward shape, the treatment does not always reach every part of the surface. If you treat furniture and mattresses, make sure they dry off thoroughly. Light or delicate fabrics can stain.

The nitrogen gas treatment is done by a contractor but is expensive, needs follow-up vacuuming, and has to be repeated frequently if you take no other precautions. It could be useful if you moved into a new home and wanted a once-off treatment to get rid of mites, then followed it up with basic avoidance measures.

If You Are Chemically Sensitive

If you are chemically sensitive, you are best advised to avoid mite-killing paint, mite-killing chemicals, and the mite-loosening solution, all of which usually contain strong insecticides or other chemicals. Nitrogen gas treatment, however, should cause no problem and may be worth trying.

The denaturing spray treatments are based on tannic acid, a natural chemical, which is tolerated quite well by some chemically sensitive people, and few reactions have been reported. You might be able to use tannic acid without problems, but there is a risk that you may not react to it until you have been using it for some time, by when your environment would be thoroughly impregnated. *If you are highly chemically sensitive, you would be prudent to avoid using denaturing sprays.* If you are mildly chemically sensitive, there is a slight risk to using them; try in a small area only at first for some months if you decide to go ahead.

Addresses of Suppliers

Allerayde
147 Victoria Centre
Nottingham NG1 3QF
Tel: 0602 240983

Cadogan Medical Co
95 Scrubs Lane
London NW10 6QU
Tel: 081–968 3311

Gem Services Ltd
Hanwell Works
Elliott Street
Silsden
West Yorkshire BD20 0DE
Tel: 0535 656010

The Healthy House
Cold Harbour
Ruscombe
Stroud
Gloucestershire GL6 4DA
Tel: 0453 752216

Medivac
Taylormaid Products Ltd
Bollin House
Riverside Works
Manchester Road
Wilmslow
Cheshire SK9 1BJ
Tel: 0625 539401

ServiceMaster Ltd
308 Melton Road
Leicester LE4 7SL
Tel: 0533 610761

Vax Appliances
Quillgold House
Kingswood Road
Hampton Lovett
Droitwich
Worcestershire WR9 0QH
Tel: 0905 795959

Moulds

Moulds are the invisible enemy of the allergy world. They are tiny plant organisms belonging to the fungus family that can usually only be seen with a microscope. Allergy to moulds often goes undiagnosed. Understanding what they are, and where they are found, can help you to understand and control often unexplained reactions.

Allergic reactions to moulds are caused by *inhaling* the minute spores that moulds release to reproduce. These are produced year-round by perennial moulds or only at certain seasons by other moulds. Inhaling spores can cause immediate reactions in the nasal passages and airways – sneezing, sinusitis, rhinitis, wheezing, constricted breathing. The perennial moulds can be the cause of year-round problems – continual mucus production, sinus headaches, rhinitis, itchy eyes, a dry persistent cough, a prolonged head cold that will not clear, glue ear or blockages of the inner ear – which may aggravate from time to time, as their concentrations increase.

Moulds can also cause delayed reactions and a wider range of symptoms beyond the nasal and breathing symptoms described above. Mould allergy has been associated with skin reactions, digestive complaints, nausea, fluid retention, arthritis and muscle pain. (>SYMPTOMS for a full description of symptoms of mould allergy.) In addition, people with mould allergy often report that their reactions are linked to mood swings and mental symptoms such as depression, lassitude, lethargy, irritability and excitability.

If you know you are allergic to moulds and want advice on how to cope, go straight to page 192. If you want information on treatments for mould allergy, >MEDICAL HELP and COMPLEMENTARY THERAPY. If you want to know more about what moulds are, where they are found and how to detect allergy to moulds, read on from here.

What are Moulds?

Moulds play an important role in nature's ecological processes. They feed on organic matter, absorbing nutrients through their cell walls, and excreting enzymes. They thus breakdown and recycle organic matter, causing dead or decaying material to disintegrate and, in its turn, release nutrients into the environment.

Moulds grow in long filaments called mycelia, branching across or into the material on which they feed. They reproduce by producing spores which are carried invisibly in the air to land on other surfaces. It is the spores of moulds which, when inhaled, cause allergic reactions. There are 100,000 known species of moulds, but only a handful are known to cause allergic reactions.

Yeasts are related to moulds, being also members of the fungus family. Yeasts reproduce by budding off cells, or by splitting, rather than by disseminating spores. Some fungal organisms can be dimorphic – they can be either yeast or mould in different conditions. Candida, for instance, behaves as a yeast when fed on a high sugar level, but is a mould in other situations.

Moulds have practical uses in industry. They are used to produce some antibiotics, and a range of acids (such as citric, malic and gluconic acid) that are used in food processing and pharmaceuticals. Some moulds are used in cheesemaking; blue cheeses are inoculated with a mould and the rind of soft cheeses like Camembert is produced by an inoculated fungus which grows on the surface of the cheese. Yeasts are used extensively in beer, wine and breadmaking. One mould, the mushroom, is eaten as a food itself. Moulds can also cause diseases in plants and humans as well as causing allergic reactions.

Where are Moulds Found?

Moulds are highly adaptable and versatile organisms. For every ecological niche, there is probably a mould which will survive or even flourish. Some survive, and produce spores under very specific conditions of temperature, moisture or light. Others, by contrast, are fairly tolerant creatures and, although they have preferences, will function happily across a wide range of environments and habitats. They feed on almost any material containing carbon – plants, leather, paper, fabric. Some can even break down the strong resistant fibres of wood and hair.

Four moulds implicated in allergy, *Alternaria*, *Aspergillus*, *Cladosporium* and *Penicillium*, tolerate a very wide range of conditions and are found worldwide. They are present in the UK throughout the year in many situations; they have peaks at certain times and in specific conditions. These are known as 'universal dominant' or 'perennial' moulds.

As a broad guide, however, most moulds like warmth and humidity.

A temperate, moist climate, like the UK's, sustains them very well. Hot, moist environments, such as swimming baths, saunas, hair-dressers, greenhouses, bathrooms, launderettes and kitchens, encourage mould growth. Very dry weather, such as the summer of 1976, or prolonged hard frosts, inhibit the production of spores, and many allergy-sufferers feel better in such conditions.

Moulds also multiply where nutrients are readily available to them, such as where well-rotted decaying material abounds. So they thrive in rubbish bins, dustbins, compost heaps, in fallen leaves and humus, in rotting wood, in hay or straw, in cut grass, in mossy dark corners, in crops. Their food does not have to be badly decayed – even a slight deterioration provides enough food potential for some moulds, early colonisers, who thrive on slightly decaying material and will cling invisibly to leaves that are starting to turn on the tree; to the skin of fruit and vegetables; to food which has just been chopped or cut; to processed food which has been opened, such as tins or jars, or a loaf of bread. Sometimes you can also find them growing visibly – grey or green growth on decaying fruit or bread.

Some of the most adaptable allergenic moulds are also found in indoor environments. Their presence is not a sign of insanitary conditions, inadequate cleanliness, or poor housekeeping. They simply thrive invisibly in particular conditions. Indoors they cling to damp surfaces in bathrooms or showers where they can feed on tiny traces of soap or human skin. Kitchen or other damp walls also provide a feeding ground from paint, glues or wallpaper. Moulds can feed on dusty objects like art treasures or old tapestries. They thrive in damp cupboards; they cling to damp clothes and shoes; to drying laundry and used tea-towels. They waft up from waste pipes, lurk under the rim of lavatory bowls and sit in pools and drops of condensation. They feed on old dusty books and paper, especially if damp. They sit in the soil of pot plants. They grow in the encouraging dark damp of pillows, duvets, upholstered furniture and cushions. They are keen on damp, poorly ventilated areas. They prefer warmth but will tolerate colder parts, even freezers and refrigerators.

The little patches of sooty grey-black deposits that are often found on window frames or in pools of condensation are perennial moulds. The pinky-grey slime that you see around sinks, taps, on tiles, lavatories and bathroom walls contains moulds.

Moulds are usually found close to the environment where they feed and grow, but their spores can be carried long distances by winds and then deposited in areas far from their source. Thus people who live in cities can be allergic to moulds and suffer attacks on days in summer and autumn when mould spores are swept into the atmosphere and carried distances by strong winds. Even though you apparently live far from their source, you can be affected by moulds in the atmosphere.

Remember, though, that although some of the allergenic moulds are ubiquitious, most of the time they will not cause you much harm. They will be producing spores quietly and gently at a level that is unlikely to cause you to react. At times, however, they produce spores in high concentrations and it is these situations that will give you severe reactions.

What Triggers Spore Release?

So what situations trigger spore release in concentrations? Usually it is some change in their environment. Sudden warming in damp conditions can stimulate spore release in an indoor environment. Using a tumble dryer, ironing clothes, drying wet towels or hanging wet laundry near a strong heat source will stimulate spore production. Bringing damp logs or a plant in from the cold will also produce mould spores. Installing central heating in an old house can bring about sudden concentrations of spores where there were few problems before. A damp spot beneath a dripping radiator valve can induce high levels of mould as the heating comes on. Keeping rooms dry and keeping a steady average temperature can do much to avoid such problems.

Climatic conditions can also stimulate spore release. A warm, humid period of weather in summer will encourage mould production on foliage, crops and plants. If there is then a windy period, the spores can be dispersed and carried even long distances. Some moulds implicated in allergy – Cladosporium, Alternaria, Botrytis Cinerea, Stemphyllium – produce spores more readily in a drying wind. They can produce explosive concentrations of spores on hot, dry days in summer.

One allergenic mould – Didymella Exitalis – is very sensitive to moisture levels in the atmosphere. Its sporulation is provoked by dew formation; between June and early September, spores are released at about midnight and reach their peak at 3 a.m. It is also provoked by thunderstorms and reaches a peak some hours after very heavy rainfall in storms.

Another moisture sensitive mould is Sporobolomyces which, like Didymella, reaches its peak on warm summer nights in humid weather. It is at its height usually at about 4 a.m. in late July and August.

Some moulds thrive better in coastal situations, others inland.

Penicillium, for instance, does well in coastal sites; *Cladosporium*, *Alternaria* and *Stemphyllium* are more prevalent inland.

Warmth and climate changes can thus stimulate spore production in airborne moulds. Disturbing and stirring up the mould's environment can also produce very high local concentrations in soilborne moulds. Some moulds, such as *Mucor* and *Rhizopus*, live in the soil and only become airborne (and thus able to provoke allergic reactions) when they are disturbed. Thus digging a garden, playing in a sandpit and ploughing a field can propel spores into the air.

Other activities, too, can expose high levels of spores. Raking leaves, mowing grass, turning a compost heap, picking fruit, sweeping a yard – all these will throw mould spores into the atmosphere in high concentrations.

How Can You Detect Mould Allergy?

You may have already recognised your own pattern of symptoms from the description above of what moulds are and where they are found.

Skin prick tests are reasonably reliable in diagnosing mould allergy (>DETECTING YOUR ALLERGIES). You can ask your GP for referral for such tests. Other ways of detecting mould allergy are to:

• analyse the seasonal pattern of your symptoms
• compare the pattern of your symptoms to high mould situations

Seasonality

Although some moulds are found year round, especially indoors, there are periods of the year when their concentrations are much higher. In the UK, unless there are unusual climatic variations, moulds will have seasonal peaks in the autumn, and in the summer months. April, May and early June are often relatively mould-free. August and September can often be good months unless the weather is warm and humid (as was the case in the late 1980s and early 1990s). In such years, there will be no real dying down of late summer moulds before the damp, rotting moulds of autumn and winter take over.

If, most years, you feel better in April, May, early June and in August and September, suspect mould allergy.

There are often significant daily and regional variations to this pattern, according to the specific conditions that cause the level of moulds to fluctuate widely, even by the hour. A sudden high dew, a change in pressure, wind or temperature can cause a local explosion of spores.

Chemical pollution combined with fog can also aggravate mould sensitivity; the damp cloud holds down the mould particles which would otherwise escape higher into the atmosphere. If you have a very capricious pattern to your reactions, these may be explained by specific climatic or local conditions, or the effect of local chemical pollution on mould levels.

High Mould Levels

Another way to detect mould allergy is to analyse in what situations your symptoms get worse. Answer the questions in the QUESTIONNAIRE below. If you answer 'yes' to a significant number, then suspect mould allergy. Try some of the avoidance measures below as well to see what difference they make.

Detecting Mould Allergy

WHEN DO YOU FEEL WORSE?	Yes	No	WHEN DO YOU FEEL WORSE?	Yes	No
In damp, cold cellars	—	—	Having a shower	—	—
Near woods and trees	—	—	Folding laundry	—	—
In dusty, fusty attics	—	—	Before and after thunder	—	—
On dewy mornings	—	—	Raking leaves	—	—
In steamy kitchens	—	—	In a greengrocer's shop	—	—
Cutting grass	—	—	Near dank, still pools	—	—
Near wet laundry	—	—	On hot, windy days	—	—
In greenhouses	—	—	Near old books	—	—
On damp, foggy days	—	—	In swimming baths	—	—
In a florist's shop	—	—	Turning a compost heap	—	—
Near canals	—	—	In damp clothes	—	—
Near dark undergrowth	—	—	In saunas or Turkish baths	—	—
Doing the ironing	—	—	Sitting on damp walls/stones	—	—
Digging the garden	—	—	Watering pot plants	—	—
At the launderette	—	—	By rotting logs	—	—
When heating is switched on	—	—	During warm winters	—	—
In a bathroom	—	—	Near freshly cut timber	—	—

How to Deal with Allergy to Moulds

You obviously cannot control the climate and the seasonal pattern of mould allergy. It helps, however, to know at least what causes you problems at certain times of year. You can keep windows and doors shut most of the time and avoid going out as much as you can at these times.

You can also try to avoid situations and places where mould concentrations are very high. Spend as little time as you can going into steamy atmospheres, such as launderettes, swimming baths, green-houses, hot kitchens and bathrooms. If gardening, avoid the really troublesome tasks of cutting grass, composting and raking leaves. Stay out of damp, dark places. If going away on holiday, look for dry places if you can; the hot, humid tropics or damp caravans or tents are probably not for you. Use medication or therapy as prescribed to help you cope in these situations (>MEDICAL HELP).

TIP

Fallen leaves in autumn are a prime source of moulds. Try to prevent a mould-sensitive child from kicking up or playing with piles of leaves.

There is a great deal that you can do to reduce the levels of moulds in your own home environment, even though there is little you can do about moulds in the world outside. There is also added value in making a major effort to control moulds in your home, in that reducing the levels at home can increase your tolerance level to moulds outside, and make you better able to cope generally where you cannot avoid exposure.

Furthermore, there is a high degree of cross-reactivity between moulds – if you are allergic to one mould, you are more likely to react to other moulds as well (>CROSS-REACTION for more explanation). Controlling the levels of moulds around you where you can helps minimise the effects of cross-reaction.

Basic Avoidance Measures

In your own home, the key ways of reducing moulds are to:

- Keep your environment as dry as you are able
- Remove obvious sources of mould spores
- Keep a constant warmth if possible

If you cannot afford the money or time to keep your whole home free of moulds, then concentrate on one or two rooms, especially your bedroom, and try and confine damp, wet activities (like drying laundry) to certain areas away from where you spend most of your time. The most useful things to do first are the following basic avoidance measures:

Dry laundry outside the home if possible. If you use a tumble dryer, locate it outside the home if you can, or at least away from the living areas, and make sure it is well vented to the outside. Put any damp cloths or towels straight on to a heat source to dry off fast. Do not leave damp towels or cloths lying around.

Dry off any condensation and damp standing on windows, walls or work surfaces – a quick wipe in the morning or after a bath or shower does the trick. Open windows and doors to air for a while – good ventilation for at least a short period each day helps to dry things out, even on damp days. Keep plugs in sinks, basin and bath plugholes – this stops moulds wafting up.

TIP

Use extractor fans if you have them when bathing, doing laundry, or cooking, to ventilate and get damp out fast.

Airing beds and keeping them dry is a very effective way of reducing mould levels in bedrooms, and away from where you breathe at night. Humans shed about half a litre (nearly a pint) of fluid in sleep each night, and moulds like damp, warm places. See HOUSE DUST MITES for suggestions on how to air beds thoroughly.

Fix obvious sources of damp and drips. If you have any persistent problems with rising or penetrating damp, or any leaking taps or pipes, then sort them out. Many millions of mould spores can be generated from small areas of damp. >BUILDING AND DECORATING MATERIALS for advice on materials.

Using gas fires or paraffin heaters can create condensation and damp problems, since they generate water when they burn. Do not use gas fires or paraffin heaters if you can avoid them. Solid fuel fires generate water, but the damp is usually drawn up the chimney and dried off, so they do not cause damp. Electric heating produces a dry heat and is advantageous. Gas central heating, and other forms of central heating, do not cause water problems. Do not use humidifiers on radiators. They can be a source of moulds and raise humidity.

Gas and paraffin cooking appliances also create damp when used, but, because they are usually not operated as long, nor as intensively, as heaters, they cause less problems with damp. If you use them, always ventilate well to clear the damp they create.

Methods of killing moulds are given on page 196.

If You Are Severely Affected

If you are exceptionally sensitive to moulds, and obliged to take extreme care, there are many things you can do to eliminate moulds

TIP

Keeping a constant warmth helps to prevent sudden surges of mould growth. A steady average, but lower temperature, is probably better than having cold and hot spots around the home, or than having a few hours a day only when the place is well heated.

from your environment. Even if this applies to you, no-one would expect you to do all of the things suggested below all of the time. They are things you might try that can be helpful. Pick and choose what seems relevant to you and do what you feel you can. These more intensive measures cover:

- Damp control
- Kitchens, bathrooms, laundry and clothes
- Plants and gardens
- Paper and books
- Foods and diet
- Antibiotics

Damp control

Keep your home as warm and dry as you can afford. The threshold for most mould growth on the organic materials on which they feed is a relative humidity (RH) of 65 per cent. As a guide, keeping the temperature indoors a steady 5°C (40°F) above the outdoor temperature should achieve this.

If you are seriously affected by moulds, your target should be to keep your environment, or at least one or two rooms where you spend most of your time at home, at between 50 per cent and 65 per cent RH. In most summers in the UK, the heat of the sun should be sufficient; heating will be required in the winter. If your house has penetrating damp, however, or is in a damp location, you will need to keep a temperature difference of more than 5°C (40°F) between indoors and outdoors, to achieve the maximum 65 per cent RH level, and may need to heat more. Use a humidity meter (from garden centres, DIY shops or jewellers) and a thermometer to guide you.

Use insulation, such as roof lining, double glazing and lined curtains, as far as you can to conserve energy and warmth (>BUILDING AND DECORATING MATERIALS for advice on building materials). Do not cut out draughts altogether; keeping your home ventilated and aired also helps to keep down damp. *Remember to air and ventilate well.*

If you have intractable problems with damp or are in a very mouldy

Killing Moulds

Use Alkaline Solutions

Most moulds dislike an alkaline environment. You can deter moulds and prevent them from growing by washing surfaces with a solution of sodium bicarbonate or Borax.

For fridges, freezers and kitchen surfaces, use a solution of sodium bicarbonate. Put one dessertspoonful of sodium bicarbonate in a bowl of warm water and wash surfaces down thoroughly. Dry off the surfaces afterwards.

A stronger agent for killing and deterring moulds is Borax. You can buy or order domestic Borax from chemists. Make a solution of one dessertspoonful of Borax in a bowl of warm water, and use to wash down bathroom surfaces, toilets, window frames or anywhere else. You can also sprinkle Borax powder neat on damp patches – say, under a sink or in a cupboard – to kill moulds.

Use Strong Chemicals

If you are not chemically sensitive, you can use chlorine bleach to kill moulds. You can also buy proprietary fungicides at chemists' or garden centres, but, again, do not use these if you are chemically sensitive (>CHEMICALS).

To use bleach, mix half a cup of liquid bleach with half a cup of vinegar. Place it in the room where you want to kill moulds, seal the room and leave for 24 hours.

Building and Decorating Materials

Many building and decorating materials (such as wallpaper paste and tile adhesives) contain fungicides to kill or deter mould growth. If you are chemically sensitive, you are best advised not to use materials containing these, but if you are also allergic to moulds, should you not use fungicide-containing materials after all? The answer is probably not. Manufacturers of fungicide-containing materials make only limited claims for the effectiveness of the fungicides. The measures outlined in this section for deterring mould growth through environmental control (particularly keeping your home aired and dry, with an even temperature) will be as effective. (>BUILDING AND DECORATING MATERIALS for details of materials to use.)

TIP

Dry damp coats and shoes off fast if you come in wet. Take care to dry wet pushchairs or prams before folding.

Using an air filter can help remove mould spores from the air. Such a machine can make a significant difference to your environment (>AIR FILTERS).

If you have very dry skin, and think that keeping things dry may make it worse, just give it a try. If moulds are indeed the cause of your problems, things will actually improve. If you have bronchial problems, it is probably better not to take the relative humidity level lower than 55 per cent.

location, say near a river or canal, you may have to consider moving house to a drier situation. If you cannot move, or have very specific damp problems, you could consider using a dehumidifier to keep down humidity and mould levels. If you do use one, you need to take great care that the dehumidifier itself is not a source of moulds. Mould spores can grow on the inside, and in the collecting containers of dehumidifiers; they are then blown back into the room with the drier air. If you use one, you must empty it frequently and keep it scrupulously clean, often wiping it down inside with a Borax solution (see page 196). The Healthy House and Medivac sell dehumidifiers designed to help allergy sufferers. Their addresses are on page 242.

If you have an intractably damp cellar, porch or cupboard, keep its door closed as much as possible, and seal it with draught-proofing material. Mould spores can seep through a house from such an isolated source, and opening a door frequently or leaving it open will blow moulds constantly through the house.

TIP

Moulds are found in house dust wherever it collects. Using filters on a vacuum cleaner can prevent moulds being dispersed around the room in the vacuum exhaust (>VACUUM CLEANERS).

Kitchens, Bathrooms, Laundry and Clothes

Keep kitchens and bathrooms as dry as you are able. If you can afford it, install extractor fans and use them whenever damp and steam are created. Use heated towel rails or radiators to dry off any damp cloths or towels as soon as they get wet.

TIP

Avoid methods of cooking that create damp, such as boiling, steaming or baking, as far as you can. Use a microwave if you can. It minimises liquid use and cooking time.

Take a shower rather than a bath to minimise water and steam creation. Dry down tiles and surfaces after a shower or bath. The pinky-grey slime found there contains mould growth. Wash with a Borax solution (see page 196) to kill or deter moulds. Use a Borax solution also to kill moulds in lavatory bowls and down waste pipes.

TIP

Be scrupulous in handling rubbish and decaying matter. Put fruit and vegetable peelings straight out into the dustbin. Empty kitchen rubbish bins each night. Wash out kitchen rubbish bins and dustbins regularly with a Borax solution. Keep dustbins away from the home if possible.

An airing or hot cupboard can be invaluable for keeping household linen and clothes very dry. If you do not have an airing cupboard, you can create a hot cupboard by wiring a small tubular space heater in a fitted cupboard or even in a wardrobe. If you run it only a few hours a day, it is cheap and it keeps clothes and linen quite dry.

Open out shower curtains to let them dry fast. Wash them frequently to remove moulds.

Do not use a steam iron. Iron clothes when very dry – they may be more creased but they will not be mouldy.

Use a tumble dryer if you can to get laundry bone dry.

Dry off clothes after you wear them, or overnight. Do not put damp clothes back in a drawer or cupboard. Moulds grow on traces of damp on clothes and will upset you if you are exceptionally sensitive. Put them in an airing cupboard, or on a radiator or towel rail overnight to dry. Dry nightwear after and before wearing. Change straight out of wet or sweaty clothes if possible.

Plants and gardens

Take care with house plants. If you are unusually sensitive to moulds, you may not be able to tolerate indoor pot plants at all. Moulds grow in the soil, and in the more humid atmosphere around the foliage.

TIP

To avoid problems with plants, put a light gravel on the surface of the soil in each pot and water the plants by placing water in a dish or saucer underneath. Take care not to let them stand in pools of water, which encourages moulds.

If you have garden beds against the walls of your home, or pots or beds immediately under windows, these can often be concentrated sources of moulds. You would be best to move beds and pots away from direct proximity to the walls, so that moulds do not rise straight into the home. Similarly, compost heaps are best kept as far from the home as possible. Water butts also are a source of moulds. Take care with siting these.

Gardening produces some of the most intense concentrations of moulds possible. If you love gardening, you will probably have to find out by trial and error what you can tolerate and what you cannot. You probably would be best avoiding many gardening tasks such as cutting grass, raking leaves, composting and heavy digging, and should stay out of greenhouses.

TIP

You could come to a deal over gardening with a friend or a family member, that you do the bits that you can for them such as weeding or pruning – in return for them doing the bits that you cannot.

Paper and books

Paper and books can be prime sources of moulds in your environment. The dusty, fusty smell that rises in libraries, or from old books, is from moulds as much as from dust.

Avoid wallpaper in your home, if possible. Moulds feed not only on the paper, but on the glues that bind the paper to the wall as well. If your plaster is in reasonable condition, there is no need to have any wallpaper at all; even lining paper is not essential. Remove old wallpaper and keep the walls simple. >BUILDING AND DECORATING MATERIALS for more advice.

To cope with moulds on books, if they cause you problems, avoid old paper as much as you can. If you are a student, do not study in a library. Avoid old filing cabinets or stores in offices. Keep books behind glass or cupboard doors, or covered with a washable cloth, to stop moulds dispersing. Kill moulds (>page 196). Vacuum books down, with filters if possible, to remove the moulds. Keep temperatures constant, and humidity at 50–65 per cent RH to prevent growth.

TIP

Moulds cling to letters and parcels delivered in autumn and winter. Air and dry them before opening, if you are very sensitive.

Food and diet

Take scrupulous care when handling and using foods if you are extremely allergic to moulds. Tiny traces of moulds grow *invisibly* on even slightly adulterated food – on chopped salads, for instance, in fruit juices or on a half-used loaf. They cling also to frozen and defrosted food, and to food that has been kept in a refrigerator for more than a few hours. If you are highly allergic to moulds, only eat food that is very recently cut or prepared. Re-heat chilled or defrosted foods thoroughly to kill moulds. Squeeze your own fruit juices.

Store foods with care. Moulds cling to fresh fruit and vegetables. Ripe fruit is particularly prone to mould growth on its skin and surfaces. Soil moulds cling to root vegetables. Store all fruit and vegetables outside the home if you can; try to avoid using your refrigerator to store them, unless you buy fresh each day. Do not eat very ripe or deteriorating fruit. Avoid fruit with the visible grey mould Botrytis. Wash all fruit and vegetables, or peel before eating to remove moulds.

TIP

Moulds adhere particularly to the skin of grapes. Soak grapes overnight in a bowl of water, or for up to a day, to remove moulds before eating. Rinse well before eating.

Moulds grow readily on dried fruit. To avoid these, either wash the fruit carefully before eating, rehydrate and cook well, or avoid altogether.

TIP

> Keep your refrigerator clear of moulds. Defrost often and wash it down in a solution of sodium bicarbonate or Borax (see page 196). Dry afterwards. This kills and deters mould growth.

You may have to avoid eating certain foods if you are allergic to moulds. If you are allergic to one specific thing, you are more prone to cross-react to things which are related to it (>CROSS-REACTION). You will not always develop such cross-reactions but you will be susceptible to related allergens, and it is prudent sometimes to take care.

Moulds are related to yeasts, and to mushrooms, which are themselves fungi. If you cross-react, you may have to take care with foods that contain yeast, or moulds, avoiding or rotating them (>FOOD AND DRINK for information on rotation diets). Details of foods containing moulds and yeast are given on page 202. A mould-free diet would avoid these foods.

If you have candidiasis, caused by an overgrowth of a fungal organism that can cause thrush, bowel disorders and other symptoms (>SYMPTOMS), you can also be allergic to the yeast Candida itself, and have allergic symptoms as well. If you want to control Candida through diet, >FOOD AND DRINK, where more details are given.

Antibiotics

Moulds are used to produce some antibiotics. Penicillin was originally discovered as a by-product of a chance mould growth that had the ability to prevent bacteria multiplying. Penicillin is produced by growing a strain of the *Penicillium* fungus. Other moulds, for instance *Cephalosporium*, are also used to produce antibiotics. If you are sensitive to moulds, you may be sensitive to mould-produced antibiotics, through cross-reaction. >CROSS-REACTION for more information.

Antibiotics are produced from sources other than moulds, however; bacteria and other micro-organisms can be used to produce them. Tetracycline and Streptomycin, for instance, are not mould-based antibiotics. Mould allergy does not therefore mean that you are allergic to all antibiotics. If antibiotics are prescribed for you, and you are concerned, ask your doctor.

TIP

Athlete's Foot is caused by a fungal infection. Some of the symtoms can be excacerbated if you are allergic to moulds and react to the fungus itself. >FIRST AID AND HOME MEDICINE for advice on treatment of Athlete's Foot.

Moulds and Yeast in Foods

Mould and yeast-containing foods include the following:

MUSHROOMS	Including truffles and morels
CHEESE	Especially blue cheeses and soft rind cheeses like Brie and Camembert. Cottage cheese does not contain mould.
BREAD AND YEAST BAKERY	Including rolls, crumpets, croissants and buns
FERMENTED DRINKS	Alcohol such as beer, wine, cider, spirits and fortified wines. Ginger beer.
VINEGAR	Plus vinegar-containing foods such as pickles, mayonnaise, salad dressings, sauces, preserved olives. Acetic acid.
MALT PRODUCTS	Whisky; beverages such as Horlicks, some breakfast cereals (e.g. Shreddies), Mars bars, many biscuits.
YEAST SPREADS	Such as Marmite.
YEAST VITAMIN PILLS	
PICKLED OR SMOKED MEATS	
FERMENTED SOY SAUCE	
BUTTERMILK	
HYDROLYSED VEGETABLE PROTEIN (HVP)	

Eat these with care, or avoid altogether. They may only cause you problems at seasons when mould levels are higher, or if you eat a lot of them. Do not automatically exclude them, but be prudent. Rotate them if you are on a rotation diet (>FOOD AND DRINK).

Pets and Other Animals

Animals, birds and domestic pets are frequent causes of allergy. Specialist doctors estimate that up to a third of people with allergies are sensitive to pets, birds and other animals. The symptoms arising are those of true allergy (>SYMPTOMS), especially nasal and breathing symptoms, itchy eyes, eczema and dermatitis. Some people who come into close contact with birds develop 'allergic alveolitis' (also known as 'allergic pneumonia' or 'bird fancier's' lung) which is a rare but serious disease.

What Causes Problems?

Reactions are caused by *inhaling* particles from pets and animals, as well as by *touching* them. So living with a pet animal or bird can be the cause of allergy, even if you are not the prime handler or carer. A number of different substances found on, or produced by, animals and birds can be allergens. These include animal fur and hair, their skin scale or dander, feathers, and the bloom on bird feathers, often given off as a fine powder. Saliva, where an animal has licked itself, you, or furniture and flooring, is also a common cause, as well as urine and faeces. Further problems can be caused by dusts and moulds found in animal cages, stalls or huts, or litter trays.

Any kind of animal, bird or pet can cause allergy, especially where you have a significant exposure to them, as with a domestic pet, or at work. Cats and dogs are thus common causes. Small mammals, such as hamsters, mice, gerbils, rabbits and guinea pigs, frequently cause allergy, and can go unsuspected. Caged birds are also often the source of problems.

If you are sensitive to horses, you may also find that you react to old furniture – sofas, mattresses, chairs – that has been upholstered with horsehair. Some vaccines are based on serum taken from horses; ask your doctor to check before you are given any vaccination.

People are known to react to clothing made of animals' fur and hair, such as fur coats, hats and collars. Angora yarns are made variously from goat hair, rabbit hair, and sometimes even cat hair. (For information on wool from sheep, >FIBRES, CLOTHING and FABRICS. For advice on leather, >MISCELLANEOUS ALLERGENS.)

Fresh feathers on birds do not cause allergy as commonly as older feathers used as filling for pillows and cushions. Here sometimes the cause can also be house dust mites and moulds rather than the feathers themselves (>HOUSE DUST MITES and MOULDS for more advice). The bloom on birds' plumage – a fine dust that rises on handling – is a known cause of allergy (>also **Feathers** in MISCELLANEOUS ALLERGENS).

If you know you are allergic to a specific animal and want advice on how to cope, go straight to page 206. If you want advice on medical treatments for animal allergy, >MEDICAL HELP and COMPLEMENTARY THERAPY. If you want to know about allergy to pets and other animals and how to detect it, read on from here.

Where are Allergens Found?

Animal allergens can disperse throughout the whole environment around them. It is not necessary to touch or handle animals or birds to be allergic to them. Pet allergens can waft through the home and, even if the animal or bird is confined to a limited area, traces of allergens can be found in other parts. If you are not very sensitive to them, this will be no problem; but if you are highly allergic, then it can be a cause of difficulty.

If a cat or dog sleeps in your bedroom at night, it could be the cause of reactions. If you allow them to sleep on a bed during the day, they can leave traces of allergens which can upset you later when you go to bed.

Pet allergens are also found in house dust and if you react to this, animal allergens may be the cause. They can also cling to clothing or surfaces where an animal has been, such as car seats, furniture, the animal's bedding, carpets and rugs, so visiting other people's homes or travelling in their cars may cause trouble. Even if you do not have a pet, people who come into your home can bring animal allergens in with them on their clothes. Again, if you are exceptionally sensitive, this can be a problem.

Animal allergens can also be an occupational hazard, depending on your type of work. Laboratory workers using animals or birds in experiments are known to develop allergy, as are zoo or circus employees, kennel workers and dog handlers. Blind people can develop an allergy to their guide dogs.

Hobbies and leisure pursuits, such as horse-riding, which bring you into contact with animals can also be troublesome. Birdkeeping is a known hazardous hobby. If you are exceptionally sensitive, even inhaling animal allergens at a distance can trigger reactions. Going to the races, visiting a circus, or watching a gymkhana, have been known to cause reactions in people allergic to horses, for instance.

TIP

If your problems started on moving house, or soon after, animal allergens from previous owners may be a cause. These can be very persistent.

If you sit next to someone wearing clothes with cat or dog allergens clinging to them, even invisibly, this can upset you. This may be the cause of problems at work, at school, at leisure activities, or even on public transport.

How to Detect Allergy to Animals

Skin tests for animal inhalant allergens are reasonably reliable at detecting allergy to animals, although results can depend on what precisely you are allergic to. If you are allergic to your cat's saliva or urine, for instance, and you have a skin test for cat hair, the result will be negative even though you are allergic. Some people also find that they can be allergic to one breed or type of animal, but tolerate others; or that they react to one particular individual animal and not to others. Tests, therefore, are not always helpful. Your doctor can refer you for skin tests.

One simple test, which you can do yourself, is the Eye Test. Stroke the animal or bird for a few minutes. Rub one eye with your hand for a few seconds. If your eye becomes itchy and swollen, then this is an indication that you are sensitive to the animal or bird.

You can also do a Sniff Test on bedding, or litter, to check if these upset you. Sniff these gently, and see if symptoms develop. (*Take care if you have a history of severe asthma attack, or anaphylactic shock.* >EMERGENCY INFORMATION *for precautions to take.*)

Another method of detecting animal allergy is to avoid the animal or bird you suspect totally for a period of a week, and see if symptoms improve. If the animal or bird you suspect is your domestic pet, and you are not highly allergic, it will be sufficient to keep the animal or bird totally outside the house, and for you or the person affected not to go near it at all during that week. Try this first. For birds, this should be a conclusive test.

If, however, this is not conclusive for animals, or if you are more severely affected, you will need to carry out a rigorous cleaning programme to clear up traces of allergens from your home before you can be sure that your domestic pet is the source of trouble. Details of what to do are given on page 207.

How to Deal with Allergy to Pets and Other Animals

How you deal with allergy to pets and animals will depend on how important they are to your life.

If You Are Not Highly Allergic

If you are not highly allergic to an animal or pet, it may be sufficient to take the following avoidance measures in your home. Make sure that the animal sleeps outside the house. Confine it, if you can, to certain areas of the home and above all keep it out of bedrooms, both during the day and at night. Groom or brush animals outside the house, or get someone else to groom them for you. Discourage animals from licking you, and particularly from licking young children and babies.

Use washable bedding for animals. Wash frequently, and beat or hose down outside the house. Vacuum or wash as frequently as you can any furniture or flooring on which the animal commonly sits. Use a washable hearth rug, and other washable flooring where possible.

Keep small mammals outside the house. Get someone else to clean out cages and litter trays if you are sensitive to these.

If you are sensitive to animals at work, using hand protection if you have contact allergies can help (>HAND PROTECTION), as can limiting your close contact as far as you possibly can. Gardeners using horse manure can react to it if they are allergic to horses, so they should use a different kind of manure or compost. Zookeepers allergic to horses have been known to cross-react to related species – donkeys, mules and zebras – and have to avoid caring for these.

If You Are Extremely Sensitive

If you are highly allergic and very badly affected by allergy to animals and birds, you may have no alternative but total avoidance even if this

TIP

Using an allergy vacuum cleaner can make a real difference. Conventional cleaners blow dusts (including animal allergens) back into the room. Allergy vacuum cleaners have special filters and allow virtually no dusts back out. Using one over a period of time will also progressively remove allergens embedded in carpets, furniture and curtains. >VACUUM CLEANERS for details.

Using an air filter can also be a help, although they will not be of benefit without other avoidance measures. >AIR FILTERS for

means giving up a much loved companion, or your current employment.

Try the avoidance measures described above first to see if they help in your home. If they do not improve things very much, do a *rigorous cleaning programme* to remove existing traces of animals and birds. Traces of allergens can adhere to carpets, flooring, even walls, even if the pet has not been in rooms for some time. Use an allergy vacuum cleaner, if you can borrow or buy one, and vacuum every surface that you can, including curtains, ceilings and walls. Wash anything movable or washable, and wash down surfaces and walls that are not. (Use low-allergen cleaning materials, >CLEANING PRODUCTS.) Wash and air clothes, and vacuum and wash down cars or anything else the animal has used. If this still does not work, you may have, sadly, to get rid of your pet.

If you are tempted to replace your pet, remember that, if you are prone to animal allergy, you can often tolerate an individual animal or bird of the same species for a while, say months or even longer, and then become allergic to it. It is probably better not to replace a pet than to have to get rid of another one to which you have become attached. This can be particularly painful for young children.

If you are extremely sensitive to animals with whom you work, it may be difficult to continue your employment, and there is little constructive advice on avoidance.

Other Preventative Measures

If you want to keep a dog, some breeds are reported to be less troublesome than others. Allergy is very idiosyncratic, however, and these may not work for you, so take care.

Many people with allergies say that dogs that require a lot of grooming are more likely to cause reactions than dogs that do not, because more hair is shed and more contact is necessary. Dogs that have shorter, wiry hair generally shed more dander than long-haired dogs, but dogs with soft, curly hair, such as small poodles' are sometimes found to be less provocative.

If you are blind and have to keep a guide dog, it may be best to choose a type of dog that sheds less hair, or needs less grooming, such as curly-coated retrievers, or cross labradors.

Be careful with children and animals at school. Small mammals are often kept in schoolrooms and these may be responsible for your child's reactions. School cats are also often allowed to roam out of school hours and can leave allergens to upset the exceptionally sensitive. Watch out for the 'school run' if your child travels regularly in a car in which dogs travel.

If you are exceptionally sensitive, be careful about where you or your child go if you visit people who have animals, or be careful with visitors coming into your home. Get them to leave coats and jackets outside the door. Research has shown that cat allergens, for instance, have been found at surprisingly high levels in cat-free homes, brought in by visitors. Beware of travelling in cat owners' cars.

When choosing holiday accommodation, ask whether pets are allowed in the place. If so, and you need to avoid them, stay elsewhere.

If looking for a new home, check whether pets have previously lived in the house or flat, and which parts of the place they have particularly used. If you have any concerns, do not move into somewhere where pet-owners lived previously. Remember that you can develop allergies to lingering allergens months or even longer after you have moved, and that you can be allergic to saliva and urine, not just to hair and fur. Be prepared to have to replace flooring and do a rigorous cleaning programme (see above) if you find that you do become sensitive to a new home.

Finally, if you have a strong family tendency to allergy to pets, it is preferable to avoid keeping a pet if you have a baby or young children. Children under two are particularly vulnerable. If you do have a family pet, then follow the avoidance measures above and keep your home as free as you can of allergens. Preventative measures with young children may help them avoid lifelong problems with allergy. If you must keep pets, try goldfish or tropical fish – maybe not as lovable as a cat, dog or small furry mammal – but allergy free!

Plants and Trees

You can be sensitive to touching, coming into contact with, plants and trees, or to touching or inhaling their products. This is caused predominantly by natural chemicals given off as vapour, or exuded by the plants and trees. The symptoms can be either those of allergy or of chemical sensitivity (>SYMPTOMS).

This section deals with sensitivity to wood and grass; to fragrances, oils, resins and terpenes from plants and trees; and on how to avoid problems.

For information on plant and tree pollens, >POLLENS. For information on fungal spores, >MOULDS. For information on latex and cork, >MISCELLANEOUS ALLERGENS.

Wood

Sensitivity to wood itself is actually quite rare. It is known for people to be allergic or sensitive to resinous woods — such as pine, cedar, iroko – which give off traces of volatile fumes from the wood. If these types of wood are sealed with varnish or paint, however, the fumes do not gas out, and the wood should not give any problem. If you appear to react to sealed wood surfaces, the cause is much more likely to be the paint or varnish used than the wood itself.

Problems with resinous woods can arise with furniture of pine or cedar, in which sometimes the inside surfaces (such as drawers or cupboards) are not sealed. They can arise from floorboards which are not sealed, but usually only when these are new and the fumes are still gassing out. Wooden pencils or crayons are sometimes made of cedar wood; the wood in their tips, being unsealed, can be aromatic and sometimes cause trouble. For avoidance measures, >page 213.

If you work extensively with wood, you can become allergic or sensitive to wood dusts – of wood of any kind, not just resinous woods. Sawn wood also harbours moulds and lichens, and these can cause allergy. These are dispersed when wood is cut or handled (say during construction or repair work), but will disappear as the wood dries out.

If you become sensitive to turpentine, the natural resin in pine wood, you may cross-react to other chemicals and plants that are chemically related to it. A description of these is given in CROSS-REACTION.

Grass

If you appear to be sensitive to grass, but your reactions do not correspond to situations or times when grass pollens are high (for full information, >POLLENS), then the cause may be grass sap or terpenes – the natural chemicals in grass that rise when the grass is growing. Some people develop problems on touching grass; others are sensitive to inhaling the vapours.

Grass sap starts to rise before pollen is produced and if you are extremely sensitive, it will bother you when you are close to grass from April, or even March, when grass starts growing, and also into the autumn until grass stops growing. Grass sap is also given off strongly into the air as grass is mown and just after. Some rush mats, baskets made of grass, and bales of hay, give off traces of grass terpenes for a while.

Fragrances, Oils, Resins and Terpenes

Fragrances, oils, resins and terpenes that occur naturally in plants and trees cause problems in two ways – firstly when touched, inhaled or eaten in their natural state, and secondly when, once extracted, they are used as material or ingredients in manufactured products.

In the Natural State

You can be affected by inhaling the volatile vapours from the plants, or by physical contact with their material, if you handle plant material extensively as part of your work (e.g. vegetable picking, flower picking or florist, food preparation), or if you have contact with plants in gardening.

Plants are usually most troublesome when they are growing vigorously. Some only give trouble if they are crushed and broken; others need not be injured. Plants with furry leaves or stems are often more problematic than others, for the chemicals are held in, and more readily given off from, the short spines. Bulbs (such as tulip or narcissi) are also known to cause reactions.

Some plants are known to be particularly troublesome, especially when handled extensively, and in cases of dermatitis. These include the following:

- primula family
- lily family (e.g. tulip, hyacinth, garlic, onion, chives)
- daffodils and narcissi
- umbellifer family (e.g. carrots, celery, yarrow)
- nettles and hops
- orange, lemon, grapefruit, dittany
- compositae family (e.g. chrysanthemum, daisy)
- ivy
- philodendron
- oleander

In some plants that frequently cause reactions, chemicals common to the plants have been identified as the specific cause. These plants are:

- artichokes
- burdock
- camomile
- wormwood
- mugwort
- pyrethrum
- feverfew

If you know you react to one of these, you should take care with others in the group.

Some people are sensitive to the fragrance of growing plants, such as roses, or to that of cut flowers.

For advice on avoidance with handling or inhaling plants, >below.

Plants as Material and Ingredients

Extracts from plants are used as ingredients in many manufactured products (including perfumes, fragrances, flavouring agents, solvents, medicines, foods, adhesives, plastics, resins, paper and fabric finishes). It is predominantly chemicals with complex structures from the oleo-resin fraction of plant chemicals that cause sensitivity – including essential oils, phenols, terpenes, resins and camphors.

Sensitivity to these is highly personal – many people tolerate natural chemicals well; some people tolerate one natural chemical and not another; other people do not tolerate any very well. It is important, however, if you are prone to chemical sensitivity (>CHEMICALS for full explanation) to treat natural chemicals as you would any other, and not to assume that they are safer or better tolerated than synthetic chemicals.

Essential oils are found in perfume essences, herbal products, in

TIP

If you want to work out if a plant upsets you, you can tape a fresh piece of the plant or its foliage to your inner arm, and follow the Patch Test procedure (>CHEMICALS).

You can also use the Patch Test or the Sniff Test (>CHEMICALS) for essential oils or products containing plant chemicals.

food as flavouring, in cosmetics and toiletries and many medical or personal hygiene products (such as toothpaste, or home medicines).

They are used in aromatherapy and as massage oils. They include oil from lavender, eucalyptus, citrus fruits, rosemary, mint (menthol), bergamot, lemon grass, cinnamon, sandalwood and vanilla. Reactions to these are known.

Resins and balsams are secretions produced by trees and plants following injury. Natural turpentine is produced this way, as is latex (>MISCELLANEOUS ALLERGENS for information on sensitivity to latex). Balsam of Peru is a chemical known commonly to cause reactions. It has an odour resembling vanilla and cinnamon. It, and related balsams, are used as flavouring agents in many food products, confectionery, drinks, and for flavouring and perfume, home medicines and toothpaste. Balsam of Peru cross-reacts with a number of common chemicals such as coal tar products (>CROSS-REACTION for details).

Rosin is a resin produced as a distillation of natural oil of turpentine. It has a very wide use in all sorts of applications from fabric finishes, through adhesive tape, to varnishes and lacquers, and sensitivity is well documented. A fuller list of its applications, and substances to which it cross-reacts are given in CROSS-REACTION.

Many natural oils and resins (such as natural turpentine and essential oils like rosemary) are used in producing building and decorating materials with no synthetic chemicals. Some individuals can be sensitive to these. >BUILDING AND DECORATING MATERIALS for sources and details of how to test in advance of use.

Linseed oil is produced by pressing from the seeds of the flax plant. It is used as a sealant in some building products and as a component of linoleum. It is relatively inert and rarely causes reactions. Linoleum is a type of flooring that causes few problems to the chemically sensitive. Forbo-Nairn manufactures lionleum which can be ordered through any carpet or flooring supplier. Their address is at the top of page 213.

Forbo-Nairn
PO Box No.1
Kircaldy
Fife
Scotland FY1 2SB
Tel: 0592 261111

How to Avoid Problems

If you are sensitive to resinous woods, use other woods wherever possible. >BUILDING AND DECORATING MATERIALS and FURNITURE for ways
in which to avoid problems in these areas.

If you work with plants, or handle them extensively, wear gloves
and a face mask to protect yourself where possible (>FACE MASKS and
HAND PROTECTION). Wear them also for food preparation and cooking
if you are extremely sensitive to vegetable and fruit juices and
vapours. Keep separate chopping boards if you or family members
have particular sensitivities.

If you are sensitive to plants in your garden, take them out and
replace them. Take care with materials, like pyrethrum, that are used
as organic pesticides. Take special care with garden or house plants
with furry leaves and stems. Always wear gloves for gardening if you
have sensitive skin (>HAND PROTECTION).

If you are sensitive to flower fragrances, avoid cut flowers or places
where they are present in numbers.

Take care with any complementary therapy that uses herbal, plant
and natural oils or remedies (>COMPLEMENTARY THERAPY).

If you think you may be sensitive to plant oils or extracts used in
processed foods, or manufactured products such as cosmetics, toiletries, toothpaste, home medicines or personal hygiene products, stop
consuming or using these for a while. Consult the main index and relevant sections of the *Guide* for alternatives to use.

Pollens

Pollens are the fine powders produced by plants, trees, shrubs and grasses to fertilise and reproduce their species. Pollens are probably the most common cause of allergic reactions.

The symptoms most closely associated with pollen allergy are those of seasonal rhinitis (also called hay fever) – sneezing, itchy eyes, runny and itchy nose, sore sinuses. Asthma, eczema and any other allergic symptoms such as headaches or joint pain (>SYMPTOMS) can also be triggered by pollens. You can get late phase reactions – symptoms developing several hours after your exposure to pollens, often at night.

Contact dermatitis can sometimes result when airborne pollens come into contact with exposed skin. These reactions can sometimes be delayed by up to a few days.

If you know that you are allergic to pollens and want advice on how to cope, go straight to page 219. Spores of fungi and moulds are the subject of a separate section. If you need information on these, >MOULDS. If you want to know more about pollens, where they are found and how to detect pollen allergy, read on from here.

What Pollens Cause Problems?

Pollens are produced in the UK from February to September. Diagram 8 shows the principal pollens causing allergy month by month. According to the area of the UK where you live, the season for each pollen will vary slightly, starting earlier in more southerly or warmer parts.

Grass pollens, with a season from May to late July or early August, are the most common cause of allergy. There are numerous species of grass which produce pollen in the UK, but only a dozen are known to be important allergens. There is a high degree of cross-reaction between grass pollens – if you react to one, you are prone to react to others.

Other pollens, such as tree, weed and crop pollens, also cause allergy, often at the same season as grass, as Diagram 8 shows. 'Hay fever', as a term used to describe the symptoms of pollen allergy, can thus be a misnomer.

_TIP_____

If you get allergic reactions in June and July, the cause can also be mould spores, not pollens at all. Mould spores are often produced in high concentrations in summer at the peak of the pollen season, and mould allergy often goes undiagnosed, or diagnosed as pollen allergy. >MOULDS for full information on mould spores if you cannot satisfactorily trace seasonal allergy to pollens.

Diagram 8: **Principal Pollen Allergens**

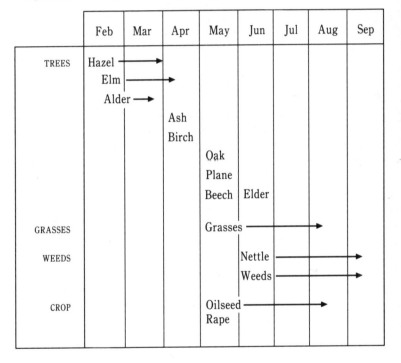

Pollens from *wind-pollinated* plants and trees cause most problems with allergy. In order to reproduce, wind-pollinated species have to produce very large quantities of pollen. The grains can, in the right conditions, be carried long distances in concentrations. This is one of the reasons why people who live in cities can suffer from allergy caused by pollens brought into the city by the wind. Grasses, nettles and the weed plantain are wind-pollinated; as are many of the common trees shown in Diagram 9.

Diagram 9: **Tree Pollens**

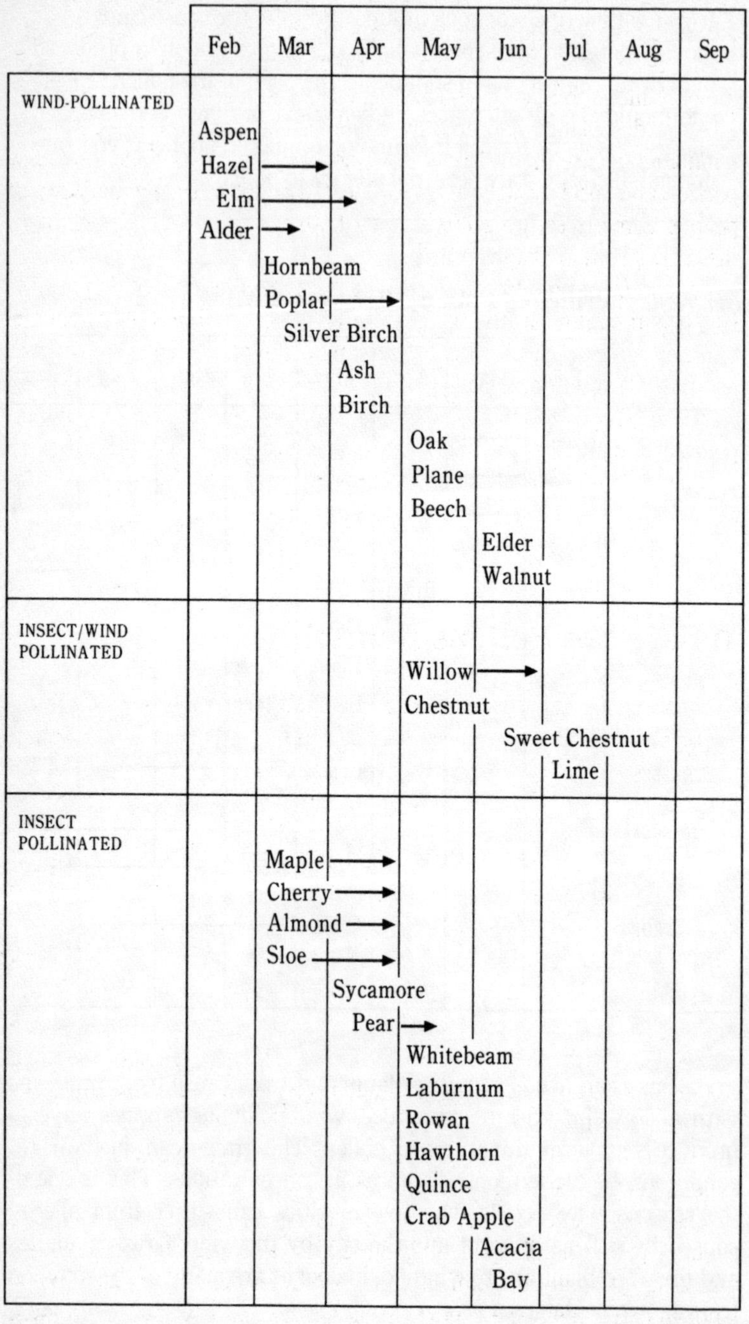

	Feb	Mar	Apr	May	Jun	Jul	Aug	Sep
WIND-POLLINATED	Aspen Hazel → Elm ——→ Alder →	Hornbeam Poplar ——→ Silver Birch Ash Birch		Oak Plane Beech	Elder Walnut			
INSECT/WIND POLLINATED				Willow ——→ Chestnut		Sweet Chestnut Lime		
INSECT POLLINATED		Maple ——→ Cherry ——→ Almond ——→ Sloe ——→	Sycamore Pear →	Whitebeam Laburnum Rowan Hawthorn Quince Crab Apple	Acacia Bay			

Insect-pollinated plants and trees, by contrast, do not have to discharge large amounts of pollen. Their pollens are only found in a localised area around them, not borne in the atmosphere. Most people do not develop allergies to insect-pollinated species and if you do, you are only likely to react if you are very close to the source of the pollen. Most garden plants, garden flowers, daisies and cut flowers are insect-pollinated, as are many fruit trees, and weeds such as dandelion, cow parsley and rosebay willow herb. These will not affect the majority of people. Some trees are pollinated by both insect and wind; details of these are given in Diagram 9.

Pollens from pine trees appear not to cause allergic reactions in the UK. It is thought that the pollens are very inert and do not trigger the immune system. Studies in Scandinavia, however, have shown evidence of allergy to pine pollens.

Oilseed rape, a relatively recent crop in the UK, is an insect-pollinated plant but, despite this, reports of allergy are increasing in localised areas where it is produced, or, for instance, from people who have driven through areas of crop fields of oilseed rape.

Where are Pollens Found?

Pollens can be carried very great distances by winds in the atmosphere. Pollen grains have been found in the air in mid-Atlantic Ocean, and have been shown to be blown up to 300 kilometres (nearly 90 miles) a day. The average maximum distance travelled is thought to be closer to 50 kilometres (about 30 miles), however, and the majority of windborne pollens fall within a few hundred metres (yards) of their source. Most pollens from insect-pollinated plants will, as described above, be found in the immediate vicinity of their plant source.

In fine, clear weather in summer, grass pollens are affected by a marked daily cycle. Most grasses discharge pollen in the early morning, and these rise in convection currents and are carried up into the atmosphere with reactions being noticeable from 7.00 a.m. to about 8.00–8.30 a.m. Some species of grass discharge pollens a second time in the early afternoon. The pollens continue to rise and collect high in the sky if the weather stays fine, and then start to fall again in early evening as the warm air descends.

The worst time for many people allergic to grass pollen is this evening period as the pollens come down. The peak occurs between 5.00 and 7.00 p.m. in country areas, or places near parks and grassland. In cities, the same evening peak occurs, but usually one to three hours later, between 6.00 and 10.00 p.m. On calm nights, there is sometimes a second peak after midnight.

Pollen counts measure the concentration of pollen grains in the atmosphere, in terms of grams per cubic metre. A count of 50 is low, while a count of 100 to 200 is high. Counts of 800 grams per cubic metre have exceptionally been recorded. The concentration of pollen in the atmosphere increases as the season goes on, reaching a peak in early July in most parts of the UK. Rain washes pollen out of the atmosphere, and a heavy shower during the pollen season often reduces the pollen count significantly.

Tree pollens are known to exhibit the same daily cycle, and the same concentration of pollen count over time as grass pollens; but weather conditions in February to May are rarely conducive, and the season for each tree pollen is much shorter than that of grass.

Chemical pollution, such as vehicle exhausts in cities, can be an exacerbating factor for people with pollen allergy, many of whom find that air pollution holds down pollens in the low atmosphere and makes their reactions worse. In addition, if you are chemically sensitive, chemical molecules adhere to the surface of the larger pollen molecules and it is believed that chemicals are thus absorbed in greater concentrations during the pollen season.

Most people with allergy to grass pollen find that their sensitivity increases as the season progresses. At the beginning of the season in May, a low pollen count of 50 or 80 may not trouble you, but later in the season after prolonged exposure and constant reaction, your tolerance becomes reduced and a low count may be sufficient to trigger a reaction. Tree pollens have the same effect, but because the season for most tree pollens is so short, the effects are often less severe.

Certain parts of the UK have consistently lower pollen counts than others. Coastal breezes blow pollen grains inland and coastal locations therefore are often favourable to people allergic to pollens. Upland areas, such as the Scottish Highlands, the Pennines, the East and West Ridings of Yorkshire and the Black Mountains of Wales, have low grass pollen counts; this is thought to be in part due to the prevalence of moor grasses which produce little pollen. The eastern side of the country, at the tail of the UK's prevailing westerly winds, has relatively high pollen counts; and South East England and East Anglia, with warmer climates, and crop and grassland agriculture, are markedly high pollen areas.

Finally, certain activities at peak pollen season can stir up very high localised pollen concentrations and are best avoided. Mowing the grass will stir up high levels of grass pollen. Pollens can also cling to long pet hair, or to clothes and human hair, if you go for a walk or drive amongst grass or trees. Pollens also adhere to laundry hanging out to dry – particularly if left out during the early evening. The pollens can then be brought indoors on the fur, hair, clothes or laundry and cause problems indoors.

How to Detect Allergy to Pollens

Skin tests are relatively reliable at detecting allergy to pollens and your doctor can refer you for these. >DETECTING YOUR ALLERGIES for full description of tests.

You can use Diagrams 8 and 9 to help you identify a specific suspect if you know that you only react at a particular time of year. If you want to identify a specific tree, shrub or weed, the names of books with good illustrations and descriptions are given on page 486.

You can also use the description of when and where pollens occur to help you work out any pattern to your reactions. If you live in a city, for instance, and get reactions in mid to late evening in summer without any apparent cause, then windborne pollens may well be the reason. If you only get symptoms after a drive through specific crops or plants, then again pollens could be the cause. If you feel better after a shower of rain at tree pollen time from February to April, or at peak pollen times in midsummer, then pollens will be the reason.

TIP

Some people are also sensitive to plant fragrances and flower scents, and to grass sap (grass terpene). These can irritate or exacerbate reactions to pollens, or be mistaken for them. >PLANTS AND TREES for more advice.

How to Deal with Pollen Allergy

When You Go Outdoors

Wear glasses, particularly wide ones which wrap around the side of the eyes. This helps to protect against pollens entering the eyes.

Avoid going out at peak pollen times during the day if you can possibly do so. On summer days these are from 7.00–8.00 a.m., and from 5.00–7.00 p.m. outside cities, 6.00–10.00 p.m. in cities. Go out during or just after rain showers if you can possibly arrange it.

Use medication, such as eyedrops and anti-histamines, if prescribed. Neutralisation and desensitisation can be effective against pollen allergy (>MEDICAL HELP). Some people find homeopathic remedies helpful. These need to be taken in advance of the pollen season (>COM-PLEMENTARY THERAPY).

Wear a scarf or hat to cover up longer hair, so that you do not bring pollens back indoors with you.

Keep windows and all air vents closed when travelling by car. Pollens are forced into cars travelling at speed. Use a sun-roof for ventilation if you have one. Some pollens even come through closed air vents and you can reduce these by taping damp surgical gauze over the vents. Spray occasionally with water to keep the gauze damp. You can also use a car filter to filter out pollens at the air intake. You can then continue to use ventilation and heating in the car. These filters are reported to be very effective at keeping out pollens. >TRAVEL for full details.

Holding a damp handkerchief or pad of cotton wool over your nose and mouth can also help when you are out of doors. It does not stop you inhaling pollens completely but it helps a little. This can be a useful aid on public transport where you may not be able to close windows or doors.

TIP

Splashing cold water into your eyes and up your nose can bring great relief to soreness and itchiness.

When You Come Back In

If you have been close to high sources of pollen, it can help to *shower and wash your hair* on returning home. *Changing clothes* can also be a help. If a dog has been out in long grass or near trees, *brush or wash it down* before it comes indoors.

When Indoors

At the height of pollen seasons, *keep doors and windows closed* as much as you can. Surprisingly high levels of tree and grass pollens have been monitored inside buildings. Keep them closed, especially at peak hours, and above all keep bedroom windows closed during the day and early evening. A good time to open windows is overnight, between 10.00 p.m. and 6.00 a.m., although on some hot nights there can be pollen peaks at around midnight.

Using an air filter can help. It will not remove all traces of allergens, but people report that using a filter can make enough difference to make life bearable indoors. >AIR FILTERS for full advice.

Some people also report that hanging damp butter muslin or damp net curtains at windows helps trap pollens, and reduce their level indoors. >FABRICS for sources.

It may not be possible to keep windows and doors closed as much as you would like at work or school. Sitting away from a window will help a little, as will holding a damp cloth to your nose.

Avoid High Pollen Situations

Do not go out at peak times, as above. Avoid mowing lawns or cutting grass in the pollen season. Do not hang laundry to dry out of doors on high pollen days, or get someone else to shake and fold it outside the home before bringing it in. Do not go for a walk across fields at peak grass pollen times. Stay away from woods or clumps of trees at tree pollen seasons. Stay away from oilseed rape fields and do not drive through them if this makes you react. Do not bring cut flowers or keep flowering plants in the house if you react, unusually, to these. Organise your garden to remove trees or plants which upset you, especially those close to windows and doors.

Avoid Long Journeys

For long journeys at high pollen seasons, InterCity trains and aeroplanes are air-conditioned and are often a better way to travel than by car or bus.

Check the pollen count before you go out or plan your day. The Pollen Research Unit (see below) provides a telephone Helpline to give information on pollen counts region by region.

Choose With Care Where You Go On Holiday

Coastal areas are generally more favourable than inland areas. Alpine or other high altitude areas are relatively free of pollens, with short pollen seasons and often with micro-climates that discourage pollen production. In some countries, such as Spain or Portugal, pollens are produced virtually all year round and you may have problems. The Pollen Research Unit has information on pollen counts and major allergens for most parts of the world. Their booklet *Holidays Without*

Hayfever is very helpful in planning holidays or travel. It is available, if you enclose a stamped addressed envelope, from:

> The Pollen Research Unit
> Polytechnic of North London
> 383 Holloway Road
> London N7 0RN
> Tel: 071–753 7010

They will also answer specific enquiries if you enclose £1 with your request.

Important Events

Important events, such as school and college exams, or sports events and school outings often take place at peak summer pollen times. In the case of exams, if you or your child are affected by allergy to the extent that your performance is reduced, make sure that the people responsible know, if necessary providing a doctor's note. Ask if you can take exams in a place better protected from pollens – say, at home so that you do not have to go outside that day. *Be assertive* if pollens make you or your child very unwell – many people view allergy as a minor inconvenience without realising how disabling it can be.

Long-Term Measures

If you are planning to have a baby, try if you possibly can to plan the month of birth of your baby to avoid significant exposure to pollen in the first six months of life. People born between September and February are much less likely to develop allergy to pollens, while those born in March and April are most susceptible. There is evidence, particularly with tree pollens, that babies exposed to high pollen counts in the first six months of life go on later to show greater sensitivity to pollens.

If you are very severely affected by pollen allergy, you may think of moving to a different part of the country. Generally speaking, upland areas, coastal parts, and the western side of the UK have lower pollen counts than other parts of the country. The Pollen Research Unit (address above) will be able to give you specific advice on particular locations if you send them £1 and a stamped addressed envelope.

Look very carefully at the immediate surroundings if you are thinking of moving house. Avoid living near any plants, trees and grasses that you know particularly upset you. Find out which way prevailing winds blow, and try and live upwind of any woods or grassy areas.

Ask the local doctors' practices if there are any particular patterns of allergies and if there are any parts of the local area which seem more favourable.

TIP

Some tree pollens cross-react with certain fruit and nuts. If you are allergic to these pollens, you may get reactions if you eat these related foods. >CROSS-REACTION for more information.

Miscellaneous Allergens

This section deals in alphabetical order with allergens or things that cause reactions that are not covered in the other main sections on allergens. It refers you on where necessary to other sections of the *Guide*. In particular, it covers sensitivity to insect bites, latex and metals.

Anaesthetics

>MEDICAL HELP

Aspirin

>CROSS-REACTION

Athlete's Foot

>MOULDS

Cork

Cork comes from the bark of a Southern European oak tree. It is an extremely inert material and even dusts produced when it is cut rarely cause reaction. If you think you react to cork used in floors, furnishings or decoration, it is more likely that you are sensitive to varnishes or lacquers used on it. >BUILDING AND DECORATING MATERIALS for more advice on varnishes and sealants.

Drugs

If you have adverse reactions to drugs, it is possible that you are sensitive to the active chemicals in the drug, or else to 'excipients', the ingredients used to tablet or formulate the drug (such as sugar, flavourings or tabletting powders – wheat, corn, potato or lactose are often used). *You should always consult your doctor about possible causes of adverse reactions.*

There is information on sensitivity to chemicals in CHEMICALS; to excipients in CHEMICALS, FIRST AID AND HOME MEDICINE, MEDICAL HELP and FOOD AND DRINK; to aspirin and to certain anti-histamines in CROSS-REACTION; to anti-biotics in MOULDS; and to anaesthetics in MEDICAL HELP.

Feathers

Allergy to feathers is common, but less common than believed, since many cases of apparent allergy to pillows, duvets or furniture containing feathers can be caused by house dust mites or moulds. Many people are not sensitive to new feathers, but are to older feathers. This may be either because older feathers become more allergenic as they degrade, or because house dust mites or moulds thrive in older feathers. (>HOUSE DUST MITES and MOULDS for how to tell if you are sensitive to these.) Some people sensitive to feathers on birds are in fact allergic to the debris or products of the bird – such as bloom on the feathers or urine, faeces or saliva (> PETS AND OTHER ANIMALS).

There is advice in BEDDING on how to tell if you are sensitive to feathers, on feather bedding in which the allergens have been rendered inert, and on alternative types of bedding.

>also FURNITURE for advice on alternative materials for furnishing.

Flour Dust

Dusts from flour are usually only a problem if you have extensive exposure at work.

Fur

>PETS AND OTHER ANIMALS

Glass and Ceramics

These are not known to cause reactions at all. If you think you are reacting to glassware or crockery, you are more likely to be sensitive to cleaning products used on them, or, if you are extremely sensitive, to traces of water. (>CLEANING PRODUCTS and WATER AND WATER FILTERS).

Glass fibre used in insulating materials can be irritant and needs care in handling, but does not cause sensitivity.

Hormones

Some women are known to be sensitive to the hormones oestrogen and progesterone. Whether this is due to a form of chemical sensitivity, or whether some other mechanism is in play, is not clear.

Neutralisation – a form of desensitisation (>MEDICAL HELP) – can be extremely effective against sensitivity to hormones, and this can relieve the aggravation of allergies and sensitivity linked to the hormone changes that affect some women.

Human Skin

>SEX AND CONTRACEPTION

Insect Bites and Stings

Allergy to insect bites and stings, especially to bee and wasp stings, can be potentially very dangerous, because a reaction to an injected allergen can be violent and rapid, sometimes causing shock or fatal reactions.

If you know that you react severely to stings, you can carry an emergency kit containing a syringe of adrenalin, which can be used in case of sudden reaction. It may also be wise to wear a disc or locket giving details of your allergy (>EMERGENCY INFORMATION) for fuller details.

In other cases of milder reactions – say to mosquito or tick bites – the reaction manifests itself usually as an exaggerated local reaction at the site of the sting or bite – a red, raised bump and flare. You can use topical anti-histamine cream to relieve these (>MEDICAL HELP). Alternatively, if you are highly chemically sensitive and react to topical creams, wiping the site with Cream of Magnesia (unflavoured from Boots the Chemist) works very well. (>also FIRST AID AND HOME MEDICINE for other treatments.)

Desensitisation – a course of injections of dilute amounts of the allergen, which prevents the body reacting allergically – can be effective against insect bites and stings and may be your most useful protection if you are highly allergic. >MEDICAL HELP for more information.

Latex

Natural latex is a milky sap produced by certain trees when they are cut. Pure latex by itself rarely causes allergy; but when manufactured into rubber, it can do, usually because of other chemicals used to produce the material. (Synthetic rubbers are not made of latex, but of synthetic materials and they too can cause sensitivity.)

If you are sensitive to rubber made of latex, it is most likely that you are sensitive to chemicals used in its manufacture rather than to latex itself. Known troublemakers include accelerators such as thiuram; solvents, such as benzene or toluene; and phenol-formaldehyde resins.

You may commonly come into contact with rubber in protective gloves, in contraceptive devices, in soles and elastic on shoes, and if you handle rubber tyres. Some kinds of teats for babies' bottles and nipple shields are made of latex (>BABYCARE for advice on this and alternatives to latex).

Hypoallergenic (low-allergen) latex excludes chemicals particularly known to cause reactions and it can be used for protective gloves, condoms and heavy duty respirators. For advice on gloves, >HAND PROTECTION. For advice on condoms, >SEX AND CONTRACEPTION. For respirators, >FACE MASKS.

If you suspect that you are sensitive to latex or rubber, the best way to test is to buy a pair of pure latex gloves (available from Boots the Chemist). Air them for a few days, then place them in a glass jar, seal it and leave for a week, then open the jar and sniff gently to see if symptoms develop. *Take great care if you have a history of anaphylactic shock or life-threatening asthma attack. >also* EMERGENCY INFORMATION *for precautions to take before testing.*

An alternative but more expensive way to test latex is to buy a latex pillow (>BEDDING for sources) and sleep on it.

Leather

If you are sensitive to leather, this could be due to tanning agents used on the leather, such as tannic acid or formaldehyde, or chromates which are salts of chromium. For more information on chromates, which are widespread allergens, >**Metals** below.

Marble, Slate and Stone

Marble, slate and stone do not cause sensitivity, except in extremely rare cases of high level exposure to dusts when they are being cut. This is virtually unknown except for people who work with these materials.

Metals

Some metals are known specifically to cause allergy – nickel and chromates (salts of chromium). These are discussed below. Otherwise, metals are not generally known to cause allergy or sensitivity. Heavy metals (such as lead or cadmium), which can sometimes be absorbed from tapwater, can cause health problems. Aluminium, too, has been linked to some cases of illness. These forms of illness are not thought to be due to the same mechanism as chemical sensitivity (>CHEMICALS). One theory is that processing or detoxifying metals in the body uses enzymes or co-factors which are needed for other detoxifying or metabolising processes. This depresses the immune system's functioning, and can exacerbate chemical sensitivity or food intolerance which are sometimes linked to enzyme defects. Thus, absorbing metals may not itself cause a specific reaction, but it may affect the body's overall tolerance of allergens, foods and chemicals.

Some people with allergies and sensitivity find that their symptoms do improve by taking care to avoid absorbing metals. Specific measures which help include using filtered water (>WATER AND WATER FILTERS) and using ceramic cookware. In extreme cases, replacement of amalgam dental fillings (which contain mercury) with fillings of other material can help (>MEDICAL HELP).

If you react to metal radiators, heaters, furniture, lampshades or light fittings, it is more likely that you are sensitive to fumes from the paint or enamel used on the surface, than to the metal itself. (>BUILDING AND DECORATING MATERIALS and FURNITURE for avoidance.)

Cookers and grills can give off fumes when used but these are usually from chemicals applied to metal surfaces, or special linings, rather than from metal itself.

Nickel

Allergy to nickel is widespread and well documented. It is particularly associated with causing contact dermatitis – sometimes at sites remote from the spot where nickel has touched the skin. This can complicate diagnosis, but as nickel allergy is reliably detected by patch testing (>DETECTING YOUR ALLERGIES), it can be quickly identified as a cause of remote reactions.

It is hard to avoid nickel in daily life. It is found in metal coins, jewellery, wristwatches, spectacles, fastenings on garments, pins and metal buttons, metal handles, wire supports in bras and other support garments. It is also found in some medical uses such as the needles of hypodermic syringes, orthopaedic implants, some prostheses, heart valves, electrodes, and in some kinds of contraceptive intra-uterine device (coil).

Tapwater can also contain nickel, leaching from pipes and boilers. Filtering water (>WATER AND WATER FILTERS) will remove this. Stainless steel contains nickel, but it is only released when in contact with water or a liquid that is acid. Cooking acid foodstuffs, such as apples or rhubarb, in stainless steel utensils can cause nickel to be released. Some detergents, and sweat, also have the capacity to release nickel from stainless steel. For these reasons, although stainless steel is usually free of problems, it is probably best avoided for cooking utensils. Ceramic utensils are a good alternative. For avoidance of nickel in daily life, it is best to try and avoid wearing metal jewellery, watches, fastenings, buttons or anything else next to the skin, or even where sweat may carry it through a garment.

Some jewellery is labelled hypoallergenic (low-allergen) but other jewellery may contain nickel (for instance, some gold jewellery). Often jewellers will not know if a certain type of gold contains nickel or not. Wearing earrings particularly pre-disposes to nickel allergy and people sensitive to nickel should only wear stainless-steel earrings (which do not release their nickel) or more costly gold earrings free of nickel. Having the ears pierced only with stainless steel needles, and wearing stainless steel earrings for at least three weeks after piercing can help protect against nickel sensitivity developing, as can avoiding piercing ears in early childhood.

More detailed advice on living with nickel allergy is given in a book called *Contact Dermatitis* (>FURTHER READING).

Chromates

Chromates are compounds of the metal chromium. They can cause allergy through contact in industrial and occupational exposure, and in daily life where chromates are used in tanned leather, in various toiletries and cleaning products, as a mordant in fixing dye to some fabrics, and a number of other uses, including in some match heads.

Sensitivity to chromates can be detected by patch testing (>DETECTING YOUR ALLERGIES).

Chromates are a significant problem in allergic reactions resulting from exposure at work. One of the most common causes is cement in the construction industry (>BUILDING AND DECORATING MATERIALS). Other occupations that are vulnerable include printing, dyeing, photography, rust-proofing, enamelling, tanning, and handling wood treated with chromates. There may be no way to avoid these problems at work, although wearing face masks and gloves (>FACE MASKS and HAND PROTECTION) can help.

For advice on CLOTHING, TOILETRIES and CLEANING PRODUCTS, >relevant sections.

Mites

The most common mite which causes problems with allergy is the house dust mite. >HOUSE DUST MITES for full advice and information. Storage mites are relatives of the house dust mite and live in stores such as warehouses, granaries, farm stores and food stores. They usually feed on grain and flour, not on human debris, and are not commonly found in homes. They need a very damp and very warm environment. You are only likely to encounter problems with these if you work or go frequently into stores in which these mites thrive. They, rather than dusts from grain or flour, may be the cause of allergy if you work in this type of environment.

Semen

>SEX AND CONTRACEPTION

Vaccinations

>MEDICAL HELP and BABYCARE

Part 5

HOW DOES ALLERGY AFFECT MY LIFE?

WHAT CAN I DO TO HELP MYSELF?

Air Filters

You can buy a range of devices which will remove particles and filter the air that you breathe. These can be of real benefit if you choose one that is effective for the things to which you are sensitive (some devices remove some allergens or substances and not others). (>below for full details.) They are cheap to run, costing little more than a light bulb to operate.

Air filters and other devices will not solve your problems on their own, however. Even the best do not totally remove allergens from your environment; they can help reduce or remove airborne particles or vapours, but they cannot remove them from surfaces or furniture, or in intense exposures. They are not a substitute for carrying out other avoidance measures – they are best used *in combination* with avoidance measures, where they often add an extra percentage of improvement which can make a real difference.

They are also helpful when you have to spend time in environments where you cannot remove allergens or substances that upset you – such as at work or when staying away from home. Again, they can add an extra percentage of improvement which can make things tolerable.

What To Look For

Air cleaning or filtering devices can do five basic things:

- mask smells, through air freshener inserts
- produce negative ions (ionise) which causes dust and other particles to be attracted to surfaces in the room
- filter out particles in a fabric filter or web
- attract particles to an electrically charged surface
- filter out gaseous vapours through activated carbon

(For information on dehumidifiers, >MOULDS.)

The various devices available often have these functions in different combinations. The basic types are described in detail on pages 236–41. Information on makes, prices and models is also given.

(For information on car filters, >TRAVEL.)

How to Choose

If You Are Chemically Sensitive

If you are chemically sensitive, you will need a device with some form of activated carbon or High Efficiency Particulate Air (HEPA) filter, since ionisers, or fabric or electrostatic filters, will not make much impact on chemical vapours. You should avoid using any optional perfume or air freshener insert in a filter; these may upset you.

If you are extremely sensitive to chemicals, only the filter models with large areas of carbon or HEPA filters – for instance, the Biotech 500, Anatomia Filtaire 300 or 600s, Enviracaire and NSA 7100A – will make any real difference.

If you are very sensitive to plastics, you need to take care with choosing the casing and materials from which the filter is made. Always run and air the device for a few days before using in the same room as you. After a few days, it should give no problems.

Some people who are very highly sensitive to chemicals say that they react to the activated carbon used in the filters. This is extremely unlikely – it is more probable that this is due to sensitivity to tiny traces of contaminants in the water used to process the carbon, or to tiny traces of particles or chemicals already adhering to the filter. If you are exceptionally sensitive, take the precaution of using a machine on trial before purchase to see how you tolerate it. Ask the supplier to put in new, clean filters before the trial, so that you do not use contaminated filters. Ask for a machine that is well aired of plastic fumes.

If you find, after using a filter for a while, that you react to it, try changing, washing or vacuuming the filters to see if this helps. If you actually react to the filter while it is on in the same room, then do not use it close to you but try using it in a room before you plan to go into it – e.g. run it in your bedroom before sleeping, or overnight in a living room or the place where you work. Even this may help a bit.

If You Are Not Chemically Sensitive

If you are not sensitive to chemicals, you will not be concerned with the need for an activated carbon or HEPA filter, or with the materials from which the device is made. You can make a choice based more on cost and convenience. Ionisers are the cheapest option, but they have a decidedly mixed performance record and they do cause dirt to adhere to walls and ceilings. For sources of supply and more detail, see page 237. Borrow one or use one on trial before purchase.

If money is less of a constraint, the middle range of filter plus ioniser devices are effective for the job or removing allergens – for instance, the Trion Electrion, the NSA 1200A, the Medivac F400 and Mountain Breeze F400.

The top price range of activated carbon and HEPA filters are generally more powerful and have much finer fabric webs to trap smaller particles, so are more effective. They will do a better job – but you may not need to go to that expense and that degree of filtering unless you are exceptionally sensitive to particle allergens.

Other Criteria

For a large room, such as an office or workroom, only the largest filters have the capacity to change the air thoroughly – the Enviracaire, the Filtaire 600S and the NSA 7100A.

If portability is an important criterion, then the Trion Electrion, the NSA 1200A, the Medivac F400 and the Mountain Breeze F400 are light and very portable. Of the filters that are more effective at removing chemicals, the Biotech 500 is the most portable.

TIP

If you need a filter for medical reasons, you should not have to pay VAT. The supplier will give you a form to complete or ask you to sign a declaration. Ionisers are not exempt from VAT.

Running a Device

Whichever device you choose, it is important to change and clean filters or accessories as often as the manufacturer stipulates. This will keep the performance of your device high. It is best to keep windows and doors closed while a filter is running. Remember to ventilate and air regularly when the filter is off.

If you are exceptionally sensitive, you may notice particles or chemical traces on the filter media before the time that the manufacturer suggests for cleaning or change. If this happens, then change, wash or vacuum the filter as soon as you begin to notice anything.

If you have used a device in a particularly heavy atmosphere, or very intensively for a while, then change or clean the filter parts straightaway to remove the traces.

Even the strongest and most effective of the filters will not instantly remove fumes or chemical vapours when they arise. If someone smokes in a room when a filter is on, for instance, it will not prevent the smoke affecting you, but the filter should clear the fumes quickly and help prevent the residues clinging to surfaces.

TIP

Filters can also be very helpful after decorating or building works have been done, to clear chemical fumes more rapidly and thoroughly.

Most filters are designed to sit off the ground, and facing without obstruction into the space of the area they are meant to clear. They will not operate properly if the space around them is cluttered.

Some people find that the noise of a filter disturbs and irritates them. In this case, run the filter before you use a room to clear the air – leave it on at home whenever you are out, or in a bedroom during the day. Most devices are very economical on electricity and cost little to run. If the filter's noise does not bother you, then run the filter as much as you want. Carry it around with you, from room to room, to work, out of the home, as much as you can.

TIP

Cooker hoods – extraction devices fitted over cookers – usually contain a layer of activated carbon. If you have one, it can help to remove fumes in the kitchen.

Types of Air Clearing and Filtering Devices

There are three basic types of air clearing and filtering device:

- air purifiers
- ionisers
- air filters and cleaners

There are also built-in, and radiator systems, discussed below.

Air Purifiers

Air purifiers are on sale in many High Street shops. They are small electrical devices, relatively cheap (about £15 at 1992) and work by drawing the room air in, and passing it through a thin fabric filter and over a perfumed insert. They are sometimes called fragrancers or vapourisers. Their main function is to mask smells and they are not very effective at removing either particles or vapours. They are generally of little benefit to people with allergy or sensitivity, and the fragrances can upset the chemically sensitive.

Ionisers

Ionisers work by producing negative ions. Dust and other particles have a positive electrical charge and are often suspended in the air. The negative ions from an ioniser neutralise the positive charge and the particles from the air are attracted to the walls and floor. The air is thus cleared by particles being attracted to other surfaces, not by them being filtered or removed. Ionisers do not remove chemical fumes or vapours.

Studies carried out on the effectiveness of ionisers in reducing the level of airborne allergens have failed to produce any evidence that they actually help allergic respiratory problems. The National Asthma Campaign does not endorse them. However, people who use them often do feel that they bring benefit. In March 1992, a *Which?* survey of 130 people who wrote to the magazine about ionisers reported that slightly more of them 'thought that their ioniser helped them, compared with those who thought it had not'. *Which?* tests also found that ionisers can clear cigarette smoke much more quickly than allowing the smoke to disperse or settle naturally.

One major drawback of ionisers is that the dirt clings to walls behind furniture and around the edges of furniture and objects. The dirt is often greasy and difficult to clean, creating permanent dark marks for which the only solution is to redecorate – a serious disadvantage if you are chemically sensitive.

The simplest ionisers are relatively cheap (from £25 at 1992 prices), light and portable. They are usually of hard plastic cases which do not upset the chemically sensitive once aired. Ionisers are also often built into other filtering devices (see below).

The *Which?* survey (March 1992) found that a number of makes of ioniser did not actually produce ions on test. The Pifco 1072 (£25) performed best on their tests.

Ionisers are readily available from electrical shops and wholefood shops. They are also available by mail order from the Air Improvement Centre, Allerayde, The Healthy House, The London Ioniser Centre and Medivac (addresses on pages 241–2).

Air Filters and Cleaners

Air filters and cleaners are electrically powered devices that cost little more than a light bulb to run. They can be run 24 hours a day if needed. They work by drawing in the air through different kinds of filters, often used in combination.

Fabric filters remove particles by trapping them in fibres, webs or pleated filters. Large particles such as dusts, moulds, pollens and fibres are readily trapped by most fabric filters; smaller particles or molecules, such as chemicals, bacteria or viruses, require much finer webs or fabrics.

Electrostatic filters charge the entering air so that particles stick to a screen within the filter which has the opposite charge. The screens are made of metal or plastic.

If you are chemically sensitive, you will need to have activated carbon filters or HEPA filters in the device you select. Activated carbon filters absorb chemical vapours and gases from the air. The activated carbon is usually held in a fabric pouch or impregnated into a fabric web. HEPA (High Efficiency Particulate Air) filters are very high performance filters. Made of semi-porous, papery-like, fibrous material, the filter medium acts like blotting paper, absorbing very tiny particles of less than 0.1 micron in size, and will take out gases and vapours.

Which model to choose?

No independent test reports have been done for air filters and cleaners. The following assessment is based on the judgement of doctors and nurses, and the experience of a range of users with allergies and sensitivity.

If you are exceptionally sensitive to particles, such as dusts, moulds and pollens, or if you are very sensitive to chemicals, you should only consider higher efficiency machines (see right).

Smaller filters

If you are not sensitive to chemicals, nor very highly allergic, most of the smaller filters will be sufficient to take out a high level of particle allergens and will be fine for most people's needs. Some of the best small filters include the Trion Electrion, the NSA 1200A, the Medivac F400 and the Mountain Breeze F400. These all have a thin layer of activated carbon filter which takes out some chemical vapours, but they are not highly effective against chemicals. For filters which are, see below.

The Trion Electrion has an electrostatic filter, a thin carbon filter and a permanent ioniser (see above). It is small, unobtrusive and very portable. It is very quiet to run and has three speeds of operation. It has a marked effect on particles and dusts, according to people who have used it. Its price (at 1992) is quoted between £80 and £100. Its electrostatic filter can be washed; its carbon filters need replacing every six months, costing £7 each. It is available from Air Improvement Centre, Beta-Plus or direct from Trion (addresses below).

The NSA 1200A is larger than the Trion Electrion but still light, unobtrusive and portable. It has an electrostatic filter, a fabric filter and a thin layer of activated carbon. It has an optional fragrancer which you should not use if you are chemically sensitive. It makes as much noise as a quiet fan heater. You can buy a carrying bag for it which is useful if you wish to carry it around with you. It has good reports from users and samplers, but it is more expensive – about £150 at 1992 prices. (At this price, a more effective, but less portable, medium-size filter [see below] would be a better buy.) Filters (£20 each) need replacing every six months. The NSA is available from Beta-Plus or NSA distributors (addresses on pages 241–2).

The Mountain Breeze F400 and the Medivac F400 also receive good reports from those who use them. (These two are virtually identical machines.) They are generally viewed to be less effective than either the Trion or the NSA devices, but nonetheless make a difference to air quality and are worth considering. They are cheaper in price (about £70), with replacement filters (£6) renewable every six months. These devices have an ioniser built-in, an electrostatic filter, and a thin activated carbon filter. They have an optional fragrancer, and three speeds of operation. They are as small and unobtrusive as the Trion, but noisier in operation. They have a stronger smell of plastic when new, but this does wear off. These are available from Air Improvement Centre, Beta-Plus, Medivac or Mountain Breeze.

Larger filters

Of the higher efficiency filters, two medium-size ones receive very positive reports, the Biotech 500 and the Anatomia Filtaire 300.

The Biotech 500 is an oblong, desktop device – compact and light, more portable than the Anatomia Filtaire 300. It has an electrostatic filter, and a thicker carbon layer than the smaller devices. It has an optional ioniser, which is useful if you want the possibility but do not want one in operation the whole time. It is very quiet in operation, with no vibration, and its hard plastic case does not give off fumes. It is noticeably effective on particles and good on chemicals. It makes a very real difference to air quality. It is large enough to clean the air effectively in a large bedroom or living room. Prices are quoted at between £110 and £135 (1992), with replacement filters costing £8, renewable every six months. It is available from Air Improvement Centre or The Healthy House (addresses on pages 241–2).

The Anatomia Filtaire 300 is made of a plastic casing which does not give off fumes once aired well. It is circular, about 30 cm (12 inches) in diameter and 23 cm (9 inches) in height. It draws in the air through round, revolving thick fabric filters, and pushes it out into the room through a thick wad of activated carbon. It has two speeds of operation. It is extremely effective for its size and price, and receives consistently the best reports for removing both particles and chemicals. Some people find it very noisy and do not like to run it if they are in same room. The noise is probably more subdued than a fan heater, but louder in volume. This device is more bulky and heavier than the Biotech 500, or the smaller filters, but is still readily portable by car, or in a strong bag.

The fabric filters need vacuuming and washing once every two to three months, unless you are very sensitive, when you should wash them as often as you need. The fabric filters need replacing every nine to twelve months and cost £7. The carbon filter needs replacing every eighteen months to two years and costs £18.

The Anatomia Filtaire 300 is priced at between £155 and £165, available from Ascot Heath, The Healthy House and Patent Filtration (addresses on pages 241–2).

The most powerful versions of filters, probably better suited to office or workroom use, are the Filtaire 600S, the Enviracaire and the NSA 7100A.

The Filtaire 600S is identical in technical design to the Anatomia Filtaire 300, with fabric and carbon filters. It is larger in capacity and size, more effective and made with a metal casing. It is available at about £400 from Ascot Heath. Filters are of similar cost to the Anatomia and need replacing at similar intervals.

The Enviracaire is round and quite bulky to move. It has a HEPA filter, thick fabric and activated carbon filters. It produces very pure air, but also a draught at ground level, and can be noisy even on low operation. It is priced at £215 (at 1992). Carbon filters need replacing every three to six months at £11 each, and the HEPA filter needs renewing every four to five years at £70. Available from Allerayde (address on page 241).

The NSA 7100A is tall and looks like a piece of office equipment. It has a HEPA filter, plus carbon filters that are thinner than the Enviracaire. It can be manoeuvred easily, being light and on castors. The air it produces is very clean, but the unit itself is made up of a slightly aromatic plastic and can be troublesome to some people with chemical sensitivity. It costs £360 (at 1992). The carbon filters need replacing every six months at £20 each, and the HEPA filter every two years at £60. It is available from Beta-Plus or NSA distributors (addresses below).

TIP

All suppliers of devices should offer you a trial period in case a machine does not suit you, or you do not find it effective. Check that you can return a machine before you make a purchase.

Other Filter Systems

For an office building or work environment, you can build in air filters, either in air conditioning systems, or into individual rooms. Consult an architect or air conditioning engineer. Air Improvement Centre and Beta-Plus can also advise on systems for workplaces.

Icleen produce filters that fit or stand over heaters or radiators. They work by filtering out particles or fumes in the air rising up from the heaters. The filters are constructed of a fabric web in a metal frame. They only function when a heater is working, but they use no electricity, make no noise and are particularly effective against particles circulating in convection currents. The filter frames can be adapted to use for storage heaters, convectors, and desktop use, such as computers. They can be wall-mounted or free-standing, and are not conspicuous.

These filters are less effective than an air filter that recirculates room atmosphere constantly, and they may have limited effectiveness against chemicals. But their other advantages may outweigh these drawbacks, and reports have said that they do make some difference. Current prices quoted are £35 per metre fitted. Replacement fabric filters cost £10 per metre – renewable once or twice a year, dependent on use. Icleen's address is given below.

Addresses of Suppliers

Air Improvement Centre
23 Denbigh Street
London SW1V 2HF
Tel: 071–834 2834

Allerayde
147 Victoria Centre
Nottingham NG1 3QF
Tel: 0602 240983

Ascot Heath (Pennine) Ltd
Throstle Bank
West Bradford
Clitheroe
Lancashire BB7 4SZ
Tel: 0200 23611

Beta-Plus Limited
The Air Conditioning Centre
Haydons Road
London SW19 8TB
Tel: 081–543 1142

The Healthy House
Cold Harbour
Ruscombe
Stroud
Gloucestershire GL6 4DA
Tel: 0453 752216

Icleen
SBP Ltd
Nash House
204A High Street South
Dunstable
Bedfordshire LU6 3HS
Tel: 0582 660491

The London Ioniser Centre
65 Endell Street
Covent Garden
London WC2H 9AJ
Tel: 071–379 7323

Medivac
Taylormaid Products Ltd
Bollin House
Riverside Works
Manchester Road
Wilmslow
Cheshire SK9 1BJ
Tel: 0625 539401

Mountain Breeze
Peel House
Peel Road
Skelmersdale
Lincolnshire WN8 9PT
Tel: 0695 21155

NSA (UK) Ltd
NSA House
1 Reform Road
Maidenhead
Berkshire SL6 8BY
Tel: 0628 776055
(Contact for Distributors)

Patent Filtration Ltd
PO Box 426
Chipperfield
Kings Langley
Hertfordshire WD4 9PJ
Tel: 09232 60993

Trion Ltd
West Portway Industrial Estate
Andover
Hampshire SP10 3TY
Tel: 0264 364622

Babycare

This section deals with the care of babies with allergy and sensitivity up to the age of two to two-and-a-half years. The questions that preoccupy parents particularly are:

- How do I know if my baby is sensitive to something?
- How do I deal with food sensitivity and feeding problems?
- What can I do to prevent problems?

These questions are the main focus of this section.

What Causes Reactions?

Milk and foods are the most common causes of reactions in babies and very young children. Babies can also be sensitive to chemicals in everyday products used on them, their clothes, nappies and equipment; and to inhalants such as house dust mites, moulds, pollens, pets and other animals.

Advice on how to know whether your baby is reacting or not is given on page 246. Detailed advice on feeding starts on page 249. Advice on other allergies and sensitivity starts on page 270.

The Benefits of Prevention

There is much that a parent can do in the first two to three years of a child's life to help prevent allergic disease or sensitivity developing later in life, or to minimise its effects. Care taken in early childhood can improve your child's chance of not developing sensitivity, and help his or her resilience if they once become sensitised to something.

Statistically, a child with one or both parents with a history of sensitivity or allergy is much more likely to develop the tendency – called 'atopy' (>DEFINING ALLERGY). Babies can be born with allergies and intolerance; they can be sensitised already in the womb, particularly to foods. Preconceptual care and care in pregnancy can sometimes prevent or minimise this and are worth finding out about if you have the opportunity (>CHARITIES).

There are things you can do to your environment by way of preparation in advance of the birth; and precautions you can take with toiletries, nappies, clothes, soap powder or any equipment you use for the
baby which can minimise the load of substances that potentially cause
trouble. See page 270 for more advice.

There are also ways of feeding and weaning babies that give them
the best possible chance of *not* developing food sensitivity. It can be
hard work sometimes, but it is much less hard (and much less distressing) than the work involved in caring for a baby or child with severe
eczema, asthma, colic or other symptoms. If there is a history of food
sensitivity in either parent, or in an older brother or sister of the baby,
special care taken when feeding and weaning is valuable, especially in
the first two years of a baby's life when you have much more control,
and you can establish eating patterns for the future.

Breastfeeding your baby and late weaning are particularly
beneficial. Doctors now urge strongly that babies born into a family
with a history of allergy are fed nothing but breastmilk for as long as
possible, preferably for the first four to six months of a baby's life.
There is evidence that this protects against babies developing all
types of allergic diseases (not just to foods), especially if it is the
mother who has allergies or carries the genes. Breastfeeding cannot
guarantee that your child will not go on to develop allergies or sensitivity, but it, and late weaning, are important protective measures.

A baby's digestive system is immature. It is more permeable and
allows more molecules to leak into the bloodstream than an adult's
would, potentially to cause reactions. As the baby matures, so the gut
matures and becomes more able to cope with substances other than
that for which it is best designed – breastmilk. Colostrum, which the
baby takes from the breast in the first days before the milk comes in,
is particularly important in helping the baby's gut to function, so even
if you only manage to breastfeed a newborn baby for no more than a
few days, you will already have done something to help.

Even just one supplementary feed with infant formula can be
sufficient to make a baby sensitive, and, although it can be hard sometimes to sustain breastfeeding for as long as you wish, every extra day
that it can be managed will count. Keep up the milk supply as long as
you can, and avoid giving supplementary bottlefeeds if possible.

Breastfeeding is not always possible or easy – sometimes because of
the baby's or mother's indisposition, because the mother has to return
to a job, or for reasons of technique. Counselling and support can help,
and local branches of the National Childbirth Trust (NCT) have
trained counsellors all over the country. Contact the NCT for your
local counsellor:

National Childbirth Trust
Alexandra House
Oldham Terrace
Acton
London W3 6NH
Tel: 081–992 8637

The NCT can offer advice with all kinds of feeding, not just breast-feeding. If you have to wean early, or if the mother has to return to paid employment and needs to express and store breast milk, help from local counsellors can be invaluable. If the mother is on a restricted diet herself, and is concerned about her ability to breastfeed, there is advice on page 254.

A further argument in favour of breastfeeding is that breastmilk contains antibodies which protect the baby's system against bacteria and viruses, and especially against diarrhoea and gastric upsets. A bout of diarrhoea in a young baby often disturbs the balance of the gut lining and makes it more permeable, so that allergy or intolerance can develop more easily from molecules passing into the bloodstream. Breastfeeding, by reducing gut infections, helps the digestive system to protect itself against food sensitivity.

Although there are many arguments in favour of breastfeeding, it is not totally free of problems, in that molecules from foods eaten by the mother can pass in tiny quantities through breastmilk, and babies can react if they are sensitive to those foods. There are ways of dealing with this, explained later in this section.

Where to Start

If your baby is totally breastfed and appears to be sensitive to sub-stances in breastmilk, see page 250 for full advice.

If your baby is totally bottlefed and you suspect he or she is sensi-tive to the feed, see page 255 for full advice. If your baby is part-breastfed and part-bottlefed, see page 256.

If your baby has just started on solids, or you want advice on how to wean before you start, see page 257.

If your baby is older and established on a diet which you suspect of problems, see page 268.

If you have a food-sensitive baby and you need help and advice on how to cope with managing both child and diet, see also page 268.

If you suspect allergies to inhalants, or sensitivity to chemicals in substances other than foods, see pages 270 and 271 respectively. Go to page 270 for advice on preventative measures if the baby, or you, or other members of your family are chemically sensitive, and react to things you use for the baby.

If you want advice on medical treatments for babies, including the use of emollients and moisturisers for severe eczema, >MEDICAL HELP.

If you want to know how to tell whether your baby might be sensitive to foods or other substances, read on from here.

How Do I Know If My Baby Is Reacting?

If you suspect your baby is ill in any way, you should *always go to see a doctor to obtain a proper diagnosis*. You should always make sure that all other possible causes, as well as allergy and sensitivity, are considered. *Never jump to conclusions yourself.*

What Symptoms Might I See?

If your baby has been sensitive or allergic from birth, it may be very difficult to work out what are symptoms, and what are just features of the baby itself. Some allergic or sensitive babies are constantly snuffly, or restless; some cry constantly, are grizzly, irritable and have difficulty in sleeping. Some have colic, excessive wind and constipation. Some have rough skin, itchy eyes and dermatitis. Some have flushed, red faces and shiny skin. With a newborn, it can sometimes be impossible to tell whether he or she is reacting or not. Unless you feel strongly that something is wrong, or the baby has clear reactions to changes in routine, it may be unwise to draw any conclusions.

If you suspect a very tiny baby of reacting, the first thing to check is its milk, whether breast or bottle (>pages 250 and 255 below. You might also investigate whether he or she is sensitive to cleaning, sterilising and laundry agents, toiletries, or other chemicals you are using (>pages 250 and 271); or to inhalants such as house dust mites, moulds or pets (>page 270).

Many babies develop the first clear signs of allergy and sensitivity at between two and six months. It is not possible to say whether this is due to some particular vulnerability or immaturity of the body's immune, digestive and other systems, or whether this simply coincides with many babies' first exposures to foods other than milk, or to other allergens, or chemicals causing sensitivity.

Eczema is particularly common at this stage of a baby's life often flaring up for a while and then disappearing, either totally or to reappear later in life. Asthma can occur in very young children; some doctors argue that babies under one year cannot develop asthma because they are incapable of wheezing. Non-wheezing asthma can be observed, however – a hoarse, dry cough unrelated to a head cold or virus, which can become productive of phlegm. Gut symptoms of allergy and intolerance are also common. >SYMPTOMS for full descriptions.

As babies grow older, it is often easier to detect their symptoms as they develop more of their own character and temperament, and a particular routine and diet. It becomes simpler to spot changes and triggers, whether it is a change of diet, a new food, a new pet, a new childminder, a change of season, new bedding, moving house, vaccinations, or a viral or gastric infection.

Table 7 gives a list of symptoms that may be due to food sensitivity in babies and children. Symptoms due to other types of sensitivity (e.g. chemicals, inhalants) include breathing and nasal symptoms, eczema, urticaria and asthma. Digestive symptoms are most likely to be caused by food sensitivity. (Colic is discussed more thoroughly on pages 250 and 251.)

Many parents whose babies go on to develop more serious symptoms as children or adults often recall that their child was unhappy

Table 7: **Symptoms That May Be Due to Food Sensitivity in Children**

Digestive System	*Nervous System*
Vomiting	Headaches
Colic (in young babies)	Migraine
Persistent diarrhoea	Epileptic fits, accompanying migraine
Diarrhoea with blood or mucus in stools	Hyperactivity
Poor appetite and failure to grow (in babies)	*Other Symptoms*
Stomach aches (older children)	Aching joints
	Muscle aches
Nose, Ears, Lungs	Rheumatoid arthritis
Runny or congested nose	Some types of kidney disease
Glue ear	
Asthma	
Skin	
Eczema	
Hives (urticaria)	

(From *The Complete Guide to Food Allergy and Intolerance* by Dr Jonathan Brostoff and Linda Gamlin)

and restless as a young baby, with mild symptoms of the kind shown in Table 8. It is often difficult to distinguish low level symptoms from an occasional head cold or virus, or from the general crankiness that babies or toddlers often exhibit when they are tired, hungry, bored, or thwarted in their desires.

It is not normal, however, for a baby or very young child to have a constantly runny nose, persistent catarrh, and blocked ears, even if they do not appear unwell with it. Many very young children do pick up colds and viruses easily, particularly if they have siblings at school or go to nursery or crèche, but colds and viruses have a clear onset and tail off and go away. Glue ear, recurrent ear, nose, and throat infections and tonsillitis are not always caused directly by allergy or sensitivity, but they can be aggravated and sustained by them, and they often disappear if a troublesome food, allergen, or chemical is avoided.

Nor is it normal for any baby or toddler to cry a great deal, to be constantly cranky, unmanageable, hyperactive, irritable, insomniac or unable to concentrate (or even intermittently so for no apparent reason). Other indicators of reactions that parents report disappear with avoidance are excessive thirst, waking at night, constant urination, and shiners (big black rings) under the eyes. Persistent nappy rash is not always caused by allergy and intolerance but it can be linked and often clears up spontaneously when problem foods or chemicals are avoided.

It is important not to over-analyse your baby and not to see problems that simply are not there, but it is equally important not to ignore indicators of this kind. In some babies and toddlers, allergy and sensitivity are temporary phenomena. They disappear totally as the child matures and are no more trouble in future life. In other children, the problems can go underground, symptoms can shift in nature – eczema goes away, for instance, but some other symptom comes in its place and can lead to more widespread problems – unless the causes are identified and avoided.

Even if your child is not seriously ill, if you are concerned about low level symptoms in a potentially sensitive child, it is worth insisting on a referral to a paediatric specialist. You run the risk that you may be cast as an over-anxious parent, but paediatricians do take allergy and sensitivity in babies seriously, and will do all they can to help or reassure you.

TIP

Reactions to food often get worse, or only occur on days when a baby is teething. These can be temporary intolerances, so wait for a few days and see if any pattern linked to teething develops.

Protecting a child in the first two years of his or her life is one of the few areas of precautionary measures against allergy and sensitivity where taking extreme care has some merit. Provided you are not obsessive or paranoid about protecting your child, and you do not place excessive restrictions on your family's life, then it is a preventative investment worth making.

Detecting the Causes

Skin and laboratory tests for food and other allergies are not always practicable or helpful for babies and very young children. Nor will they identify food intolerance or chemical sensitivity (>DETECTING YOUR ALLERGIES).

For detecting the causes of reactions to milk (breast and bottle) and foods, see **Feeding Your Baby** (below).

If you see seasonal variations in your baby's symptoms, the causes may be seasonal allergens, such as pollens or moulds. >POLLENS and MOULDS for more help.

If your baby or toddler gets reactions only at night, these can be delayed reactions to allergens inhaled during the day, such as moulds, pollens, or pets and animals. Food reactions in very young children are very rarely delayed, but waking in the night, discomfort and restlessness are often due to food sensitivity continuing into the night. The most common causes, however, of night time reactions are house dust mites in bedding or soft toys (>HOUSE DUST MITES), fibres or chemicals in bedding (see below and BEDDING).

Symptoms can sometimes develop some months after a change in the baby's environment, so look back a few months and see whether there was a recent change, such as a new soap powder, new childminder, new pet or new bedding.

If there is no obvious potential cause of reactions, try investigating foods first, and then follow the avoidance measures below for chemicals and inhalants to see if they make a difference.

Feeding Your Baby

For All Babies Who Do Not Yet Take Solids

If your baby appears to react to milk (breast or bottle) and is not yet taking any solid foods, make absolutely sure that there is nothing else he or she is taking or absorbing that might be the cause. What else is your baby ingesting? Think of any juice, drinks, medicines, vitamin drops, toothpaste. What about any cream or oil that you use on your nipples if breastfeeding? Stop giving or using any of these, with doctor's advice, and see if things improve.

If the parents, other members of the family or visitors smoke in the house, then stop, and wash and air the home well. Colic, for instance, has been linked to exposure to tobacco smoke. If the baby goes to a childminder, nursery or crèche, where smoking is allowed, then take the child out of that environment for a while to see if things get better. Move the baby to another childcare place if necessary.

If you have any suspicion that the baby may be chemically sensitive, take care with chemicals used where the baby may take them in with the milk. Do not use chemical sterilising tablets for bottles – use a steam steriliser or boil all bottles and teats for 20 minutes. (Do this for bottles used for boiled water and for expressed breastmilk as well.) Try a teat made of different material – you can buy them made either of soft brown latex or of clear silicone. Some babies react to one type and not to another. Similarly with nipple shields, if you use them – try either latex or silicone, or do without them if you can.

Do not use creams, ointments or toiletries on your breasts or nipples if breastfeeding. Wash them just in water. If you get sore or cracked nipples, wiping them with a little expressed breast milk and leaving them to dry for some time in the open air is as effective as any other healing measure.

If the baby takes boiled water, try using filtered or bottled water (Evian, Buxton or Malvern for preference) as this can help. The chlorine and other chemical traces in tapwater can upset some babies. >WATER AND WATER FILTERS for full advice. Boil and prepare whatever water you use with the usual hygiene precautions.

If you are taking drugs while breastfeeding, check with your doctor whether you could discontinue these.

If you want to take further preventative measures against chemical sensitivity, and to investigate allergies other than to food, see pages 270–8.

If Your Baby Is Totally Breastfed

It is possible for tiny traces of foods to pass into the baby's system from the mother via breastmilk, and a sensitive baby can react to these. If this is the cause of the baby's sensitivity and you are able to leave the right things out of your diet, or reduce their level sufficiently, then the baby will stop reacting. It sounds simple but the problem is knowing where to start.

If you are the mother and have food sensitivities yourself, it is important to keep in mind that the baby is not necessarily sensitive to the same things as you are. Babies inherit the tendency to sensitivity, not the specific allergies or intolerances that you or your family may have. If you and the baby turn out to be sensitive to the same things, it may be no more than a coincidence. You have to investigate the baby independently of yourself.

Adjust the morning feed pattern

So where do you start? If the baby has evening colic, one of the most likely causes is thought to be a form of lactose intolerance whereby the baby is able to cope with small frequent feeds, but not the large first morning feed that most babies take. The volume of this can overwhelm the baby's supply of the enzyme lactase which breaks down the milk sugar lactose. The morning feed reaches the intestines by evening and causes the symptoms at that time.

There are a number of ways in which you can adjust the baby's feeding pattern to see if it helps evening colic. You can try waking the baby up early to give a very early morning feed, smaller than usual. Giving a little boiled water (see page 250 for advice) before the first feed also helps to quench the baby's thirst and appetite a little, and means he or she takes less milk at the first feed. If you have plenty of milk, giving the whole feed from just one breast seems to improve things, rather than swapping to the other breast after a set interval. Giving shorter, more frequent feeds and using just one breast, thereby reducing the milk supply, also seems to help.

Select a food to omit

If the baby does not have evening colic, or if the above measures do not work, then the next step is to select a food or drink to leave out of the mother's diet. The most common causes of babies' reactions to breastmilk are the foods that most frequently cause food allergy and intolerance, namely cow's milk (including cheese, butter and yogurt), wheat, eggs, yeast, corn, nuts, pulses, fish and citrus fruit.

How to choose?

If your baby has ever had a supplementary cow's milk formula bottle feed – even just one – then cow's milk would be a strong suspect. Corn is also often found in infant formula milk (cow's milk and soya formulas) so may be a candidate. If your baby was given a supplementary dextrose drink (usually corn-based) while in hospital, that is another reason to suspect corn.

If your baby has never had any supplementary feed or drink, then prime candidates for suspicion are foods that the mother ate in large amounts in pregnancy, perhaps binged on or craved particularly, or those which the breastfeeding mother is now eating in large amounts or craving particularly. ('Foods' here includes *any* substance or drink you ingest – including tea, coffee, alcohol, sweets, snacks, drinks, cakes, herbs, spices, oils, fats and chocolate.)

If there are still no obvious candidates, then keep a Foods Diary for a few days, writing down absolutely everything you consume and the time, and noting down the time and nature of any of the baby's symptoms, to see if there is any correlation. Some foods that the mother eats will break down rapidly, and be absorbed almost straightaway or within a couple of hours into the bloodstream and into the milk – fruit juices, drinks, many fruits and vegetables, often sugar. Other foods, such as grains or proteins, break down more slowly. Their molecules may not reach the mother's bloodstream for up to eight to twelve hours later, and may not affect the baby for a further few hours.

So if your baby reacts first thing in the morning, before the mother has eaten, and after his or her first feed, it may be due to foods eaten by the mother at lunch or supper the day before, slowly breaking down. If the baby reacts mid-morning, after the mother has had breakfast, it may perhaps be due to drinks such as juice, tea or coffee, or to milk or fruit going straight into the system.

Sometimes no clear pattern of timing emerges from a Foods Diary and, in that circumstance, you probably just have to pick one prime suspect (such as cow's milk, wheat, corn, eggs or orange juice) and reduce the amount you eat or leave it out of your diet totally to see. It is best to test out only one food at a time to be sure of your results.

Cut down on a chosen food

As a first step, it is sometimes sufficient simply to cut down on the amount of a particular food that you eat rather than to eliminate it totally from your diet. Try this first: reduce the amount you eat of your chosen food for two days. See if the baby improves at all.

(If you are reducing the amount of cow's milk you take, the first step is to stop taking cow's milk as a drink, in cooking, or in tea or coffee. Avoid using it in sauces, baked dishes or puddings. Continue taking a little, but not too much, in yogurt, butter or cheese, if you like, as these are sometimes tolerated better. Continue, if you want, to take any processed foods such as margarine or biscuits, which usually contain small traces of milk products.)

Leave a food out totally

If reducing the level of any food has little effect, you should go further and leave the chosen food totally out of your diet totally. If you do this for common foods, such as cow's milk, wheat, eggs, yeast, corn and soya, it can mean drastic changes to your diet and usually entails leaving out most processed and manufactured foods.

If you want to leave one of these totally out of your diet, there is full advice on how to do it in FOOD AND DRINK. There is also advice on what substitutes to use, on nutritional balance and precautions to take against new sensitivities developing in the baby.

Babies with a tendency to food sensitivity can become sensitive to foods that are introduced into a breastfeeding mother's diet as substitutes (e.g. to goat's milk or soya milk used as an alternative to cow's milk) and you need to take care not to binge on or overuse any foods you use as substitutes in case this happens. So, even if a mother is not food sensitive herself, she needs to observe the preventative guidelines given in FOOD AND DRINK on using substitutes.

TIP

If leaving out these foods seems hard at first, an easier route, and one that women sometimes try before they turn to total exclusion of cow's milk, etc., is to leave out some common culprits which are less fundamental parts of the diet, and see if baby improves. You could choose one of these food groups at a time and leave it out for two to four days to see what happens. Move on to another if you get no response.

Try leaving out *one* of the following groups at a time:

- Tea, coffee, cocoa and chocolate
- Alcohol
- All sweet and fizzy drinks, sugar, sweets, biscuits and bakery
- Orange, grapefruit, lemon and other citrus fruits and juice
- Onions, garlic, leeks, spring onions
- Spices (NB curry)
- Cabbage, broccoli, sprouts, cauliflower, kale, spring greens

---

Some babies are sensitive to chlorine and other chemicals from tapwater passing in breastmilk. The mother could try as an alternative using filtered or bottled water (Evian, Buxton or Malvern for preference). Use the chosen water for drinking, making hot drinks and soups, and for all cooking purposes. For more information on water, >WATER AND WATER FILTERS.

A breastfeeding mother needs to take care of her own diet. Consult your doctor about any intentions you have to leave out common foods, and about the need for any vitamin and mineral supplements.

It can sometimes take several days for the benefits of exclusion to be seen on a breastfeeding baby. So give each food (or group of foods) time to show results.

If you have severe problems

If your baby is very severely affected, or if you get no results from selective exclusion dieting by the mother, a doctor may recommend that the mother goes on to a full exclusion diet. This is rarely done during breastfeeding, because it can affect the mother's wellbeing and strength, and should only ever be done under close medical supervi sion.

If nothing helps your baby, and you and your doctor are still confident that breastmilk is at the root of the problems, it is probably better nonetheless for the baby to keep breastfeeding, and to delay weaning off the breast for as long as possible. A food-sensitive baby has a higher probability of having problems on infant formula feeds (even non-cow's milk-based) and on solids than on breastmilk.

If you have to give a supplementary bottle feed, or want to wean from breast on to a milk formula, it may be better to give a soya milk formula feed than a cow's milk-based formula to help prevent sensitivity. Soya is not totally free of problems, but it is less allergenic than cow's milk formula. Your doctor will be able to advise you on what best to do. (See also page 255 for information on bottle feeds.)

If you are breastfeeding on a restricted diet

It is perfectly possible for a mother on even a very restricted diet to produce and breastfeed a sturdy, healthy baby. Babies are very efficient and ruthless survival machines, and they take the nutrients that they need from the mother. The mother needs to make sure that she looks after herself, and eats as much and as well as she is able, in order to maintain her own nutritional status. Take a doctor's advice about the need for any supplements.

Make sure that you eat enough, even if you have a restricted choice of foods. Eating a little and often, especially in the early days when the baby feeds almost constantly, helps keep up your energy and blood sugar levels. If you are on a rotation diet, that should be no obstacle to breastfeeding, but you may find you have to juggle or shorten your rotation a bit, especially in the early days, to meet your hunger and feeding needs.

Make sure that you eat well in the early part of the day and at lunch

– the milk supply in the late afternoon and evening is often much more plentiful if you take plenty of protein, and large meals at breakfast and lunch. This may help you avoid the need for supplementary bottlefeeds. Drink a lot of water or other fluids; it can make a real difference to the milk supply.

If your baby develops sensitivity to your breastmilk and you have to start leaving out even more foods from an already restricted diet, make sure you take care of yourself properly. It is important to get your baby well, but it is also crucial to keep yourself well. Keep a balance between his or her needs and your own.

Contact your local branch of the National Childbirth Trust (national contact address on page 245) for any support or counselling you need with breastfeeding.

If Your Baby Is Totally Bottle-fed

If your baby is totally bottle-fed, make sure you have taken basic precautions against other things that the baby may be ingesting before you investigate its feed (see page 249).

If your baby is on a cow's milk formula feed, the first thing to try is giving smaller, more frequent feeds. This may help babies who are intolerant of lactose, the sugar found in milk, for the reasons explained on page 250 in connection with breastfeeding.

If this does not work, you can try alternative formula milks, with your doctor's advice. Soya-based milks (e.g. Wysoy, Nutrition Soya) are most people's first option; these are readily available in chemists' shops, and are sometimes a good solution for babies sensitive to cow's milk. Use a soya milk formula for at least a week to see if your baby settles – if he or she is clearly worse straightaway, see your doctor at once – but if the baby has been having colic, diarrhoea, or other gut disturbance, it can take a couple of weeks for these symptoms to clear.

Some babies also start to react to soya formulas, either straightaway or after some time. If this happens, there are other special formula milks that you can try. These are available on a doctor's prescription. One type is based on chicken, highly processed to make it digestible (e.g. Chix). Another type is called hydrolysed formula, and is based on cow's milk and corn, treated with digestive enzymes in order to break down and pre-digest allergens. Examples of these are Pregestimil and Nutramigin. These are sometimes tolerated by even highly allergic babies.

If you have a lot of problems with bottle-feeding, it is worth working your way through the alternative formulas, as one may suit where others do not. Each time you try a new one, give it a week to show effects if you can, unless the baby reacts strongly against it early on. *Consult your doctor as you try each one.*

A goat's milk formula milk for babies has recently been introduced in the UK. There is no current evidence that it is of benefit to babies sensitive to other milks. *Do not use it without consulting a doctor.*

Other so-called hypoallergenic brands of cow's milk formula are soon to be marketed in the UK. Hypoallergenic does not mean they are 'safe', only that cow's milk allergens have been modified to make them better tolerated. These may not be tolerated by extremely allergic babies and have been known in the United States to cause anaphylactic (shock) reactions. *Always consult your doctor* before using any of these to be sure it is advisable for your baby. Only use them on prescription and under supervision. Do not buy over the counter.

If you can find nothing that suits your baby, the only option, if your baby is very unwell, will be to breastfeed – either to relactate if you have already breastfed, or to start now. This can be difficult, especially after a few weeks, as hormone production changes, but it can be done. Doctors and the NCT (address on page 245) will give you support and advice.

If this does not work, and your baby is already a few months old, there may be no alternative to early weaning, of stopping bottle and milk feeds altogether. This is the least attractive of all options. An allergic or food-sensitive baby should be weaned as late as possible under any circumstance, and the mainstay of the diet of a very young baby of only a few months should still come from the nutrients in milk. *You will need specialised guidance on early weaning from a dietitian and doctor.* The advice on weaning below is designed for babies, preferably at six months old, still with some form of milk as a substantial component of their diet, not for very early weaning.

If Your Baby Is Part-Breastfed, Part-Bottlefed

See page 249 for advice on precautions to take before changing the nature of the baby's feed.

If your baby is part-breastfed and part-bottlefed, the preferred course of action is to stop the bottle feeds, and build up the breastmilk supply, so that the baby is once again totally breastfed. Local NCT breastfeeding counsellors (address on page 245) can advise you on how to do this. If the baby still has problems with breastmilk, see page 250 and follow the steps for identifying what foods in the mother's diet might be the cause.

If you are not able to build up the milk supply enough, or there are other practical obstacles (such as mother's job) to total breastfeeding, you should go to page 255, above, and follow through the steps advised for sorting out problems with bottle-feeding.

How to Wean

This advice is designed to be helpful to you if you are just starting to add solids to a baby's milk diet, or if you have already started a young baby on solids and are finding that the baby is reacting to the new foods. For early weaning of a severely ill baby intolerant of all kinds of milk, you need a doctor's advice (see page 256).

Wait As Long As You Can

Ideally you should aim to give no foods, drink or juices other than milk or water to a baby with a history (or a family history) of food sensitivity before the baby is six months old. Even very big, sturdy babies can be totally satisfied by a milk diet until they are that age, or even later. Delay weaning as long as you can. If you have problems keeping up breastmilk supply, ask local NCT counsellors for help (contact address on page 245).

Doctors, dietitians and health visitors sometimes give conflicting advice about the need for vitamin and iron supplements for babies. Not all doctors are convinced that supplements are necessary for a baby on a milk diet. Some doctors advise against giving anything by mouth to potentially sensitive babies, unless absolutely vital. *Consult your own doctor*. See also page 275 for advice on supplements well tolerated by babies with sensitivity.

Some babies do demand to be weaned earlier than six months, showing their need by unsatisfied hunger and more frequent feeding. If your baby clearly really needs food other than milk, and you cannot meet its needs with milk, then do start weaning earlier, but try to delay it as long as you can and do not start before four months if you can manage it.

How to Introduce a Food

Use the method outlined below to establish the baby on a solid diet which he or she tolerates when first weaning, and use it in future as the child grows up, *whenever you introduce anything new* that the baby or child has not eaten or swallowed before. Use it even for medicines, sweets, toothpastes or vitamins and minerals.

If your baby is already on a mixed solids and milk diet, and is reacting to the solids, you can start weaning from scratch using the same protocol. Stop the baby's existing solid foods and start from the beginning with single-food testing as outlined.

If your child is already a wilful toddler with an established diet and preferences, see page 268 for a way of testing foods that is less likely to result in tantrums and explosions.

When you introduce a food (or drink) to a baby for the first time, it helps to introduce it by itself, so that you can tell as clearly as possible how the baby tolerates it. The best way to do this (whether you are just starting a baby on solids for the first time, or whether you are trying to sort out a diet for a baby already on solids) is to give the chosen food by itself as one meal of the day and preferably as the only food of the day.

Testing foods

Give the chosen food as the first meal of the day after a milk feed. A 'food' in this context mean an individual food, given as food or drink, without any flavouring, salt, pepper, oil, fat, sweetening, sugar, sauce, gravy or anything else. Water can be used for cooking. So you cannot usually give processed baby foods (dry or in jars) or juice. You have to make your own foods. If you give potato, for example, you give nothing but plain potato, boiled, baked or mashed with water – without frying or roasting fat, butter, margarine or milk. A fruit given as a juice is also an individual food, so only give water to drink. For advice on how to serve some foods, see pages 265–6, below. >also FOOD AND DRINK for information on how to serve common foods as single foods.

If the baby shows no sign of any adverse reaction after the first meal, offer the food again at the next meal of the day, and again a third or fourth time if the baby shows interest. If your baby is hungry or seems to enjoy it, give as much as he or she wants, or as much as you think sensible.

If your baby is on an established diet and will not weather eating just one food for the rest of the day, then give him or her their usual food for the rest of the day, omitting any foods that you propose to test in the next three days, and omitting any processed baby foods (dry or in jars). In particular, leave out the most common allergens – cow's milk and products, wheat, eggs, yeast, nuts, pulses, citrus fruits.

Note down any changes that you observe in your baby during the day, the following night or next day. Babies are more likely than adults to react fast to a food and to show symptoms, signs of discomfort or being unsettled or unwell, within a few hours of eating or

TIP

If your baby has ever had a history of severe or anaphylactic (shock) reaction to anything, or if you want to be extra careful, try the Cheek Test before giving a food by mouth. Smear some juice or fat from the food on to the skin on the baby's cheek half-an-hour before a feed. If the baby has any symptoms, especially swollen lips, difficulty in breathing, or hives, do not give the food. Contact a doctor straightaway.

drinking a food, although they can be wakeful the night after; eczema, for instance, sometimes develops the next day or in the days after eating a problem food.

Vomiting, diarrhoea, sneezing, runny nose, eczema, asthma, colic or unexplained crying are clear signs of a reaction. *If your baby has any difficulty in breathing, always contact a doctor immediately.*

Some parents can identify a baby's reaction from less clearcut signs (such as bright red face, snuffly nose, big black rings under the eyes, red spots, irritability, sleeplessness, restlessness), which often precede or accompany more severe symptoms.

Take vomiting and diarrhoea seriously. Some people will tell you that it does not mean anything for a baby to throw up food or have diarrhoea when first weaning, or even as a toddler trying new foods. If he or she tolerates a food well, however, it should not cause any vomiting or diarrhoea, nor is it a good idea for a potentially food-sensitive baby to have gastric upset. *If you have any doubts about a food, leave it out of the diet until the baby is older* and try it again when the baby may have matured enough to be able to digest it properly. Do not tolerate so-called toddler diarrhoea.

Wait four days before retesting

If the baby shows no sign of reaction after the food tested on the first day, wait four days before retesting that specific food. On the fifth day, repeat the test process. A baby may not react to a food the first time around, but may have been sensitised by that first eating. So test the food systematically second time around as well. If the food then seems fine, include it on your list for the baby's permanent diet.

The reason why you wait four days to retest is that it gives your baby's system time to clear a food. Any symptoms which might be masked by eating every day then become clear when the baby eats the food again. In addition, eating a food at a fixed interval in this way (called 'rotation') can help control mild allergy and intolerance by

moderating the baby's system's exposure and controlling any overload. It helps to prevent sensitivity developing. (>FOOD AND DRINK if
you want to know more about the purpose and management of rotation diets.)

Test the next foods

On the second day of introducing foods, try a different food from the
first day, follow the same test and monitoring process, and wait for a
four-day period before testing that food again. Follow the procedure of
testing and waiting four days with four foods, one per day, consecu-
tively.

By Day Nine, unless your baby has reacted to any of the first four
foods, you should have identified four tolerated foods which can form
the core of the baby's diet. If this is the case, see page 261 for advice
on how to build up and expand your baby's diet.

If your baby reacts

If your baby has reacted to a food during the day of testing it, (first or
second time around), *do not repeat it.* Try and get through the day
without giving another new test food – it may not be easy to work out
which food the baby is reacting to, and will confuse the results.

If your baby is first weaning and reacts to a number of foods that
you try, keep trying different foods on a four-day rotation until you
find four foods that suit. Try not to give foods more frequently than
once every four days – a food-sensitive baby may start to react to
foods that he or she tolerated well if they are eaten too frequently. Ask
a doctor for advice as you go on, particularly if you start running out
of foods to try and you have a very hungry baby shouting for food.
Ask for specialist help if you need it – some health visitors and GPs
are very experienced and helpful with highly sensitive babies.

TIP

If your baby appears to start to react to foods for unexplained reasons, one of the causes may be cross-reaction between related
foods. If you have a very sensitive baby, read FOOD AND DRINK
and CROSS-REACTION before planning a weaning programme.

If your baby is on an established diet and is only testing single
foods at the first meal of the day, you may get confusing results if he
or she is reacting to foods in the normal diet, eaten during the rest of
the day. The only way to sort this out may be to go to a full rotation
diet. Consult a specialist doctor and >FOOD AND DRINK.

How to build up a diet

If you are weaning a baby on to solids for the first time, most babies will be happy at first on a very simple diet and you should feel no great pressure to expand their diet or increase the range of foods they eat. Once you have identified four foods that the baby tolerates well, follow the advice above on how to keep these on a four-day rotation – one food per day – as the core of the diet. Give these on a four-day rotation for a few times round to be sure that the baby is well, then introduce new foods singly as the first meal of the day using the protocol above. See page 262 for advice on which foods to introduce at what age.

You can then either give the new food for the rest of the day if the baby seems fine, or go back to the usual food for that day of the rotation. Repeat a second time round four days later to check a new food, then add new foods to the diet as suits. Build up and expand the diet slowly, month by month, following the timetable in Table 8.

Table 8: **Weaning Foods**

First Weaning Foods	Next Weaning Foods	Not Before Nine Months	Not Before Twelve Months
Potato	All fruits	Rice	Wheat
Carrot	(except citrus	Oats	Yeast
Sweet Potato	fruit)	Rye	Corn
Avocado	Other vegetables	Millet	Sugar
Parsnip	(except cabbage		Cow's milk (and
Swede	family)		products)
Turnip			Goat's milk
Aubergine			Sheep's milk
Banana			Meat
Buckwheat			Poultry
Sago			Eggs
Tapioca*			Beans, pulses
			peas
			Fish
			Nuts and seeds
			Citrus fruit
			Cabbage family
			Tapioca**

*For totally breastfed babies
**For part or totally bottlefed babies

Babies often tolerate foods better eaten singly – just on their own, rather than combined – so do not be in a hurry to combine foods. The longer you can keep your baby well, and not reacting to foods, the stronger and better his or her system will function.

Many babies will stay quite happily on a rotated diet, at least until they are well over 12 months and become more wilful. Provided they are getting plenty of a milk that they tolerate, and your doctor or dietitian is happy with their nutritional balance, keep to a rotation diet until the child really refuses it.

If the baby's diet seems eccentric, do not worry if he or she is happy and healthy and your doctor has no worries. Babies will happily eat things that they need and like, that adults would never consider eating. Babies on restricted diets have been seen to devour large bowls of sago, tapioca or buckwheat cooked just with water, and be totally satisfied and happy.

As the baby gets older

Once a baby gets to about 12 or 15 months old, he or she usually becomes less tolerant of the sort of weaning diet described above. Babies at this stage often want and need less of a milk diet, ask for foods with more variety and texture, and are keen to start feeding themselves. They become much more aware of what other people are eating. They develop memory, wants and wishes and become aware of the rotation if they are on a rotation diet.

How you deal with introducing foods now depends a great deal on the temperament of the child, your family situation, any childcare arrangements, and, importantly, on how sensitive the child actually is. If the child is extremely sensitive to foods and has very few foods that he or she tolerates, then you may have to continue with as strict a routine as you can manage. You may find, however, that a child who has been weaned carefully gets stronger as he or she matures and better able to cope with foods that previously were not tolerated. It is worth trying foods again on a 15-month old child that were not tolerated when first weaning, *unless the child has had a very severe reaction, and your doctor advises against it*. This may help you expand the diet. If the child is less severely affected, you may not need to keep to too strict a routine and can run a more flexible diet with less rigorous introduction of foods.

Which Foods to Introduce?

When your baby first starts weaning, he or she does not really need solids so much for specific nutrients, or vitamins and minerals, as for

TIP

If your baby goes to a childminder or childcare place, it is probably better not to get them to do food introduction for you, but do it yourself first meal of the day or on days when the baby is at home. They can help with monitoring symptoms if you give them guidance on what to look for.

If the child has meals at a childcare place or childminder, give them their own foods to take with them.

variety of taste, filling up the tummy, and a few extra calories. Vegetables, most fruit and some of the less allergenic grains meet these needs very well, as well as keeping the baby off the most highly allergenic foods.

It is best to leave certain foods out of the baby's diet totally for as long as possible – until the baby is at least 12 months old and preferably longer. If you can avoid the highly allergenic foods for as long as possible, you will give him or her an excellent start. Babies' resistance and tolerance of allergenic foods does increase – a baby's system matures and strengthens, and he or she is much less likely to become sensitive to a troublesome food the older he or she is when first introduced to the food. So avoid certain foods totally for as long as you are able.

Table 9 shows categories of foods in the order in which they are usually best tolerated for weaning. First weaning foods should be cooked or puréed with water, unless they can be eaten raw like avocado and banana. (Instructions for making purées of unusual grains are given on pages 266–7.) These foods have been chosen for first weaning because they are much less likely to cause sensitivity, and because they fill up the tummy and meet the baby's hunger. (Some very sensitive babies do react to these, so do not persist with them if your baby is sensitive – simply use them as the first ones to try. See page 264 for more advice.)

Tapioca is sometimes an ingredient in cow's milk formula feeds and your baby may be sensitive to this if he or she has ever had a cow's milk formula feed. Do not try this until your baby is over 12 months old if your baby has ever taken a cow's milk formula bottle feed.

After the filling fruit, vegetable and unusual grains, you can then try other fruit and vegetables, such as apples, pears, courgettes, tomato. After nine months, you can try the less allergenic grains – rice, oats, rye and millet. See page 267 for advice on drinks, snack foods and variety in this kind of weaning diet.

Save the highly allergenic foods – wheat, cow's milk, eggs, etc. – until babies are at least 12 months old and for as long as you can thereafter.

If your baby runs into problems on the suggested weaning programme, and starts reacting to the less troublesome foods, or else is very hungry, then you may be obliged to bring forward some of the more troublesome foods earlier than you would like. If you do this, then leave foods such as wheat, eggs, cow's milk, yeast and corn to the very end of those you try. Try lentils, soya, meat, poultry, fish and nuts before the others, and maybe sheep's milk, unless your doctor advises strongly against it.

TIP

Never overload a potentially food-sensitive baby with too many new foods at once, or too many allergenic foods. Keep to a varied, spaced out and simple diet. Babies' digestions can usually cope better with simple demands.

Most babies are extremely happy on this kind of weaning diet, having known no different, until they are 12–15 months old. You need not worry, provided they are still getting plenty of breastmilk or bottle formula milk, are generally well and healthy, are keeping to their projected height and growth charts, and your doctor has given you any vitamin and mineral supplements that are necessary.

TIP

Do not be tempted, if you have very few foods that baby tolerates, or if baby shows a particular liking for something, to allow the baby to eat lots of that food every day. This can pre-dispose a food-sensitive baby to develop allergy or intolerance of that food. Craving and addiction can also be a symptom of food sensitivity (>FOOD AND DRINK). Keep the diet spaced out and varied.

Some babies and toddlers develop sudden passions or aversions to particular foods and they can also develop temporary intolerances – due to viruses, gastric upsets or sometimes coinciding with teething. Allow for these temporary preferences and intolerances – foods and preferences will come and go in and out of a child's diet. Stay flexible and ready to try new things.

Appetite also can go up and down day by day. Temporary loss or surge of appetite is a normal feature in toddlers.

If you can keep up breastfeeding for 12 months or longer, then stick to it. If you have to wean from the breast from nine months onwards, you may be better to wean the baby on to a soya milk formula milk rather than a cow's milk formula (see pages 254 and 255).

If you wean from the breast after 12 months, you may still find that a soya milk formula suits your baby better. You do not have to give it in a bottle – you can give it in a cup or as an ordinary drink.

If your baby has been on a cow's milk formula without problems, continue giving this for as long as you wish – many young children tolerate an infant formula much better than they tolerate ordinary cow's milk.

When you first try cow's milk on a breastfed child who has never eaten it before, try heat-treated milks as follows. Either use a cow's milk infant formula, or bring cow's milk to the boil, simmer for five minutes, and then cool, or you can use diluted evaporated milk. Heat treatment modifies the proteins and can make cow's milk less likely to cause allergic reactions.

If your child is lactose intolerant, >FOOD AND DRINK for foods which he or she may better tolerate. >FOOD AND DRINK for advice and precautions to take with cow's milk substitutes, goat's milk, etc.

If your child is very severely sensitive to any form of cow's milk, goat's milk or soya, one other option is nut milks (>FOOD AND DRINK). Sheep's milk is less prone to cause reactions than cow's or goat's milk (>FOOD AND DRINK for more advice). Always get a doctor's and dietitian's advice if your child has a very restricted diet.

If your baby has multiple food sensitivities, he or she may be advised to go on a rotation diet. A full explanation of what this is can be found in FOOD AND DRINK.

Weaning Recipes and Diet

Here you will find instructions for cooking the following foods for weaning:

- Amaranth
- Buckwheat
- Millet
- Oats
- Rice

- Rye
- Sago
- Tapioca
- Vegetable and fruit juices

On page 267, advice is given on snack foods and fillers for babies on unusual or rotation diets. On page 268, there is information on sources of organic babyfoods.

If your baby is chemically sensitive, use filtered or bottled water (>WATER AND WATER FILTERS). For sources of unusual foods by mail order, >FOOD AND DRINK.

Amaranth

Serve puffed amaranth, mashed with a little water.

Buckwheat

40 g (1½ oz) buckwheat flakes
300 ml (½ pint) water

Stir the flakes into the water in a saucepan and bring to the boil. Simmer for 5 minutes, stirring occasionally.

To cook in a microwave, put the flakes and water in a large, covered bowl. Heat at full power for 1½ minutes. Stir, then heat at full power for a further 1½ minutes. Leave to stand for 10 minutes. Make sure that the mixture is cool enough before serving.

Millet

65 g (2½ oz) millet flakes
300 ml (½ pint) water

Mix the flakes into the water in a saucepan. Bring to the boil, stirring all the time, until the porridge thickens. Turn off the heat. Cover tightly and leave to stand in a warm place. Thin with water if necessary before serving.

To cook in a microwave, follow the instructions for Buckwheat (above).

Oats

40 g (1½ oz) porridge oats
300 ml (½ pint) water

Stir the oats into the water in a saucepan. Bring to the boil and boil for 1 minute, stirring.

To cook in a microwave, follow the instructions for Buckwheat (above).

Rice

Either cook ordinary rice (white, for preference) in water and liquidise with boiled water to a fine purée, or give ricecakes or plain rice puffs (Kallo brand available from wholefood shops). (Baby must be able to chew to take these.) Alternatively, cook 50 g (2 oz) rice flakes in 300 ml (½ pint) water, following the instructions given for Buckwheat (above).

Rye

Give Ryvita Original Crispbread if the baby can chew, or soak the crispbread in water, mash it a little and give it by spoon.

Sago

25 g (1 oz) pearl sago
300 ml (½ pint) water

Mix the sago and water in a saucepan. Bring slowly to the boil, stirring constantly, then cover and allow to simmer gently for 5–10 minutes, stirring frequently. The mixture will turn clear and soft when ready. Add more water if necessary.

Tapioca

20 g (¾ oz) pearl tapioca
300 ml (½ pint) water

Follow the instructions given for Sago.

Vegetable and fruit juices

You can make your own vegetable and fruit juices by simmering a 25–50 g (1–2 oz) piece of vegetable, or 50 g (2 oz) dried or fresh fruit in 600 ml (1 pint) water, then straining for a thin, flavoured drink, or liquidising for a thicker juice.

Fennel, carrot and parsnip can be popular drinks. Try also apricot, fig or prune fruit drinks.

Snack Foods and Fillers

One of the difficulties for a young baby or toddler on a restricted diet is finding foods which will meet hunger between meals and which are portable and attractive. Dried fruits are useful – chopped for very young babies. Try apricots, sultanas, dates and dried peaches. Green Farm Foodwatch sell dried fruit free of preservative and oils (>FOOD AND DRINK for address).

For more chewy, crunchy snacks for a teething youngster, try raw chopped vegetables, such as carrot or celery.

For biscuity snacks, try oatcakes, rye crispbread or ricecakes. Some wholefood brands of potato crisps (e.g. Bensons and Hedgehog) specify the oil used for cooking the crisps.

For titles of useful books, >FURTHER READING.

Organic Babyfoods

Organic babyfoods in jars are made by Babychain, available by mail order, or from Morrison's supermarkets; by Mother's Recipe range from Boots the Chemist; and by Johanus, from The Green Catalogue by mail order.

> Babychain
> Product Chain
> Ascot Management
> PO Box 433
> Reading
> Berkshire RG3 3DE
> Tel: 0734 56955

> The Green Catalogue
> Badgworth Barns
> Notting Hill Way
> Weare
> Axbridge
> Somerset BS26 2JU
> Tel: 0934 732469

If Your Baby Is Established On a Diet

If your baby is weaned, established on a diet and appears to have food sensitivity, you will find it helpful to read the section on FOOD AND DRINK. It will help you to understand the advice you will be given about sorting out what your child reacts to, and the advice on diet you may receive. In particular, you will need to understand the difference between food allergy and intolerance, the basic principles of exclusion dieting, precautionary measures against developing new sensitivities, and what substitutes you can use for common foods you may have to leave out of your child's diet.

As anyone who has tried it will tell you, sorting out food sensitivity is tricky enough, before you add to it the difficulty of dealing with a wilful and assertive one- to two-year-old. There is no easy way through it and it would be naive, even insulting, to claim that there is. Perhaps the best advice to share is to try not to place too high standards on yourself or your baby, accept that you probably will not be able to go about it the way you would really like, and learn to value any achievement you make, however small.

The real battles come over leaving out foods to which the toddler is accustomed, and over persuading them to eat alternatives. With leaving out foods, it makes it easier if the foods that the child wants to eat but cannot, are simply not around, and that other family members should not eat them either, at least in front of the child.

It sometimes works to go for a subtle, rather than a direct, approach, by simply substituting other foods without comment – such as corn flakes, porridge oats or a rice cereal for a wheat cereal, or goat's or sheep's yogurt or cheese for cow's milk versions; or offering rye crispbread or oatcakes rather than wheat biscuits or bread; or oat flapjacks instead of biscuits.

It can sometimes help if you try excluding or testing foods when something else is going on – a day out, a special picnic, or going away on holiday – so that a new and different food becomes part of the new experience.

Subtle strategies of this kind can work well but often do not pass muster with toddlers, who have an unerring instinct for a strange food that you are trying to foist on them. (They have an even keener instinct for rejecting costly foods, and ones that take a lot of finding and preparing!) Most parents arrive very quickly at the point of confrontation and rows (and frequently screams for a longed-for food).

If you decide it is important that you carry through the process of exclusion to prevent your young child eating a food, then you must start out as you mean to go on. It helps enormously to be firm, clear and consistent – not to bully nor plead. Explain as far as you can (and as far as the child can comprehend) the reasons why (to stop you getting spots, to help you breathe, to stop your tummy ache, etc). Do not manipulate – if you do so, the child invariably manipulates you in return.

Toddlers can rarely deal with the logic of future consequences for their present actions, and sophisticated concepts of moral responsibility. However, most toddlers have a sound grasp of pragmatic reality. If that reality is that you will not budge, and that they are not going to get that food, and that there is an alternative to eat which meets their hunger, then they will accommodate themselves to that reality even if they sulk and miss a meal or two. It may take a few days, even longer, of rows; and the rows will return for a while when they see the food they want; but if you stick to it, they will eventually come around.

Do not give in once you have started, as it will be even more difficult to restart. Do not over-compensate by pampering or offering treats – it sets up a dangerous precedent and irritates siblings. Just be matter-of-fact and firm.

If you have to compromise, and a child will not keep to a rotation diet or stay off a food, then do the best you can, keep his intake to a minimum and do not punish yourself, nor the child, nor other family members with your guilt and anxiety. Do the best you can in difficult circumstances.

As a child grows up, his or her capacity to understand increases greatly. It is quite surprising to hear a child of three or four say 'No milk – no spots' in a matter-of-fact way, when the same child kicked and screamed for milk only a short while before. That understanding is sown when the child is emerging from babyhood – set the right habits of thinking in toddlers, even if at the time you despair of their capacity for reason.

Allergy to Inhalants

Babies can be allergic from birth, or develop allergies later, to inhalants such as house dust mites, pollens, moulds, pets and other animals, or fibres, such as wool. If you want full information on any of these, go to the relevant sections of the *Guide* for detailed advice on full avoidance measures. Below you will find advice on precautionary measures to protect a potentially allergic baby.

Babies (and people generally) with allergies sometimes have a predisposition to develop further allergies. It can help to prevent this by taking general precautions to reduce the load of allergens on a young baby, particularly in the first two years of life. >MULTIPLE SENSITIVITY for fuller information on the value of avoidance.

Precautionary Measures

For bedding, using pure cotton blankets, which are washable at high temperatures, helps protect against house dust mites. Duvets are more difficult to dry and air, not usually washable at high temperatures, and are best avoided. Wool and feathers are more allergenic than cotton and best avoided.

Do not put a newborn baby on a sheepskin sleeping rug, to protect against allergy to wool. Allergy to cotton is rare but if your baby is allergic to cotton, >FIBRES and BEDDING for more information.

Wash all bedding regularly (including the mattress if using a synthetic one, see page 276), and keep it aired and dry to keep house dust mites and moulds under control. Turning back blankets to air and placing a hot water bottle in a cot a few hours before bedtime helps to keep bedding dry. Avoid cot bumpers which obstruct ventilation and can harbour dust mites. Keep all rooms well aired, dry and ventilate well. Damp and poor ventilation encourage house dust mites and moulds.

Avoid keeping any pets if you can until a child is at least two years old. If you do keep a pet, prevent it sleeping on the baby's cot, in the baby's room, or where the baby crawls or plays most of the time.

Use filters on a vacuum cleaner, and 'damp dust' (>VACUUM CLEANERS and HOUSE DUST MITES for instructions). This prevents virtually all allergens (house dust mites, pet allergens, pollens, moulds, fibres) being dispersed back around the room during the cleaning, and gradually clears allergens embedded in furnishings and flooring.

TIP

Dry out buggies or prams before folding or storing. This helps protect against invisible mould spores developing (>MOULDS).

Sensitivity to Chemicals

For a full explanation of what chemical sensitivity is, >CHEMICALS.

For precautions to take with bottle-feeding equipment, teats and nipple shields, smoking, creams and ointments used by breastfeeding mothers, water for drinking or bottled feeds, >pages 249 and 250 above. For emollients and moisturisers >MEDICAL HELP.

The avoidance measures for babycare that follow cover the following topics:

- Toiletries, ointments and home medicine
- Laundry agents
- Nappy changing
- Vitamins, medicines, vaccinations and toothpaste
- Clothing, fibres and fabrics
- Baby equipment and furniture
- Buying and using secondhand
- Toys, books and games

You do not need to carry out all of these avoidance measures. Select the ones which seem easiest or most helpful. Only if your baby is very sensitive, or if you or other members of the household are very sensitive to things you use for baby, do you need to take comprehensive measures.

Toiletries, Ointments and Home Medicines

Avoid using any toiletries, shampoos, soap, bubble bath, cream, ointments, medication, oil or anything else on a baby. Babies can be washed and kept perfectly clean in nothing but water. You rarely need shampoo nor soap until they become rumbustious, mudseeking toddlers – and then only when essential.

TIP

Do not use baby wipes. When going out, carry a damp cloth with you in a plastic bag or jar. >NAPPY CHANGING, below.

If you need a shampoo or soap, >PERSONAL HYGIENE for choices. Those given are entirely suitable for babies and children.

TIP

Babies can be sensitive to cosmetics, perfumes, aftershave or toiletries that you or other carers or family use. Stop using things if you think this might be the case. Check what a childminder or relatives who care for the child might be using. >COSMETICS, TOILETRIES AND SKINCARE and PERSONAL HYGIENE for advice on substitutes.

For sun protection, it is best to avoid using anything at all on extremely sensitive baby skin. Cover up with hats, long sleeves and thin leggings or socks in the sun. If you have to use anything, use a hypoallergenic brand (>COSMETICS, TOILETRIES AND SKINCARE) for names. For sunburn treatments, >FIRST AID AND HOME MEDICINE.

TIP

If your baby has eczema or extremely sensitive skin, playing in sand or saltwater can be very uncomfortable. Carry a hand water spray bottle with you and spray the skin gently to wash off sand easily from sore skin.

For scratch mitts and flat-seamed clothes suitable for babies with severe eczema, >CLOTHING for sources.

For nappy rash, >**Nappy changing**, below.

To treat cradle cap, olive oil is usually well tolerated. Massage it into the scalp; leave for two to three days, rubbing in more oil twice a day; and then shampoo and rinse thoroughly. Repeat after a week's interval, if required.

For cuts, bruises, sunburn and other mishaps, >FIRST AID AND HOME MEDICINE for full information.

TIP

Try to avoid exposing a chemically sensitive baby to traffic fumes. When you cross roads with the baby in a buggy, do not allow the baby to sit close to vehicle exhausts inhaling fumes. Cross at lights or pedestrian crossings. Choose a buggy with a higher level seat or use a pram. (>also TRAVEL.)

Laundry and Cleaning Agents

Use relatively trouble-free laundry agents for all baby items, nappies, clothes, bedding and towels. In CLEANING PRODUCTS, you will find the names of several products well tolerated by chemically sensitive people – all these are suitable for babies as well as for adults. Above all, do not use perfumed or biological agents.

TIP

If your baby is very sensitive to laundry agents and sleeps at childminder's, nursery or crèche, send your own sheets and blankets to use. Alternatively, send a pillowcase which can be laid over any surface on which the baby sleeps.

Use low-hazard cleaning products around the home (>CLEANING PRODUCTS), and do not use disinfectants, especially on surfaces from which babies eat, or air fresheners. Use plenty of hot water to deal with any baby messes, and ventilate to clear smells. (>**Nappy changing**, below, for information on disinfecting nappies.)

Nappy Changing

Some babies, and carers, are sensitive to disposable nappies. The simplest and cheapest alternative is to use cotton Terry towelling washable nappies, sold by Boots the Chemist and Mothercare among others. Do not use sterilising agents for soaking. For disinfecting and killing smells, you can use one tablespoonful of Domestic Borax (available from Boots the Chemist) per nappy bucket. Do not use one-way liners, or other nappy liners.

For waterproof nappy protection, plastic nappy pants give off fumes at first, but do not do so once washed a couple of times. Wash and air before use. Tie-on plastic pants, sold by Boots the Chemist, give off less fumes than pull-on pants.

Other options, especially if you are sensitive to plastic pants, are re-usable one-piece nappies which can be disinfected with Borax as above and washed. These have a 100 per cent cotton lining and some form of waterproof layer or cover – usually a synthetic fabric or fibre, but kept away from baby's skin. Boots the Chemist sell one brand called Bumkins. Other mail order suppliers of cotton re-usable nappies are:

Coochies
Baby Business Ltd
12 Park Hall Road
London N2 9PU
Tel: 081–442 0491

Earthwise Baby Nappies
Seedbed Centre
Vanguard Way
Shoeburyness
Essex SS3 9QX
Tel: 0702 589055

The Green Catalogue
Badgworth Barns
Notting Hill Way
Weare
Axbridge
Somerset BS26 2JU
Tel: 0934 732469

Kooshies
Clare Blight
Packer's Cottage
Albion Street
Exeter
Devon EX4 1AZ
Tel: 0392 219560

If you have to avoid all types of plastic or synthetic fibre, The Green Catalogue sell Dappers which are very thick 100 per cent cotton nappies which have no waterproofing layers – damp but pure! If you or your baby are allergic to cotton, they also sell 100 per cent wool re-usable nappies.

If you cannot face rinsing and laundering re-usable nappies yourself, contact The National Association of Nappy Services to give you the name of a local nappy hire service:

The National Association of Nappy Services
23 London Road
Loughton
Milton Keynes MK5 8AB
Tel: 0908 666968

If you or your baby are sensitive to sterilising agents or laundry agents, do not use laundered nappy services, or else take care. Check what agents your local nappy hire service uses on their nappies.

Do not use baby wipes on baby's bottom. Use damp cloths at home, or take a damp cloth or natural sponge with you in a toilet bag as part of the change-kit.

For nappy rash, the best treatment is to leave a naked bottom out in the air, and to change nappies very frequently. Nappy rash often clears spontaneously if food or chemical sensitivity is sorted out. If you really need a soothing cream on chapped, sore parts, Calendula homeopathic cream works well: use sparingly and infrequently as it is alcohol-based. Do not use it on broken skin or eczema.

Nappy change mats are usually made of plastic-covered synthetic foam. Avoid using these if you can, as they can give off strong fumes, especially when new. If you do use one, wash it well before use and air to remove fumes. See below for advice on using second-hand equipment. As an alternative to change mats, use a towel on a waterproof floor or surface. You could also use a towel over a waterproof plastic cot sheet, which gives off less fumes and is less troublesome than a change mat. Wash these a few times and air before using. These are useful to carry with you for changes outside the home.

Vitamins, Medicines, Toothpaste and Vaccinations

Take care with anything that a potentially sensitive baby ingests, absorbs or swallows. Only use medicines or vitamin supplements if your doctor considers them absolutely essential, and use low-allergen versions where possible. Medicines, such as anti-histamines, can be prescribed in low-sugar syrups without colourants.

Some vitamin supplements are tolerated well by some highly sensitive babies (e.g. Abidec, Seravit, calcium lactate or calcium gluconate) and a paediatrician will be able to give specialist advice. If you are giving homeopathic remedies, >COMPLEMENTARY THERAPY for advice.

If you use anything, introduce it like a food, using the protocol described on pages 257–62. Use only once every four days at first, unless your doctor advises otherwise.

TIP

Do not use gripe water. It contains alcohol and some babies react to it. Excessive wind can be due to food sensitivity (>FEEDING YOUR BABY, above).

Do not use toothpaste for a baby. Sodium bicarbonate used as a toothpowder is totally satisfactory (>PERSONAL HYGIENE). You can give fluoride in drop form in distilled water. Introduce as advised above.

TIP

Babies highly sensitive to plastics can react to plastic dummies. Avoid using these if you suspect them.

For vaccinations, some doctors advise delaying diphtheria, whooping cough, tetanus and polio immunisation until the baby is four months old, rather than three months old, to reduce any risk of adverse reaction. The sera prepared for these vaccines are extremely pure and very rarely cause adverse reaction. As an extra precaution, a nurse or doctor should take the baby's temperature immediately before to ensure that he or she has no fever or other illness.

The measles, mumps, rubella vaccine given at 12 months is based on the embryo of hens, and can sometimes cause problems to babies who are very highly sensitive to eggs. Take your doctor's advice before the vaccination is done.

Clothing, Fibres and Fabrics

Use synthetic fibres, materials and fabrics as little as you can near the baby (>CHEMICALS for full explanation). If you buy a synthetic or foam mattress, wash it well and air before use to disperse any fumes. Alternatively, get a pure cotton cot mattress (>BEDDING for sources). Avoid synthetic duvets: use pure cotton blankets for preference (>BEDDING). For sources of pure cotton baby clothes of all kinds, >CLOTHING.

If you or your baby are allergic to cotton, >BEDDING, CLOTHING and FIBRES for alternatives.

Baby Equipment and Furniture

If buying new, buy whatever you can of natural fabrics, materials and metal – cotton, wood and metal have many advantages. Avoid foam

TIP

Do not put a newborn baby into a newly decorated room.
Decorate and air the room well in advance of the birth, using rela-
tively trouble-free materials if possible (>BUILDING AND DECORAT-
ING MATERIALS).

padding on chairs, mats and mattresses if you are able, or air well and
wash before using. Avoid new chipboard veneered furniture if you
can. For full explanation, >FURNITURE and CHEMICALS.

If you have to buy things of synthetic materials, (such as a buggy or
pram), buy well in advance and let them air before use. If buying secondhand or using equipment passed on to you, >below for precautions
to take.

For waterproofing a cot, bed or pram, waterproofing sheets of plastic are well tolerated if washed several times before use, which disperses the fumes. Wash just in water or in a solution of sodium
bicarbonate or Borax – one tablespoonful per bowl or machine.

Most baby goods suppliers sell wood and metal cots and chairs. It is
also possible to find pure cotton baby carriers, and bouncing chairs.
Kiddycare sell a pure cotton babies' sleeping bag with a pure cotton
lining. Contact:

> Kiddycare
> Burgie Hall Cottage
> Forres N36 0QU
> Tel: 034 385 379

Kids In Comfort sell a 100 per cent cotton baby sling. Contact:

> Kids In Comfort
> 118 South West Avenue
> Bollington
> Macclesfield
> Cheshire SK10 5DS
> Tel: 0625 576386

Buying or Borrowing Secondhand

Buying or borrowing equipment or toys secondhand, or using passed-
on equipment, can often be a good solution for the chemically sensitive
since fumes from new synthetic materials have usually worn off well.
You need to take care, however, that anything you use has not been

washed or cleaned with cleaning or laundry agents that you or your baby do not tolerate. Ask what has been used on anything you are thinking of acquiring. Take extra care with baby clothes and nappies – in particular, avoid anything washed in biological agents. Wash and air anything you buy before using yourself.

If you or your baby are sensitive to pets, animals, house dust mites, or tobacco smoke, also check that anything you buy is free of the things that upset you.

Toys, Books and Games

Hard plastic toys are rarely a problem for the chemically sensitive once they have been washed and aired for a while. Buy, open up and air toys before giving to baby to play. Washing plastic toys in a solution of domestic Borax or sodium bicarbonate (one tablespoonful to a bowl of warm water) helps speed the process of airing.

Wooden toys sometimes give problems with fumes from paints and varnishes when new. Again, allow them to air when new, or wipe with a solution of Borax or sodium bicarbonate.

For full advice on preventing and controlling house dust mites in soft toys, >HOUSE DUST MITES. Buy washable soft toys wherever possible and wash and air frequently. If you or baby are very sensitive to synthetic materials, make or knit soft toys in cotton, and stuff with kapok. >FIBRES for a description of kapok. Kapok is stocked by branches of John Lewis and Woolworths. For other stockists, contact the manufacturers:

Abbey Quilting Ltd
Selinas Lane
Dagenham
Essex RM8 1ES
Tel: 081-592 2233

Air new books before use to remove fumes.
For more advice on toys and games, >CHILDCARE.

Bedding

Most of us spend a third or more of our lives in bed. For the greater part of that time, our noses and mouths are pressed hard against bed-clothes and mattress, inhaling substances that can cause reactions.

Sorting out your bed can reduce the load on your system and make you better able to tolerate substances when you meet them elsewhere during the rest of the day. It really is worth the effort to get it right.

This section deals with how to work out what is causing your reactions to bedding, including all your bedclothes, pillows and mattress. There is advice on the best choice of bedding, whatever you react to, and details of sources of supply. For information on beds, >FURNITURE.

The most common symptoms caused by your bedding are nasal, breathing, sinus and skin symptoms, but headaches, nausea, joint and muscle pain are also common. Do not exclude bedding as a cause of trouble because you have unconventional symptoms (>SYMPTOMS and DETECTING YOUR ALLERGIES).

Before You Start

If you feel worse when you lie down in bed, or on waking first thing in the morning, the most likely cause is house dust mites, rather than the material of your bedding. Doctors have estimated that 80 per cent of people with any sort of allergy, and up to 90 per cent of asthmatics, are sensitive to house dust mites. Before replacing any bedding or pro-ceeding any further in this section, >HOUSE DUST MITES and follow the advice there.

Your laundry agent or fabric conditioner may also be the cause (>CLEANING PRODUCTS).

Mould allergy is another frequent cause of reactions to bedding. Moulds grow invisibly even on slightly damp bedclothes and mat-tresses. You can control them by keeping beds warm and dry. >MOULDS for fuller details.

If a pet sleeps on your bed during the day, this may also cause you problems later when you use the bed. >PETS AND OTHER ANIMALS for further advice.

What to Choose?

Synthetic and latex materials are conventionally described as non-allergenic and are often recommended by doctors in the belief that they do not cause allergy and that house dust mites do not thrive in synthetic materials. This advice is misleading. Synthetic and latex are useful as an alternative to wool and feathers, which commonly cause allergy, but people who are chemically sensitive often react to synthetics and latex (including plastic mattress covers as well as the bedding itself). >CHEMICALS for a full explanation of chemical sensitivity.

Synthetics and latex also harbour dust mites. To thrive, mites need warmth, moisture and human skin, bacteria or moulds as food. Bedclothes, pillows and mattresses of synthetics and latex provide these just as natural materials do. Some synthetic bedding can be washed and this helps in controlling dust mite allergy in that the mite's faecal pellets (which are for most people the allergens) are washed out. But mites are not themselves killed by washing at the low temperatures necessary for virtually all synthetics. So they can survive the wash and continue producing faecal pellet allergens. Synthetic and latex bedding are therefore not an automatic choice for people with allergies and chemical sensitivity. They are a good choice if you are:

- allergic to wool, feathers, cotton or other natural fibres
- not chemically sensitive

TIP

Do not use a plastic or vinyl mattress cover even if you do not react to plastics. It prevents the mattress airing, keeps in damp and aggravates house dust mite problems. Use a small plastic sheet under the area that needs protection against bedwetting.

You can buy anti-dust mite bedding covers which are designed to prevent dust mites thriving and to stop allergens passing through. These are reported to be very effective. Using special covers on your existing bedding is a cheap and easy alternative to replacing all of it. Also available are anti-dust mite pillows and duvets in special synthetic materials that can be washed at 95°C (200°F). This will kill dust mites outright. (>pages 288–9 for stockists.)

If you are chemically sensitive, you are unlikely to be able to use any of these anti-dust mite products which are of pure synthetic or synthetic/cotton blend materials. Try using a mattress cover or under-sheet of pure cotton or pure wool which will help to protect you in part (but not totally) against dust mite allergens.

Pure cotton bedding is a good choice for most people with allergies and chemical sensitivity. It is less likely to cause allergy than other natural materials, especially wool and feathers. Moreover, pure cotton blankets can be washed at over 60°C (140°F), which will kill dust mites. Avoid pure cotton bedlinen labelled 'Easycare' or 'Crease Resistant' if you are chemically sensitive as these will be chemically treated.

If you are allergic to feathers, you can buy modified feather and down pillows and duvets which have been specially treated to remove the allergenic quality of the feathers. These have a lifetime moneyback guarantee, should you react to the feathers or the treatment at any time. (>also **Feathers** in MISCELLANEOUS ALLERGENS.)

If you need to replace your mattress, choose a pure natural fibre mattress if you are chemically sensitive. If you are not chemically sen-sitive, you have the option of a latex or synthetic mattress.

If you have multiple allergies, you could try more unusual and expensive materials, such as linen or silk, or unusual products such as wool pillows or wool or silk duvets. Go to page 284 for advice on how to cope, and what to try. If you want to know more about fibres, >FIBRES.

If you are chemically sensitive, see page 286 for more detailed advice. If you are allergic to cotton, see page 287.

If You Do Not Know Where to Start

If you do not know where to start, your simple course of action is to:

- Take precautions against house dust mites (>HOUSE DUST MITES)
- Use the Pillow Test (see page 110) to work out what fibres you react to before making any major changes
- Do not replace everything at once. Try out one piece (e.g. a pillow-case or pillow) of a new material to see how you go
- Use anti-dust mite bedding and covers if you tolerate synthetics
- Use pure cotton bedding unless you are allergic to cotton
- Test out bedding in small samples before making any major pur-chases

Allergy and chemical sensitivity are very idiosyncratic. What works for one member of your family or for a friend may not work for you.

So keep an open mind, stay flexible, take it one step at a time, and with luck you will not waste time and money. Use the Pillow Test (see page 110) to test out materials before deciding what to buy. Borrow bedding from relatives or friends to test them out before replacing yours. Buy one pillowcase, or one pillow rather than a whole set at once.

It is often enough just to replace the bedclothes that immediately surround your head, where you inhale. Some people find, for instance, that if they replace their pillow or pillowcase, or use an anti-mite pillow cover, it can be enough to stop problems. Another trick is to place a piece of fabric which you tolerate over the top of the sheet, duvet or blanket where you breathe in. If this works, you may not need to replace sheets or duvets. It is also a good way of testing out fibres fully before making a major purchase.

How to Investigate Your Bedding

If you really want to be sure of what you are doing with your bedding, and to avoid expensive mistakes, there is no alternative to a systematic approach. Diagram 10 is a step-by-step flow chart, guiding you through the questions you need to ask at each stage, and what your choices are.

The three crucial questions you will need to answer to find your cheapest and easiest options are:

- Am I allergic to house dust mites?
- Am I sensitive to chemicals?
- Am I allergic to cotton?

You can answer these either by doing the Pillow Test (see page 110) to test out synthetics, latex and cotton, or by going to the relevant sections of the *Guide* (>HOUSE DUST MITES, CHEMICALS and FIBRES).

A Shortcut

If you are daunted by such a systematic approach, a shortcut is to go straight to question three and to test pure cotton, either by doing the Pillow Test, or by using a few pure cotton items for a while.

Why pure cotton?

Pure cotton is not totally safe from allergy, nor is it an automatic choice for avoiding allergies, but it is often the best choice for a number of reasons. Pure cotton bedding is for most people the easiest and

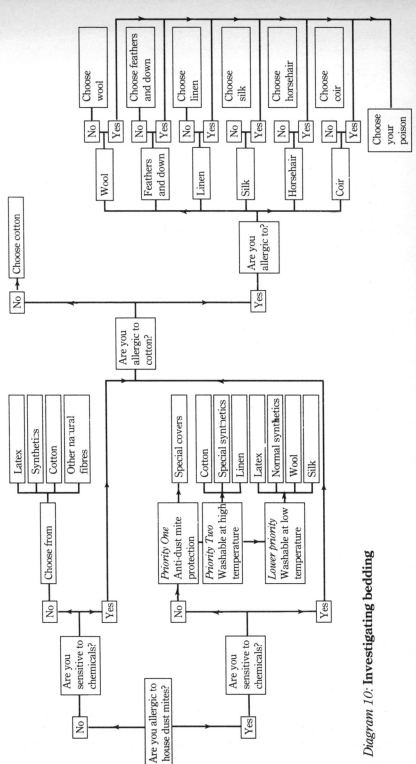

Diagram 10: **Investigating bedding**

cheapest alternative if they are chemically sensitive. It is a good option for avoiding house dust mites because cotton blankets can be washed at high temperatures. It is cheaper and more practical than wool, linen or silk. It is less likely to cause allergy than wool or feathers. Allergy to cotton is known, but is not common. Test it out before you make any major move and if you react to it, use alternatives.

If Life Gets Complicated

If you follow through the chart and find that you have multiple sensitivities and react to many things, you will have to find a way of choosing between materials that upset you, without spending a fortune trying expensive things. Read on from here on how to cope with multiple allergies and where to find unusual products.

TIP

Be careful to check the material of covers of pillows and duvets if you are buying new ones.

You can buy the fillings for duvets and refill an old one. This can be cheaper as a means of replacing old dust mite-full duvets, or of using a different material. Limericks sell these fillings (address below).

If you can only use pure cotton bedding, a sleeping bag liner in pure cotton can be useful to take with you if you go away on holiday, on visits or for work. The Healthy House sell these (address on page 292).

If You Have Multiple Allergies

If you have multiple allergies, you may already have discovered them through trial and error. If you have already tried a variety of different kinds of bedding, the best advice is *do not throw anything away – it may come in useful one day*.

Many people with multiple allergies find that they tolerate one material for a while, then start to react to it. If they leave it out and use something else for a time, they can often go back to the previous bedding and use it again – at least for a period. It is a way of managing multiple allergies – to give your system a break and not to overload.

So if you find yourself reacting to something that has been fine for a while, do not feel desperate and that the end has come. Just put it away for a bit and try again later. >MULTIPLE SENSITIVITY for more advice on dealing with multiple allergy.

If you suspect multiple allergy but don't know where to start, follow the step-by-step approach in Diagram 10 and the advice in **If You Do Not Know Where to Start** above (page 281).

What to Try

If you begin to feel desperate, having tried a range of the obvious and cheaper materials, you could try more unusual and expensive options.

Linen and silk can cause allergy, but allergy to these is less common, mainly because people rarely wear them. The less exposed you are, the less likely you are to react. Linen and silk bedlinen is extremely expensive and less practical to wash, but you can improvise by using a linen tea-towel or a silk scarf as a pillowcase, or as a cloth to cover blankets or duvet where you breathe in. If you can afford to buy new bedding, sources for linen and silk bedding are given below, including a source for silk-filled duvets. In FABRICS, you will find sources for linen, furnishing silks and silk wadding if you want to make your own quilts or covers.

If you tolerate wool, you can buy wool-filled pillows and wool duvets (sources below). You can also improvise by using a wool sweater or rug as a pillow, or folding it over your upper bedclothes to protect where you inhale.

You can sometimes find herb or hop pillows in gift shops. They usually have other fillings, such as kapok (>FIBRES) or cotton, as well as the herbs or hops. Some people tolerate these well.

Choose Your Poison

If you really cannot find anything you tolerate well, even the most expensive options, then you are left with the grim prospect of choosing your poison – being forced to choose the option that upsets you the least and using that one. It might be a combination of different materials – a pillow or pillowcase of one material, and sheets or duvet of another – or whatever suits you. You may eventually go back to something you originally discarded, such as polycotton, pure nylon or feathers – they may upset you but not as badly as other things. Alternatively, you could try rotating – use one set of bedding for a while, or for one week at a time – so that you never build up very severe reactions to one particular material. It can be hard work, so only do it if it is worth the effort for you.

If You Are Chemically Sensitive

If you are chemically sensitive generally, or if you know you are specifically sensitive to:

• Nylon
• Polycotton blends
• Latex
• Acrylics
• Other pure synthetics

you should avoid using synthetic, latex or synthetic blend bedding, mattresses and pillows.

You are unlikely to be able to use any of the anti-dust mite bedding covers and systems available which use synthetic or synthetic blend materials. Use instead a pure cotton or pure wool mattress cover or undersheet which will protect in part against dust mites.

Do not dry-clean bedding. Do not buy bedding which cannot be washed, unless you have multiple allergies and have no option.

You also need to take care when choosing bedding of natural fibres. Be sure to check:

• Covers
• Fabric treatments and finishes

With pillows and duvets, check that covers are not made of synthetic or synthetic blend fabrics. With sheets, duvets and pillowcases, avoid any labelled 'Easycare' or 'Crease Resistant' since these will have been treated with a chemical, usually a formaldehyde resin, which can cause reactions. You can buy unbleached and untreated pure cotton sheets; sources are given below.

Sources for Indian cotton bedspreads and candlewick bedspreads which are untreated are given below. If you wish to make your own bedcovers, >FABRICS for sources of untreated cotton fabrics.

To comply with fire regulations, pure cotton mattresses must be treated with fire retardant chemicals. Cotton wadding for mattress and futon fillings is invariably treated with boric acid. This can irritate if you handle the powder itself, but it does not give off fumes and does not cause sensitivity reactions. It is well tolerated by people with chemical sensitivity.

Pure cotton ticking, used for the mattress or futon cover, also has to be treated for fire retardancy. Water soluble phosphate salts are often used on mattress and futon covers and these do not cause sensitivity (although they can cause irritation to fabric production workers if handled excessively). Back coatings and other chemicals are sometimes also used, and these sometimes cause sensitivity. A variety of chemicals can be used – some are well tolerated and others are not: they are often specific to one fabric manufacturer, made to their own formula.

The mattresses supplied by the firms named below are all well tolerated by chemically sensitive people, and are as low-hazard as you can obtain within current fire regulations. Some of the futons made by the firms listed below use back-coated covering fabric, which is more likely to give problems. Check what fabric has been used before you buy a futon.

For more information on chemicals used in fire retardant treatments, >FABRICS.

TIP

If you are very highly chemically sensitive, you may be better off keeping an old mattress rather than running the risk (however remote) of reacting to a new one. If you do buy one, air it very well before use and do not throw away the old one for a few months, or even longer, before you are sure you tolerate the new one.

If You Are Allergic to Cotton

If you are allergic to cotton but not chemically sensitive, you have the choice of synthetics and latex as well as of other natural fibres. If you are chemically sensitive as well as allergic to cotton, you will have to look to other more expensive natural fibres, such as wool, linen and silk.

If you have to use cotton because of multiple allergies, avoid very flocky cottons, such as candlewick bedspreads or terry towelling, which irritate more. You may be better able to tolerate smooth woven cottons, or T-shirt fabric. Try using a T-shirt as a pillowcase or to cover the upper part of your bedding. Look for a cotton jersey mattress cover (sources overleaf).

Sources of Supply

Table 9 shows what type of bedding can be bought in which materials. The sources of supply which follow cover:

- Anti-dust mite and modified feather products
- Pure cotton bedding
- Wool, linen and silk bedding
- Synthetic and latex bedding and mattresses
- Cotton mattresses

Addresses of all suppliers are given on pages 291–2.

Table 9: **Bedding and Materials**

BEDDING

CAN BE MADE IN	Anti-dust Mite Bedding	Mattresses	Pillows	Duvets	Blankets	Mattress Covers	Sheets, Duvet Covers and Pillow cases
Synthetics	✔	✔	✔	✔	✔	✔	✔
Latex		✔	✔				
Horsehair		✔					
Coir		✔					
Feathers and Down			✔	✔			
Modified Feathers and Down			✔	✔			
Cotton		✔				✔	✔	✔
Polycotton	✔						✔
Wool		✔	✔	✔	✔	✔	
Linen						✔	
Silk				✔			✔

Anti-Dust Mite and Modified Feather Products

The following companies are suppliers of anti-dust mite bedding and covers: Allerayde, Derpi, Green Farm, The Healthy House, Medivac and Slumberland. See pages 291–2 for addresses.

The anti-dust mite covers allow ventilation of pillow and mattress, and evaporation of damp without allowing dust mite allergens to pass. They are made of pure synthetic, or synthetic and cotton blend materials. Medivac and Green Farm supply anti-dust mite pillows and duvets which are washable at home at high temperatures. All of these products are sold free of VAT to people who need them on medical grounds. Derpi offers a further discount to people who are members of allergy charities.

Fogarty manufacture Superfil feather and down pillows and duvets in which the filling is treated with a special coating which stops the escape of any fibres which might cause allergy. The outer wrappings are 100 per cent cotton. Fogarty offer a lifetime moneyback guarantee if you react to them. The products have been selling since the early 1980s and none has yet been returned. The prices are similar to ordinary feather and down pillows or duvets.

Pure Cotton Bedding

The following are suppliers of all kinds of pure cotton bedding, including untreated, unbleached sheets and pillowcases; blankets, bedspreads and mattress covers: Cologne & Cotton (sheets and pillowcases), Cotton On (blankets), Freemans (sheets, pillowcases and candlewick bedspreads), HL Linen Bazaars (sheets, pillowcases, unbleached undersheets, jersey mattress covers and blankets), The Healthy House (sheets, pillowcases, duvet covers, blankets and unbleached mattress covers), Keys (sheets, pillowcases, unbleached mattress covers and undersheets, and candlewick bedspreads), Limericks (most cotton bedding requirements, plus sheeting by the metre), Littlewoods (sheets, pillowcases, blankets, jersey mattress covers, fleece underblankets and candlewick bedspreads), Nice Irma's (Indian bedding and quilts). For cotton mattresses, see below.

Wool, Silk and Linen Bedding

The following are suppliers of wool, linen, and silk bedding: Green Farm (wool pillows, wool and silk duvets), HL Linen Bazaars (wool underblankets and blankets), Harrods (silk sheets and pillowcases), The Healthy House (wool underblankets), Keys (wool blankets, pillows and duvets), Limericks (wool underblankets, blankets and pillows; linen sheets and pillowcases), Orvis (wool pillows). Some of the prices are terrifying – be warned!

Synthetic and Latex Bedding

The following are suppliers of synthetic bedding, including latex and other pillows, duvets, and pure nylon sheets: Celic (duvets, blankets, bedspreads, quilts, nylon sheets and pillowcases, and mattress covers and underblankets), Foam for Comfort (latex mattresses and pillows; foam mattresses), Freemans (latex and synthetic pillows, mattress covers, underblankets and duvets), HL Linen Bazaars (latex and synthetic pillows, mattress covers, underblankets, duvets, blankets and bedspreads), Keys (latex and synthetic pillows, mattress covers, underblankets, duvets, blankets, bedspreads, quilts; nylon sheets and pillowcases), Limericks (latex and synthetic pillows, mattress covers, underblankets, duvets, blankets, bedspreads and quilts), Littlewoods (latex and synthetic pillows, mattress covers, underblankets, duvets, blankets and bedspreads). Polycotton bedlinen has not been included because it is so widely available and easy to find.

Pure Cotton Mattresses

The following firms supply mattresses with pure cotton fillings and covers, and pure cotton futons (Japanese sleeping mats): Burgess Bedding (mattresses), Futon Express, Futon Furnishings, The Healthy House (mattresses and cot mattresses), Hypnos (mattresses), Pennine Futons, York Bedding Company (mattresses and cot mattresses).

The filling of pure cotton mattresses is usually composed of cotton wadding with coir fibre, a natural fibre which rarely causes reactions. Pure cotton futons are filled with cotton wadding alone.

The Healthy House can supply pure cotton cot mattresses. The York Bedding Factory can make them to order.

If you are chemically sensitive, see page 286 for information on fire retardant treatments used on pure cotton mattresses and futons.

Addresses of Suppliers

These firms supply by mail order unless otherwise stated.

Allerayde
147 Victoria Centre
Nottingham NG1 3QF
Tel: 0602 240983

Burgess Bedding
Hope Mills
113 Pollard Street
Manchester M4 7JA
Tel: 061–273 5528

Celic Ltd
PO Box 7
Ashburnham Road
Bedford MK40 1DL
Tel: 0234 354811

Cologne & Cotton
74 Regent Street
Leamington Spa
Warwickshire CV32 4NS
Tel: 0926 332573

Cotton On
29 North Clifton Street
Lytham
Lancashire FY8 5HW
Tel: 0253 736611

Derpi Dustop
39 Spring Close
Portswood
Southampton SO2 1FZ
Tel: 0703 586709

Foam for Comfort
401 Otley Old Road
Cookridge
Leeds LS16 7DF
Tel: 0532 678281

Fogarty
Havenside
Boston
Lincolnshire PE21 0AH
Tel: 0205 361122

(Manufacturers; contact for
stockists)

Freemans plc
139 Clapham Road
London SW99 0HR
Tel: 071–735 7644

Futon Express
Woodman & Wolfe Ltd
23–27 Pancras Road
London NW1 2QB
Tel: 071–833 3945

Futon Furnishings
5 Lincoln Road
East Finchley
London N2 9DH
Tel: 081–444 7249

Green Farm
Burwash Common
East Sussex TN19 7LX
Tel: 0435 882482

HL Linen Bazaars
Churchbridge
Oldbury
Warley
West Midlands B69 2AS
Tel: 021–541 1918

Harrods
87 Brompton Road
Knightsbridge
London SW1X 7QL
Tel: 071–730 1234

The Healthy House
Cold Harbour
Ruscombe
Stroud GL6 4DH
Tel: 0453 752216

Hypnos
Station Road
Princes Risborough
Aylesbury
Bucks HP17 9DN
Tel: 08444 2233

(Manufacturers; contact for
stockists)

Keys of Clacton Ltd
132 Old Road
Clacton-On-Sea
Essex CO15 3AJ
Tel: 0255 424351

Limericks Linens
Hayle
Cornwall TR27 6BR
Tel: 0736 756054

Littlewoods Warehouses Ltd
Staley Avenue
Crosby
Liverpool X L70 2TT
Tel: 051–949 1111

Medivac
18A Water Lane
Wilmslow
Cheshire SK9 5AA
Tel: 0625 539401

Nice Irma's Mail Order
Ground Floor
Spring House
Spring Place
London NW5 3BH
Tel: 071–284 3836

The Orvis Co Inc
The Mill
Nether Wallop
Stockbridge
Hampshire SO20 8ES
Tel: 0264 781212

Pennine Futons
Cellars Clough Mill
Manchester Road
Marsden
Huddersfield
West Yorkshire HD7 6NA
Tel: 0484 846748

Slumberland Medicare Ltd
Bee Mill
Shaw Road
Royton
Oldham OL2 6EH
Tel: 061–628 5293

The York Bedding Company
Garden Place Factory
Hungate
York Y01 2NZ
Tel: 0904 626425

(Manufacturer; contact for
stockists)

Building and Decorating Materials

This section contains information about building and decorating materials to help you make choices about materials if you have to do building work, repairs or redecoration at home. Few people have any control over materials used at work or school, but if you do have any say, try to persuade people to use the methods and materials suggested here.

If you are looking for a solution to a specific problem, see pages 300–14 for an alphabetical list of suggested materials. For information on car maintenance, >TRAVEL. If you want some initial background on building and decorating materials, read on from here.

What Causes Problems?

The main causes of reactions to building and decorating materials are chemicals contained in them: these are specifically described in more detail below. The symptoms resulting are those of chemical sensitivity, such as breathing problems, skin symptoms, headaches, nausea, digestive problems, and mental symptoms. These and other symptoms are set out fully in SYMPTOMS.

Other causes of reactions to building materials can be chromates in cement, and brick dust if you have significant exposure to these (>MISCELLANEOUS ALLERGENS). Some people can be sensitive to wood, but this is exceptionally rare unless, again, you have heavy exposure (>PLANTS AND TREES).

Some materials used in building and repair work are irritant and need handling with care – using gloves, overalls or face masks to prevent contact or inhaling. These materials do not cause sensitivity but irritation to skin and airways for anyone who uses them intensively. Such irritant materials include glass fibre, dusts from steel wool and sandpaper, plaster and rubble dust, and sawdust and chippings. Toxic materials also need handling with care when applying them; unless these give off fumes or are solvent-based, they should not cause sensitivity after a period of airing.

If you are extremely sensitive to moulds, wallpaper can be the source of reactions. Moulds grow invisibly on paper, especially in damp conditions, and they can feed also on the cellulose pastes used to fix wallpaper. >MOULDS for more information.

Which Chemicals to Choose?

Many chemicals in building and decorating materials will cause sensitivity at the time when they are applied or for a short period of airing thereafter, but will not cause reactions, even to the very sensitive, once they are aired. It is important to bear this distinction in mind as you read the advice that follows.

If you are extremely sensitive, you may not be able actually to use the materials suggested below yourself, or you may need to avoid the room or building where they have been used for a while. If you are less sensitive, you will probably be able to use the materials yourself and a little airing will be sufficient for you to be able to use the place.

All the alternatives proposed are ones which are well tolerated in the long term, once aired, even by the extremely sensitive, and which, importantly, actually do the job required.

Avoid Known Hazardous Materials

Some chemicals are particularly associated with chemical sensitivity, and give out fumes and gas at a low level for a long time after they have been applied. Even small levels of such vapours can be enough to cause reactions. These persistent chemicals include organic solvents which have a wide range of building uses (notably in gloss paints, varnishes, stains, some paint strippers, various wood and damp treatments) and formaldehyde, found in particle board, melamine, paper, and some types of cavity wall insulation. Other persistent chemicals – such as organochlorines, used in fungicides and pesticides; plasticisers; vinyls; rot treatments; some coal-tar based chemicals, such as asphalt and creosote – also give out fumes over the life of the building.

All the materials suggested on pages 300–14 avoid these persistent chemicals wherever possible.

Choose Less Troublesome Alternatives

Some kinds of materials do not cause sensitivity, and are best used wherever possible. Ceramic tiles, glass, marble, stone, rock, gravel, sand, brick, plaster and plasterboard do not cause reactions. If you have a very heavy exposure to them, you may get irritation, and you may exceptionally become sensitive to the dusts, but not to the material once in place. If you work in the building trade, and have constant exposure, then sensitivity is known but it is still rare (see page 300).

Cements are made by heating limestone and clay, which are then ground with gypsum. Portland cement is the main cement used in construction. It is mixed with sand and gravel to form concrete, and with sand to form mortar. Cements are also used as adhesives. Cements, concrete and mortar do not cause sensitivity, but they can burn on contact and need to be handled carefully. Chrome salts from the earth's crust – chromates – contaminate cement accidentally during manufacture and these are known to cause allergy to building workers who handle cements extensively. >MISCELLANEOUS ALLERGENS for more detail.

Metals very rarely cause allergy and sensitivity when used as building materials. >MISCELLANEOUS ALLERGENS for more information.

Wood and cork rarely cause sensitivity. If you think you react to them, the cause is more likely to be varnishes or lacquers covering the surfaces than the material itself. See **Varnishes** (below) for more detail. >also PLANTS AND TREES if you want further information on wood and cork.

Water-based materials are generally much less troublesome than solvent-based ones. Many alternatives are now available and they are often equal or better in performance to solvent-based products. Product choices are given below.

Some *toxic materials* do not cause any problems if handled with care. Unless they give out fumes or are solvent-based, they will not cause sensitivity. For some building uses, toxic materials can be the only solution to decay, collapse or reconstruction. They are proposed below only where their use is essential.

Some *synthetic materials*, such as plastic pipes, window frames, covings or polystyrene tiles, will not cause sensitivity unless they are very new, or unless they get heated and then give off fumes. Virtually all chemically sensitive people can tolerate aired-off plastics used in these situations. >CHEMICALS for information on sensitivity to plastics.

Take Care With Natural Chemicals

Some building and decorating materials are now available which are based on natural chemicals, such as natural turpentine, rosin, vinegar, plant and vegetable oils, and linseed oil. Some of these are natural organic solvents and are known to cause sensitivity as their vapours are given off. (>PLANTS AND TREES for more information.) Some people tolerate these better than synthetic organic solvents, but other people react to them. Take care with natural chemicals until you are sure how you react to them.

Turpentine and rosin cross-react with a number of chemicals (>CROSS-REACTION) and should be treated with care. Linseed oil evaporates fast and is generally trouble free.

Sources of natural chemical-based materials are given below.

How to Detect Sensitivity to Building Materials

It is difficult to detect whether you are sensitive to building materials already used or applied in your home or other environments. Changes in your symptoms when you go into different places, or if you stay away from home, can be indicative, but not always conclusive, evidence of sensitivity to materials.

You can be tested by patch testing or sublingual tests for allergy or sensitivity to specific chemicals (>DETECTING YOUR ALLERGIES). There are also two environmentally controlled units in the UK, which are as chemical free as possible, where rigorous testing for chemical sensitivity can be done. >MEDICAL HELP for details.

You can use the Tile Test (opposite) to test specific materials to see if these induce symptoms, but the only reliable way of finding out in your own environment whether materials around you upset you is to remove and replace potential hazards. However, for most people this is impracticable, as well as costly and disruptive. At work or school, it is invariably impossible. Unless you are absolutely confident that materials are the key source of trouble for you, it is wiser first to reduce chemicals from other sources around you – cleaning materials, toiletries, personal hygiene products, clothing, furniture, bedding, flooring before you make significant changes to your decoration or building.

If, thereafter, you determine that you need to change the materials,

The Tile Test

This is a way of testing materials to see whether they cause you to react once they are well aired. You can use it also to help you choose between products to see which suit you best.

You only need a small amount of product to test, so if you can borrow some from a friend, persuade a supplier or shop to give you some to test, or get a sample from the manufacturer, it will be sufficient. Even if you cannot get a sample to test and have to buy a full-size product, it is worth doing the Tile Test before you use a material extensively, in case it does upset you badly. It may waste money but it might mean less pain long-term.

To do the test, take a spare or old shiny ceramic tile. (You can also use an old saucer, glass or cup if you want.) Scrub it clear of any dirt or grease, and wash, rinse and dry thoroughly. Dab or paint a 2.5 cm (1 inch) square of the material you want to test on the surface of the tile and allow to dry. Mark alongside it with a code letter or number, and keep a record of what it is. Leave the tile with its sample to air for one week.

After a week, lift the tile to your nose and sniff gently (just in case of strong reaction). See if any symptoms develop. Monitor symptoms for 10 minutes. If you have no symptoms, then the sample is likely to be acceptable in practice.

If you have symptoms, leave the tile to air for a second week and repeat the test. If you have no symptoms this time round, the product is likely to be acceptable to use. If you have symptoms, again, wait for a further week and try again. Keep repeating the test, up to six weeks if necessary, until you no longer get symptoms.

If you continually have severe symptoms, then avoid the product. If your symptoms keep reducing, then it is worth trying unless you can test and find a better alternative.

Take great care when doing the test if you have a history of life-threatening asthma attack or of anaphylactic shock. >*EMERGENCY INFORMATION for precautions to take before testing.*

Do Not Overload When Testing

If you are testing a number of products to find which suits you better, you will get better results if you test them on separate tiles (or pieces of tile). Do not test more than three products per day and leave an interval of at least half an hour between tests. Grade on a scale of one to five the severity of your reactions to each.

Test Blind If Possible

It can also help if you do the tests with the help of another person who sets up the tiles for you and keeps the code of the products a secret from you, so that you have no idea what you are testing. This is called single-blind testing.

---

or if you are obliged to redecorate or do repair work, use low-hazard materials as suggested below and see, after a period of airing, whether your symptoms improve.

How to Avoid Trouble

Here are some guidelines on how to avoid trouble when using building and decorating materials, or if having work done. If you work in the building trade, see page 300 for specific advice.

Avoiding Trouble at Home

Even if you have decided that you need eventually to replace the materials around you in your home, *go gently* if you remove or replace them. Unless you are in the unusual position of being able to move out while work is done, and stay out until the place is aired, then do one room or one major task at a time. Give it time to air and give your system time to cope without overload.

If you are a tenant, negotiate with your landlord over what he or she can do for you. You may have to pay yourself for the work you need. If you cannot afford to do a lot of work, then do one room, preferably the bedroom, or your 'oasis' (>CHEMICALS), and do it thoroughly, rather than do everything partially.

Allow rooms to air for as long as you possibly can, even up to a few weeks, before using them again. Decorate or do work before going on a visit or on holiday, for instance, and air well on return, or ask a neighbour to open windows and air the home while you are away.

Do not decorate or do work in a new baby's room close to the delivery date; decorate it months before if you can, and if your superstition permits. New babies are more vulnerable than adults to chemical load.

Redecorate infrequently to keep the load, and the inconvenience, down. Get someone else to redecorate or do work for you if you possibly can. If you cannot afford to pay for work to be done, then look for friends who are keen on DIY, and offer to do something for them in return – other household jobs, or car-washing or window cleaning, for instance. Ask your voluntary services or charities if there are groups, such as scouts' groups, who could help you out.

If you do work yourself, protect your skin and airways with overalls, gloves and face masks (>HAND PROTECTION and FACE MASKS). Sander and Kay sell pure cotton work overalls by post (address below). Ventilate thoroughly while working and take frequent breaks. Wash hair and bathe or shower immediately after doing work.

Use low-hazard materials as far as possible. Details are given below. Use solvent-free materials wherever possible. Avoid using wallpaper or lining paper, especially if you are allergic to moulds. Avoid using particle board (see below) if you are able to.

If you are starting from scratch, or replacing old structures or materials, use materials which are inert, such as ceramic tiles, cork, cement, glass, marble, stone, most woods, or materials which do not need repainting, such as metal or varnished wood. Doors, window frames, skirtings, wall panels and cupboard doors can be made from unpainted wood, sealed with a clear varnish which needs redoing very seldom. >PLANTS AND TREES for choice of wood, and see **Varnishes** (below). Ceramic tiles can be used for floors, work surfaces, even walls. Kitchen work surfaces can also be made from sealed wood, stainless steel or tiles.

Do not paint or repaint radiators. They give off stronger fumes when hot and can be persistent sources of chemical vapours. If already painted, do not redecorate. Leave them be, even if shabby. If you have to repaint them, use a water-based metal paint (see **Paints** below).

If you have persistent damp problems, these can aggravate allergy to moulds and to house dust mites. It is important to get them sorted out and treated; there are ways of doing this which are relatively trouble free (see page 302).

If you have cavity wall insulation of the urea-formaldehyde foam type, this is a potent source of formaldehyde vapours, especially when new. There is no practicable or economic way to remove this, and if this affects you badly, you may have to move house. If extensive woodworm or rot treatments have been carried out in the building, persistent chemicals remain and there may also be no alternative to moving if you are badly affected.

If you are planning to move flat or house, check what chemical treatments, if any, have been done to the place. Beware of urea-formaldehyde cavity wall insulation; see whether fitted furniture and other places where particle board has been used are newly installed. Ask what type of damp-proof course is in place. Check what type of

TIP

Registered disabled people can apply to their local authority for grants for alterations to their home, under the Local Government Housing Act. These can be awarded to people with allergies needing work done if you are registered disabled. >FINANCIAL HELP for more advice.

lagging is round the central heating pipes. Use the information in the alphabetical list of materials below to help you know what to look for.

Avoiding Trouble Away From Home

There is often very little you can do at work, at school, at friends' houses or social gatherings, or in public buildings to avoid materials that upset you. Above all, try to avoid places when building or decorating work is actually being done. Ask for notice to be given if work is to be done at work or school, so that you can arrange to be off for a few days.

If you work in the building trade and are sensitive to the materials you use, then your life will be very hard. You may have no say at all in the choice of materials you use. The Health and Safety Executive is increasingly active in the field of hazards from building materials and can provide specific guidelines on basic precautions to take when using them. These will not always prevent low-level exposure sufficient to cause sensitivity, but may be important information for you to bring to the attention of an employer or contractor, if you are concerned that adequate care is not being taken. Consult the telephone directory to find your local branch of the Executive.

Alternatively, the building union UCATT produces health and safety information and recommendations for handling and working with hazardous materials. Contact UCATT at the address below.

What to Use

The following topics are covered below:

- Adhesives and Pastes
- Chipboard
- Damp-proofing Treatments
- Fillers
- Floor sealants
- Grout
- Hardboard
- Insulation

- Mould Treatments
- Paints
- Paint strippers
- Particle and Other Boards
- Paving
- Plywood
- Putty
- Rot treatments
- Stabilisers and Sealants

- Varnishes
- Varnish Remover
- Veneer and Sheets
- Wallpaper
- Wiring
- Wood
- Wood Preservatives
- Wood Stains
- Woodworm Treatments

The materials suggested below, once aired off, are the best choices available for the chemically sensitive. *Always use with care.* Use the Tile Test (see page 297) before using extensively if you want to be extra cautious. Ask manufacturers to send you Technical Data Sheets to be absolutely sure of product contents. These are usually clear and easy to understand for the non-expert.

Most of the materials proposed are for internal use since these are where most problems arise. External materials are constantly aired and only certain situations (e.g. paints, roofing, wood treatments and paving) really need care. These are included where useful.

Adhesives and Pastes

Many adhesives and pastes are based on organic solvents such as toluene and other hydrocarbons. These give off persistent vapours and are best avoided. Many also contain fungicides or mould inhibitors which can cause reactions.

For use on tiles, cement-based adhesives without fungicide are a good choice. One product name is Evostik Cemfix, available in shops.

For wood and paper, and for use on other materials, such as cork and fabrics, PVA (polyvinyl acetate) without fungicide is relatively trouble-free. Brands of this include Polycell Super Bond, Evobond Building Adhesive, and PRITT Child's Play. Copydex is a PVA adhesive which is latex-based; avoid it if you are sensitive to latex.

Epoxy resin adhesives (such as Araldite) work by a chemical reaction caused by mixing two compounds. Fumes are given off at the moment of mixing, but not over the life of the bond, and they are generally well tolerated.

For wallpaper and other papers, cellulose pastes made up with water are well tolerated. Look for one without chemical fungicides: Polycell Classic Interiors is one such brand. The Healthy House and Livos supply cellulose paste without fungicide by post (addresses on pages 315–6).

TIP

Using products without fungicides will not cause you undue problems if you are allergic to moulds as well as chemically sensitive. Fungicides are of limited effectiveness, especially in damp conditions. >MOULDS for more advice on deterring and killing moulds.

Chipboard

See **Particle and Other Boards**, below.

Damp-proofing Treatments

Injection damp-proof courses work by injecting chemicals into the fabric of the building above ground level to form a chemical barrier which deters the passage or rise of damp. Many building societies will not now grant a mortgage on a building without such a course.

The main ingredient of the damp-proofing liquid is silicone, which does not cause sensitivity. This is held, however, in an organic solvent and with a catalyst which continues to work throughout the life of the building. Damp-proofing firms can provide a solvent with a catalyst which contains acetic acid (vinegar) and acetate of glycerol, which are much less aggressive than other chemicals. Ask for these if you are installing or replacing a damp proof course.

Bitumen is often used as a solid damp-proofing layer when new floors are laid, or as part of a sealing layer in brick walls or masonry. The fumes from this can cause sensitivity when it is being laid, but once dry and aired, it does not give off persistent fumes and does not cause problems in this use.

Plastic sheeting is often laid under floors or as a sealing layer between courses of bricks or masonry. The plastic sheeting usually airs off fast, and is also well sealed by flooring or plaster. It does not therefore cause sensitivity.

Other damp-proof treatments are barrier chemical treatments, which involve placing a sealed plastic or rubbery membrane between the damp site, usually a wall or floor, and the inner surface. These are best avoided, because isocyanates, which are known to cause symptoms on use, are used in liquid rubber preparations.

Fillers

There are various kinds of fillers. Two basic kinds are reasonably trouble-free – acrylic fillers used to fill gaps and cracks, providing a

TIP

Dry-lining a wall with an insulating layer can help solve persistent condensation problems on external walls (see Insulation,
below).

hard surface once set, and cellulose fillers used to fill finer holes, providing a less hard surface.

Acrylic fillers can give off fumes on use and can cause sensitivity at
the time, but do not usually cause problems over their life. Brand
names are Unibond, Evo Seal, W. H. Smith Do It All Acrylic Filler.

Cellulose fillers cause no sensitivity problems, although the dust can
irritate. Brand names of these include Polyfilla and Tetron. Most DIY
chains have their own-label cellulose filler.

Expanding fillers are based on a foam which hardens once in place.
They contain isocyanates and are best avoided. Exterior fillers contain
resins and can cause reactions. Use only if essential.

Floor Sealants

For varnishes and lacquers to seal wood and cork floors, see
Varnishes and Lacquers, below. If you need to seal quarry tiles,
use linseed oil. This is available by post from Livos (address on page
316). You can also use linseed oil as a sealant on cork floors, as well as
varnishes and lacquers.

Grout

Grouts for tiling often contain fungicides and these types are best
avoided. Grouts are either cement-based or epoxy-based. These can
burn or irritate the skin on contact when using them, but do not cause
persistent sensitivity. Cement-based grouts are less troublesome on
use. Cement-based grouts without fungicide include Polycell Tile
Grout, Evostik Wall Tile Grout and Evostik Floor Tile Grout. The
colourings in coloured grouts are usually minerals and do not cause
sensitivity.

Hardboard

See **Particle and Other Boards**, page 308.

Insulation

Various materials are used in cavity wall insulation, in which insulating material is placed between the outer and inner wall of a building. One such material is urea-formaldehyde foam (UFF) which is injected into the cavity and forms a foam which adheres to the wall surfaces. UFF is only ever used on existing buildings, not at time of construction. It releases formaldehyde vapours for some considerable time after, at low levels but sufficient to cause sensitivity reactions. This type of cavity wall insulation should be avoided. It is not practicable to try and remove it.

Use of UFF has been controlled more closely by Building Regulations since 1985, due to concerns about health risks and bad publicity, and is very unlikely to have been installed after 1985. It was most in use in the 1970s to the mid-1980s.

Polystyrene is also commonly used in cavity wall insulation, as is mineral wool. These do not give off fumes in everyday circumstances and are well tolerated. Polystyrene insulation can be installed in an existing building in bead form. Polystyrene in other forms, and mineral wool can be installed in cavity walls only at the time of construction.

For dry-lining walls with an insulating layer, you can use polystyrene block bonded to plasterboard, or mineral wool secured to plasterboard.

For insulating and lagging water and heating pipes, two types of material are commonly used. One type consists of foamed plastics, often polyurethane, which give off fumes when new, or when warm, and which are best avoided. Use fibreglass wool as an alternative that does not cause sensitivity. It can scratch and irritate skin and airways when handled, so use hand and face protection.

For roof insulation, glass and mineral fibre wools are commonly used. These do not cause sensitivity but again can irritate the skin and airways on handling. Formaldehyde is applied to virtually all roof insulating material but not in high concentrations. If the material is in a well-sealed, or totally sealed, roof space, the formaldehyde should not cause any problem. Untreated roof insulating material can be manufactured, but is not usually available at wholesalers and cannot be ordered in the small volumes needed for domestic use, so, for all practical purposes, is not available. Always use hand and face protection when handling irritant insulating materials.

Hot water tank jackets do not normally cause problems once aired off. Keep cupboard doors well sealed and shut.

Mould Treatments

Most treatments for mould growth are based on chlorine bleach, or other powerful chemicals. If you are not chemically sensitive, bleach is effective, but if you are chemically sensitive, it is a risky chemical. Borax does not cause sensitivity and can be effective where mould growth is not serious. >MOULDS for how to apply.

Mould growth results from persistent condensation and damp. It is a good idea in the long term to solve the problems at source by eradicating the damp or keeping the place as dry as you can, rather than using chemicals to remove the symptoms. >MOULDS for more information on how to keep your environment free of moulds.

Paints

The basic components of any paint are resins which form the protective coating or film that any paint gives to its surface; solvents or liquids to hold the resins and other ingredients before and as the paint is applied; chemical driers which help the drying process; and pigments to give colour. Specialist paints contain a variety of chemicals according to their use – some external wood paints may contain fungicides, for instance, or textured paints for walls and ceiling contain fibres or grains.

The principal cause of problems are solvent- or oil-based paints which give off fumes on application, and over their life. Water-based alternatives are increasingly becoming available for most applications, and should be used wherever feasible.

Some people tolerate paints based on natural solvents and chemicals, which have some performance advantages over water-based paints. Details of these are given on page 307.

Other components of paint vary a great deal, according to brand and type of paint, and their acceptability to people with chemical sensitivity can also vary a great deal – sensitivity can be idiosyncratic with paint, just as with other chemicals. A choice of paints is therefore given below wherever possible. Use the Tile Test (see page 297) to choose the better one for you. If the Tile Test is not possible, paint a small area first as a trial before major work is done.

Gloss paints

Water-based gloss paints for indoor use are produced by Dulux (who also produce a water-based satin paint), by Ark, by B & Q, and by Green Paints. The first two are available from DIY shops, the third from B & Q stores, and the fourth can be ordered through the trade or direct from Green (address on page 315). None of these firms provides small samples for testing. Water-based primers are available for all water-based gloss paints.

Indoor water-based gloss paints do not generally achieve a high gloss finish like solvent-based paints and they are less sturdy in use; they chip and wear more readily. They dry very fast, however, and, although they give off fumes at first, from the acrylic resins that form the permanent coating, they are well tolerated. Other advantages are that brushes can be cleaned, and the paint thinned, with water; organic solvents such as turpentine or white spirits are not needed at all.

Crown Paints make a low taint, solvent-based gloss paint which has the high gloss finish and wear advantages of solvent-based paints, but which has a low level of fumes. This is often acceptable to chemically sensitive people. This can be ordered through the trade or via DIY shops (Crown's address is on page 315). They do not provide small samples.

See page 307 below for natural solvent-based gloss paints.

For outside woodwork, water-based gloss paints are also available, made by Sandtex (Exterior Gloss Paint), Sigma (Sigmatorno), Solignum (Solocote AQ), Jotun (Demi Dekk) and Sadolin (Superdec). Some of these are only available to order through the trade (the manufacturers' addresses are given below). The Sandtex exterior gloss water-based paint has, according to *Which?* surveys, consistently out-performed other paints, including solvent-based ones, over five-year tests.

Emulsion paints

For use on internal walls and ceilings, all emulsions or vinyl paints are water-based, but some are more troublesome and less well tolerated than others.

The brand names of emulsion paints change frequently, as do the formulations in minor ways, so it is not easy to indicate specific paints. At the time of writing, Dulux and Crown both make their brand of simple vinyl matt emulsion called Vinyl Matt Emulsion which can be bought in most shops. Major chains such as B & Q or Do It All sell their own brand Vinyl Matt Emulsion. Ask for current Technical Data Sheets to check contents.

As general guidance when buying emulsion paint, look for as simple a paint as possible. Matt paints are generally better tolerated than others. Avoid paints which are said to be non-drip, easy-to-apply or one-coat, for they are likely to have higher vinyl content, to contain polyurethane or other chemicals, or even to contain solvents. Generally speaking, a simple, water-based vinyl matt emulsion, needing more than one coat (and usually cheaper) will be a better choice. Simple emulsions of this type are best not used in kitchens or bathrooms, or anywhere else where condensation levels are high. They offer less protection against damp, dirt, cooking residues and moulds. In these situations, either tile walls, or use a water-based satin paint such as Dulux Water-Based Satin which is suitable for these conditions.

Masonry paints

For exterior walls, it is not possible to find a masonry paint which is free of fungicide. If you have to use one, get someone else to apply it for you. The following are water-based acrylic masonry paints: Dulux Weathershield Fine Texture Masonry Paint or Dulux Weathershield Masonry Paint, Sandtex Matt and High Cover Smooth Acrylic, Crown Stronghold and Smooth Stronghold, and B & Q Textured Masonry Paint and Smooth Masonry Paint. The Sandtex paint has very low levels of fungicide and small samples are available from them for the matt paint. As an alternative, you can use a cement-based masonry paint, such as Snowcem Cement Paint.

Metal paints

For metal paint, you can use any exterior or interior water-based gloss paint, as above, provided that the metal has been properly primed. Livos sell Duro metal primer which is linseed oil-based, and can be used on iron and any other metals. You can obtain a water-based metal primer from B & Q, Dulux, Green and International Paint but it cannot generally be used on iron. It will cause the iron to rust unless the metal is very clean and totally free of any rust or corrosion. Water-based metal primers are thus best used only on non-ferrous metals such as zinc, aluminium, brass or copper.

Natural paints and varnishes

You can obtain paints and varnishes for all applications which are based on natural solvents, oils, resins and other chemicals. Some people with chemical sensitivity tolerate these well; others do not. You are best advised to treat these as cautiously as you would any other chemicals, unless you know that you are not sensitive to plant terpenes, oils and resins (>PLANTS AND TREES). Use the Tile Test (see page 279), if you can, before using them extensively.

Materials of this kind are supplied by The Healthy House and Livos, who will also give you thorough advice on what to choose and any potential problems. Some of their products avoid specific natural chemical allergens. Livos will supply small samples for testing. (Addresses on pages 315–6.)

Paint Strippers

Paint strippers are of two basic kinds – organic solvent-based ones which dissolve paint, and caustic strippers which are applied as a paste, allowing the paint then to be peeled away. Avoid using solvent-based strippers as significant fumes are given off on use. Using caustic strippers is probably preferable to using a blowtorch, where you will have to deal with the fumes of the blowtorch and of the paint or varnish being burnt.

Caustic strippers are based on caustic alkalis, and can burn the skin on contact, but do not cause sensitivity. Take all usual precautions with face, hands and body when using irritant materials and handle all waste carefully.

Langlow make Safer Paint and Varnish Stripper which is water-soluble, and does not contain caustic soda, or methylene chloride. It is less irritant than other caustic strippers, but still requires careful handling. It is available from DIY shops, and Do It All (Langlow's address is on page 316).

Particle and Other Boards

Particle boards, of which the most common is called chipboard, are made of chips of wood bonded together by adhesive resins, usually formaldehyde resins. They are used in many applications in building and furniture-making, often as a base for wood veneer, and as a base for plastic or melamine decorative finishes. They provide the structure for most fitted kitchen and bedroom cupboards, the core for work surfaces and can be used for partitions, wall and ceiling linings, and for flooring.

These boards have a high resin content relative to other building boards, and can give out significant amounts of free formaldehyde, especially when new, or when being cut or installed. If you have relatively small amounts of chipboard in your home, say only in the kitchen, and if it is not new, then it will probably not bother you too much. But chipboard can be a problem if you are exceptionally sensitive to formaldehyde, if you have large amounts in your home, or if you have newly installed chipboard – say in a new floor or fitted kitchen, for instance.

Unless chipboard bothers you a great deal, it may be better to leave it in place, and allow it to gas out over time, rather than to go to the expense and risk of replacement. If chipboard is exposed anywhere, or if it is used as flooring, sealing it with varnish (see page 312 for choice) will reduce the level of fumes escaping. Fit an impervious floor covering such as linoleum (see page 183), rather than carpets, to reduce vapours.

If you decide to replace chipboard, or have to have work done, then wherever possible use alternatives without formaldehyde resins, or with lower resin contents.

Alternatives to particle board

For wall and ceiling linings, you can use plasterboard which is made from a layer of gypsum dried and hardened on paper. This does not cause sensitivity. You can also use hardboard in some uses (see below for details). For solid floors, you can use concrete, wood or stone.

In general, it is better to avoid built-in furniture, or surfaces with veneers if you can, since these will usually be constructed with particle boards. If you instal fitted furniture, do so on solid wood frames, and use glass or solid wood doors and sides. If you need to replace a fitted kitchen and cannot afford to use solid wood throughout, one way to cope is to leave the old gassed-out chipboard frame in place, and to replace doors with glass and solid wood doors. Alternatively, you could use boards such as fibre building boards, plywood or block-board. These are much less troublesome than particle boards and cheaper than, and sometimes technically preferable to, solid wood.

Fibre building boards (such as hardboard, medium board or soft-board) are made with a natural bonding process, using the lignin present in wood fibres as an adhesive. They contain no formaldehyde resins and generally very few chemical additives (except for some which contain bitumen as a water repellent – avoid using these). They can only be produced in relatively thin widths – up to 4 mm ($^{1}/_{8}$ inch) – and thus have limited applications, such as linings for walls or ceilings, or thin work on furniture. Medium-density fibreboard (MDF) is a particle board, not a fibre building board and has a high resin content.

Plywood is made from thin sheets of wood, usually softwood, bonded together with resins under heat and pressure. The grain of each sheet is set at right angles, so that it provides a very strong and stable material at low thicknesses. The resins used are formaldehyde resins, at very much lower concentrations than those used in particle board. Plywood uses a different process of manufacture and if the manufacture has been correct, it does not release free formaldehyde as particle boards do and thus can be used without problems. A well-aired plywood sheet, used in moderate quantities, should not give problems. Plywood is available in thicknesses similar to chipboard and has similar applications.

Blockboard is made by glueing a veneer with resin to a core of solid wood blocks, usually of softwood. Like plywood, formaldehyde resins are used but, if manufacture is correct, do not release free formaldehyde at all. Blockboard can be used for kitchen cupboards and built-in furniture.

TIP

If you are sensitive to pine wood (see below), you can obtain plywood or blockboard made of hardwood from DIY shops. If you want to specify a particular wood, you can order woods of your choice through the trade.

Paving

Stone slabs, bricks, concrete and gravel used for paving will not cause sensitivity. Take care with tar or asphalt paths and drives; the asphalt can give off persistent fumes, especially in hot weather, and is best avoided if possible.

Plywood

See **Particle and Other Boards** (above).

Putty

Putty is made either of linseed oil and chalk, or of acrylics. Use the linseed oil version for preference. It can irritate the skin, and gives off mild fumes at first but is unlikely to cause reactions over time. Vapours from linseed oil evaporate fast and putty is usually problem-free. Brands of linseed oil and chalk putty include B & Q, available from their stores, and Vallance, from DIY stores. Livos sell a linseed putty by post.

Rot Treatments

Treatments for dry and wet rot are usually composed of a fungicide, dissolved in an organic solvent. Timber treatments often contain an insecticide as well. Treatments for dry rot on brick and stonework contain a fungicide, or sometimes bleach. The fungicides used are unpleasant toxic chemicals, including phenols and tributyltin, and they, plus the solvents used, can cause persistent sensitivity. Avoid them if you possibly can.

Treatments of this kind are usually sprayed or applied on site. If you absolutely have to use them, make sure you are not around while they are being used, and air the building well, if necessary staying somewhere else for some time before returning.

Use alternatives wherever possible. Timbers affected by rot can often be cut out and replaced with timber treated in advance. Ask for timber which has been vacuum-impregnated with salts of copper, chromium and arsenic, and ask for it to be aired for some time before use. These are toxic salts which are forced into the timber through vacuum treatment. These salts do not cause sensitivity over the life of the building. This treatment is available from all major rot treatment firms and is accepted by building societies to meet conditions of mortgage. Timber of this type can also be used for fencing, doors, window frames and other external timber applications.

Some hardwood timbers are more resistant to rot than softwoods such as pine. Use a resistant hardwood if you can, although they are more expensive and now less available because of concerns over rainforest depletion. The choices include greenheart, iroko, cedar, padauk, white oak, teak and hickory.

If you cannot cut out timber and replace it, and need to apply something on site, use Boric Salt powder which again is solvent-free and fume-free, although it is toxic and needs handling carefully. It will not cause sensitivity, but can irritate on use. This is available from Livos and from The Healthy House.

In the long term, the best way to avoid rot problems is to control moisture and damp levels. Deal with rising damp (see **Damp-Proofing Treatments**, above) and any leaks in the structure. Keep buildings as warm and dry as you can afford, and ventilate well. >MOULDS for more advice on damp control.

You should also read **Woodworm Treatments**, below, as many treatments for rot are combined with these.

Stabilisers and Sealants

Stabilisers and sealants are used to stabilise the surface of flaking or crumbly walls or plasterwork. Polyvinyl acetate (PVA) without fungicide is relatively problem-free (see **Adhesives and Pastes**, above). You can use Polycell Super Bond or Evobond Building Adhesive as a stabiliser and sealant; these are available in DIY stores. You can also use Cuprinol Stabilising Solution, a water-based acrylic solution without fungicide, available to order through the trade or DIY shops.

Varnishes

Most varnishes for floors, wood and cork surfaces, doors and furniture, are solvent-based. Polyurethane varnishes also give off isocyanates on use, and can be unpleasant to apply. The fumes of the solvents usually disperse after several weeks and, unless you are exceptionally sensitive, they are not troublesome over years of use. If you are very sensitive, you are best advised to avoid them.

One alternative is to use Bona Kemi Pacific Strong Floor Seal (available to order through the trade), a two-part sealer which works by chemical reaction at the time of application and does not give off persistent fumes. It protects fully against grease and water and can be applied in heavy use areas. (Address on page 315.)

Another option is to use water-based acrylic varnishes such as Cuprinol Enhance and Ronseal Solvent-Free Varnish, available in DIY shops. These give off mild fumes on use and shortly after, but pose no problem long term. These are solvent-free, dry very fast and brushes clean off with water.

Water-based varnishes like these do not protect fully against water spills, grease or fat, even with several coats, and they do not wear well on heavy use. They are thus not really suitable for floors in kitchens, bathrooms, stairs, or entrances; or for work surfaces or furniture that get splashed.

One solution for these areas is to use Bona Kemi Pacific Strong Floor Seal, as above. Another option is to apply one or two coats of polyurethane varnish to give water and greaseproofing, and then use a water-based varnish for the final coats. This keeps fumes under control.

For exterior wood, Ronseal Fencelife, a water-based acrylic wood treatment, can be used as a sealant.

For information on shellac, French polishing and other lacquers used on furniture, >FURNITURE.

For natural solvent-based floor varnishes, see **Paints** (above), for advice and sources.

Varnish Remover

See **Paint Strippers** (above).

Veneers and Sheets

Veneers are thin layers of wood glued to a thicker surface, often particle board. The particle board is often the cause of reactions to veneers (see **Particle and Other Boards**, above), rather than the veneer itself.

Melamine and plastic sheets used as a covering on particle boards can give off fumes when new, but usually air off well. Again, the particle board is the more likely source of problems.

Wallpaper

Wallpaper, including lining paper, is best avoided if you are highly sensitive to moulds as moulds grow on it. Wallpaper also contains chemical finishes, such as formaldehyde, rosin and vinyls which will affect you if you are exceptionally chemically sensitive. Again, it is best avoided.

For wall finishes, use plaster with simple emulsion paint, or tile walls where appropriate.

For stripping wallpaper, use a steam stripper rather than solvent strippers.

Wiring

Some people who are extremely sensitive to plastics can react to plastic-covered electric wiring if it heats up. If this affects you, contain wiring behind skirtings if possible. Alternatively, you can contain wires in steel conduit, or use mineral-insulated copper cable (MICC). The latter option is usually cheaper.

Wood

Wood very rarely causes sensitivity (>PLANTS AND TREES for full details). If it does, the cause is most likely to be solvents from varnishes or paints used to seal the wood. Fresh wood used on building sites is often mouldy. It can cause reactions if you are highly allergic to moulds. Once dried out, the moulds will disappear.

Some extremely sensitive people react to woods which contain natural resins, such as pine or cedar. These problems can be avoided, either by using non-resinous woods – for example, birch, beech, ash or oak – or simply by sealing the resinous wood with a few layers of varnish. Seal with varnish also the insides of pine or cedar cupboards and drawers. This is usually enough to stop problems (see **Varnishes**, above).

Wood Preservatives

Boric Salt powder can be used as a wood preservative (see **Rot Treatments**, above). Linseed oil can be applied to preserve benches or surfaces used outside. For fences and other garden surfaces, Ronseal Fencelife is a water-based treatment without fungicide which protects external timber. Avoid using creosote, which can cause persistent sensitivity. For timber proof against rot, see **Rot Treatments**, above.

Wood Stains

Most wood stains are based on solvents such as naphtha. Use the following alternatives for preference. For internal use, Cuprinol Enhance and Ronseal Solvent-Free Varnish (water-based acrylic varnishes as above) are available in coloured as well as clear versions. Organic pigments are used as the colouring agents and are usually trouble free.

Livos sell Bela wood stains – water-based wood stains based on natural plant dyes – and will provide small samples to test. Available by post from Livos (address below).

For external use, Ronseal Quick Drying Wood Stain is a water-based acrylic stain, without fungicides, with iron oxide pigment. Avoid any products labelled preservative wood stains – these will contain fungicides.

Woodworm Treatments

Woodworm treatments are usually based on organic solvents, and contain unpleasant chemicals, such as lindane or dieldrin, as the pesticide. Permethrin is an alternative pesticide to these chemicals. It is naturally derived and less hazardous generally to humans, but it is still toxic and known to cause sensitivity. Do not use any treatment unless you have to. Take avoidance precautions as in **Rot Treatments** above.

The better course of treatment is to remove and replace affected timbers if you can afford to. Some hardwoods are more resistant to worm attack than softwoods, so use these if you can (see page 311). Follow the advice in **Rot Treatments** (above) on the type of timber to request if you are replacing timber.

Addresses of Suppliers

Ark
PO Box 18
Melbourn
Royston
Hertfordshire SG8 3JQ
Tel: 0763 263132
(Manufacturer; contact for
stockists)

B & Q plc
Portswood House
1 Hampshire Corporate Park
Chandlers Ford
Eastleigh
Hampshire SO5 3YX
Tel: 0703 256256

Bona Kemi
Cementone Beaver Ltd
Tingewick Road
Buckingham MK18 1AN
Tel: 0280 823823
(Manufacturer; contact for
stockists)

Crown Berger Europe
PO Box 37
Crown House
Hollins Road
Darwen
Lancashire BB3 0BG
Tel: 0254 704951
(Manufacturer; contact for
stockists)

Cuprinol Ltd
Adderwell
Frome
Somerset BA11 1NL
Tel: 0373 65151
(Manufacturer; contact for
stockists)

Do It All Ltd
Falcon House
Dudley
West Midlands DY2 8PG
Tel: 0384 456456

Dulux ICI Paints
Wexham Road, Slough
Berkshire SL2 5DS
Tel: 0753 534225
(Manufacturer; contact for
stockists)

Green Paint
Hague Farm
Hague Lane
Renishaw
Sheffield S31 9UR
Tel: 0246 432193
(Manufacturer; contact for
stockists)

The Healthy House
Cold Harbour
Ruscombe, Stroud
Gloucestershire GL6 4DA
Tel: 0453 752216

International Paints
24–30 Canute Road
Southampton SO9 3AS
Tel: 0703 226722
(Manufacturer; contact for
stockists)

Jotun
Henry Clark Ltd
16 Alston Drive
Bradwell Abbey
Milton Keynes MK13 9HA
Tel: 0908 321818
(Manufacturer; contact for
stockists)

Langlow Products Ltd
PO Box 32
Asheridge Road
Chesham
Buckinghamshire HP5 2QF
Tel: 0494 784866
(Manufacturer; contact for
stockists)

Livos
Tony Robinson
PO Box 103
Warwick CV34 6QZ
Tel: 0926 400821

Ronseal
Roncraft
Chapeltown
Sheffield S30 4YP
Tel: 0742 467171
(Manufacturer; contact for
stockists)

Sadolin Nobel UK Ltd
Sadolin House
Meadow Lane
St Ives
Cambridgeshire PE17 4UY
Tel: 0480 496868
(Manufacturer; contact for
stockists)

Sander and Kay plc
Mail Order House
101–113 Scrubs Lane
London NW10 6QU
Tel: 081–969 3553

Sandtex
Akzo Coatings plc
135 Milton Park
Abingdon
Oxfordshire OX14 4SB
Tel: 0235 862226
(Manufacturer; contact for
stockists)

Sigma Coatings Ltd
Sigma House
Tingewick Road
Buckingham MK18 1ED
Tel: 0280 812081
(Manufacturer; contact for
stockists)

Snowcem PMC Ltd
Snowcem House
Therapia Lane
CroydonCR9 4EY
Tel: 081–684 8936
(Manufacturer; contact for
stockists)

Solignum
Thames Road
Crayford
Kent DA1 4QJ
Tel: 0322 526966
(Manufacturer; contact for
stockists)

UCATT
UCATT House
177 Abbeville Road
Clapham
London SW4 9RL
Tel: 071–622 2442

Vallance & Co Ltd
Bruntcliffe Avenue
Leeds 27 Trading Estate
Morley
Leeds LS27 0LL
Tel: 0532 537211
(Manufacturer; contact for
stockists)

Childcare

This section deals with the special problems that caring for a child with allergies and sensitivity brings. It covers:

- How do I know if my child has allergies?
- Preventative measures
- How to manage a highly allergic or sensitive child

For advice on caring for a baby up to two to two and a half years old, including feeding and weaning advice, >BABYCARE.

>MEDICAL HELP for information on drug treatment and use of inhalers, and emollients and moisturisers.

How Do I Know If My Child Has Allergies

The basic approach for working out what your child might be allergic or sensitive to is little different from that required for adults. To do this properly, you need to understand what allergy, intolerance and sensitivity are, the likely symptoms, and the methods of detection, including medical tests. It will help to read the following sections of the *Guide* first:

> DEFINING ALLERGY
>
> SYMPTOMS
>
> DETECTING YOUR ALLERGIES

You should always consult a doctor if you suspect allergy or sensitivity in a child.

The particular difficulties of dealing with children lie in the fact that it is sometimes hard for a child to identify any symptoms or changes they experience, and to articulate them. It is often up to the person caring for the child to learn to spot the signs of reactions, and to interpret the child's behaviour. In addition, it can be very difficult to get the child to co-operate in elimination and testing, particularly with special diets. This often requires a degree of subtlety and deviousness on the part of the carer to test things properly.

Where a child's symptoms are obvious, and particularly if they are those of true allergy – asthma, eczema, rhinitis, urticaria, etc.

(>SYMPTOMS) – there is little doubt about diagnosis. Some children with allergy and sensitivity have lower-level and more diffuse symptoms, and these are often overlooked by both carers and doctors, especially when they manifest themselves in behavioural symptoms. Symptoms of this kind most commonly accompany food intolerance and chemical sensitivity.

If you suspect your child is sensitive to foods, see page 247 for a list of symptoms which may be due to food sensitivity in children. In FOOD AND DRINK, you will also find a box entitled 'Am I Food Sensitive' (see page 123), which describes various character traits and behaviour which are commonly found in food sensitive children and adults.

In CHEMICALS and SYMPTOMS, you will find a description of some of the most common characteristics of people with chemical sensitivity.

Parents often describe children who are subsequently found to be sensitive to foods and chemicals, or to have multiple allergies and sensitivity, as being very restless, demanding, irritable, difficult to manage children, with unpredictable moods, tempers quick to flare and readily tired.

Other low-level symptoms which subsequently clear up when allergens or troublesome foods and chemicals are identified and avoided can include a constantly runny nose, persistent catarrh, and blocked ears. Children do pick up colds and viruses easily at school or elsewhere, but colds and viruses have a clear onset, and tail off and go away. No child should have the symptoms of a head cold permanently or for weeks on end.

Glue ear, and ear, nose and throat infections, and tonsillitis, are not always caused directly by allergy or sensitivity, but they can be aggravated and sustained by them. These conditions often clear up spontaneously when allergy or sensitivity is dealt with.

Constant urination, waking at night, general aches and pains, puffiness, excessive hunger or thirst, mood swings, sudden excitability, are all low-level symptoms which often accompany allergy and sensitivity in children.

Hyperactivity in children has been linked in some cases to food and chemical sensitivity (see opposite).

Preventative Measures

Doctors who practise in the field of allergy and sensitivity urge strongly that preventative measures help children with a family history avoid developing severe problems themselves, or stop problems getting worse. This is especially important when a child is very

Hyperactivity in Children

What is Hyperactivity?

Many young children – even older children and adolescents – are highly active – being mobile, easily bored, restless, in need of stimulation and often difficult to manage and wilful. This sort of behaviour, while stressful to deal with, can be disruptive but is controllable (usually through extra stimulation, activity or attention) and entirely normal.

Hyperactivity – sometimes called hyperkinesis – is different, in that the child's behaviour does not respond readily to extra stimulus or attention, and that the degree of activity and restlessness is truly excessive.

Hyperactive children display some or all of the following characteristics:

- Cranky and irritable
- Constantly mobile, rushing from one thing to another
- Very short attention span, poor concentration
- Failure to make and maintain eye contact
- Excitable, explosive and impulsive moods
- Disruptive, erratic, wilful, and disobedient
- Clumsy and lacking in co-ordination
- Accident-prone, touches everything, creates havoc
- Lacking in verbal fluency, writing difficulties
- Poor hand/eye co-ordination, drops things
- Needs very little sleep, wakes constantly
- Excessive thirst
- Uncooperative, disruptive, failing at school
- Self-abusive (picking at skin, hair, etc.)
- Aggressive, sometimes bullying
- Moodiness and vagueness
- Often spurns affection and comfort

Boys are more commonly diagnosed as hyperactive than girls; this may be that less physical symptoms in girls, such as short attention span, clumsiness, and moodiness, may go unnoted.

Hyperactive children often displayed problems when babies, such as colic, sleeplessness, constant crying, head-banging, feeding problems, resistance to comforting and affection, failure to thrive. For more information on babies, >**BABYCARE**.

Some children grow out of their hyperactivity. In others, it continues, sometimes worsening in adolescence. Some adults have persistent problems, often being restless, disruptive, and anti-social.

What Causes Hyperactivity?

Research has shown that a proportion (20 per cent) of cases of hyperactivity are clearly linked to true food allergy – IgE-mediated reactions to food (>DEFINING ALLERGY and FOOD AND DRINK).

Allergy and sensitivity to other substances also play a strong role. From clinical practice, doctors estimate that between 50 per cent and 80 per cent of hyperactive children are allergic or sensitive to other things as well, including pollens, house dust mites, moulds, pets and other animals, common chemicals and food additives. Many hyperactive children have multiple sensitivity.

The role of food additives in hyperactivity has received a great deal of attention, and the Feingold Diet, excluding certain food additives, together with aspirin and naturally occurring salicylates (the active chemical in aspirin), is widely publicised. Some children do extremely well on the Feingold Diet; but only a small proportion of hyperactive children respond that well – most show some but not great improvement. Higher levels of improvement are found when all types of allergens, foods and chemicals (including food additives) causing reactions are identified and avoided.

Food additives (particularly E102, tartrazine, a colouring) do, however, play a significant role in hyperactivity, and, although not the prime cause, need to be considered seriously. Research has shown that hyperactive children seem to be deficient in a specific enzyme – PST-P – the role of which is to detoxify various chemicals produced naturally in the body during metabolism and digestion. Certain food colourings can block or limit the working of this enzyme, and hence be damaging to an individual who is already lacking in adequate levels of the enzyme. Reactions to certain food additives may thus be due to intolerance due to enzyme defects, rather than to true allergic mechanisms.

What To Do About Hyperactivity

A significant proportion (50–80 per cent) of cases of hyperactivity can respond to identifying allergy, food and chemical sensitivity, and to avoidance measures. Not all respond, in part because it is very difficult to avoid everything you need to if a child has indeed multiple sensitivities, and in part because it can be difficult to gain the child's co-operation.

Get a specialist doctor's advice before embarking on trying to identify food or other sensitivity. Make sure that you have a proper diagnosis of your child's condition, and specialist guidance.

Many parts of the rest of this book will be helpful to you if you are trying to sort out what your child reacts to, and how to avoid things. FOOD AND DRINK gives a basic methodology for detecting food sensitivity. In each section on the major allergens, there is advice on basic avoidance. For simple advice on reducing the load of allergens generally, see page 37.

There is a charity which offers help and advice specifically for the hyperactive child – The Hyperactive Children's Support Group. They can provide invaluable support, and put you in contact with fellow carers to meet and talk to. They also offer advice on their own dietary programme, based on the Feingold Diet, which, as noted above, can be extremely effective for a small proportion of hyperactive children. Contact the HACSG at:

> The Hyperactive Children's Support Group
> 71 Whyke Lane
> Chichester
> West Sussex PO19 2LD
> Tel: 0903 725182

>also FURTHER READING for useful books.

---

young. A basic preventative programme is outlined on page 37. Preventative measures for babies are given in BABYCARE.

If you know what your child reacts to, go to the relevant sections, e.g. HOUSE DUST MITES, CHEMICALS, MOULDS, PETS AND OTHER ANIMALS, etc., for full advice on prevention. If you know your child is sensitive to specific things, such as soap powder, clothing, footwear, or toiletries, consult the main index or go to the relevant section (>CONTENTS) to find the advice you need.

How to Manage a Highly Allergic or Sensitive Child

If you have a child who is extremely ill, you should read MEDICAL HELP for information on drugs and other treatments. Some of the allergy charities give extremely helpful advice and support on caring for children. >CHARITIES for full advice.

The issues dealt with here are:

- Avoidance and elimination, including special diets

- School-life
- Toys and games
- Support for the carer

Avoidance and Elimination

Some of the worst problems with caring for a child are caused by avoidance and elimination, particularly over food elimination and special diets.

There is no easy answer on how to manage a child on an elimination diet when foods are being tested, or on a special permanent diet which excludes problem foods. It can also be very hard to have to get rid of a much-loved pet, or for a child to give up a loved activity, such as swimming.

Perhaps the best advice is to start as you mean to go on; to be as firm, clear and consistent as you can, and not to go back on your word or appear to waver. Explain, as far as the child is able to comprehend and in practical terms, *why* you are doing things – 'because you get spots', 'to stop your tummy hurting'. Even very young children can be sensible if they see practical consequences.

Do not bully, plead, cajole, manipulate or over-compensate – most children can spot when you are feeling vulnerable and will exploit it. Just be matter-of-fact and do your best.

Do not be provoked, either, by other siblings playing off the situation – deal with them as fairly as you can, quash any taunting or teasing, and make sure they get enough attention – they may act badly if they feel neglected. Do not over-compensate, either – they too have to learn that life sometimes can be unfair and does not deliver exactly what they want.

Try and make a special diet as flexible and normal as you can. (There are some tips on ways of doing this in FOOD AND DRINK.) Have the confidence to ignore any pressure from family or friends to conform or not to give unusual foods – if the child is well on his or her special diet, that is your justification.

One of the most difficult areas is to establish rules on things that a child can or cannot do – especially things to eat and drink. If you operate a total ban on some things (e.g. playing with friends' pets, buying sweets, eating ice creams, going swimming or eating biscuits) then you have to trust the child to observe them when out of your sight.

If you are fairly sure that the child is breaking the ban but lying about it, it may be better not to have an absolute prohibition. One option is to allow treats or outings at regular intervals, so that there is less emotional friction around the issue. Although the child may be doing things that upset him or her, at least you know the extent of the damage and the child is sharing in the responsibility for his or her actions.

For full advice on avoidance measures, >the following sections:

CHEMICALS   PETS AND OTHER ANIMALS

FIBRES   PLANTS AND TREES

FOOD AND DRINK   POLLENS

HOUSE DUST MITES   MISCELLANEOUS ALLERGENS

MOULDS

>also all sections in Part 6 for advice on things like first aid, toiletries, clothing, soap powder, etc. For information on precautions with vaccinations, >MEDICAL HELP.

Food fads can also be tricky to handle. Food sensitive children often have strong food cravings or obsessions, and aversions to other foods. Craving, addiction or aversion to a food is often an indicator of allergy or intolerance (>FOOD AND DRINK). However, food faddiness is also common to many children – most children have periods of strong preference and aversion, and go through phases in which they will only eat certain things, or phases in which they use refusal of food you offer as an emotional tool. Managing food fads can be exhausting at the best of times, without adding to it the need to stop a child eating a food that clearly does him or her harm.

Again, there is no easy solution, except that if you decide that your child *must* stop eating a particular food in the interests of health, then you will have to carry it through firmly and take the storms that will follow. If you are concerned that your child does not eat enough or has the wrong balance of nutrients, be reassured that studies have shown that children left to themselves to choose what they eat select foods which give them a proper balance of nutrients – even if they only eat one food for a day or more.

A child who is hungry will eventually eat, and although you may have to endure two or three (or more) terrible days when you first take out a loved food out of a child's diet, a child will eventually co-operate if you are firm and do not weaken.

It helps a great deal if other family members do not eat the deprived food in front of the child (and do not tease him or her about it). But often this cannot be managed and you will have to sit things out.

School-life

You may need special help and collaboration from staff at school if your child is made ill by things he or she encounters there. The best way to achieve this is, again, to be matter-of-fact, combined with offering staff as much practical help as you can in sorting things out. If you want them not to use certain polishes or cleaners in your child's vicinity, for instance, it helps to be able to propose or even give them an alternative. If you want your child not to wear certain parts of the uniform, for example, it helps to offer them an alternative which is likely to be acceptable. Be assertive, but not aggressive or over-emotional. The staff may privately consider you over-fussy, but if your child genuinely will be better for something being done or avoided, you are right to insist. Do not ask for things which are not strictly important, and try to get the staff not to differentiate your child – to treat him or her as normally as possible.

Your child's needs will vary according to his or her allergies or sensitivity. Some of the things over which you may need to take care are food and drink. It may be easier for a child sensitive to foods to take a packed lunch each day, rather than eat school lunches, and to take his or her own water or juice for break-time drinks.

If your child is sensitive to chemicals, he or she may be sensitive to cleaning products, polishes or disinfectants used in the school. If you suspect these, either ask for them not to be used in the places where your child goes, or offer substitutes (>CLEANING PRODUCTS).

If your child is sensitive to solvents, check that paints and glues used in schools are not solvent-based. Oil paints should be avoided, but water-based paints will be no problem. PVA adhesive rarely causes problems. Ask that felt-tip pens are water-based, rather than solvent-based.

If your child is sensitive to synthetic fabrics and materials, >CLOTHING for sources of school clothing in pure cotton.

Swimming can cause a child sensitive to chlorine and other disinfectants to react, and may be best avoided if your child appears unwell or worse afterwards. Other sports activities may affect your child – on damp days outside in winter if allergic to moulds, or on summer days if allergic to pollens. Ask for alternatives to outdoor activities if your child is severely ill. If pollens *are* the problem, exam time in summer can be difficult for your child. >POLLENS for more advice on how to handle this.

If school pets or animals are kept, or allowed to roam, in schoolrooms, these can affect a child highly allergic to pets. See if this can be changed or controlled.

If your child goes on any school trip or holiday, make sure that staff have details of any medication, special diet or other requirements. Send supplies of unusual foods with the child, if necessary.

TIP

The National Asthma Campaign and National Eczema Society run special activity holidays for children. >CHARITIES for addresses.

If your child has very sensitive skin, take a hand-held water spray to the beach to spray off sand and salt. >FIRST AID AND HOME

Toys and Games

If your child is allergic to house dust mites, >HOUSE DUST MITES for advice on precautions to take with soft toys.

If your child is chemically sensitive, it is a good idea to air plastic and painted toys as much as possible when new, in order to air off any fumes as fast as you can. Wash if possible in a solution of domestic Borax or sodium bicarbonate (one dessertspoonful to a bowl of warm water) to hasten the loss of fumes. Hard plastic toys do not cause reactions at all once aired. Air books and paper as well before use if you can.

Avoid solvent-based products such as glues and pens. PVA adhesive is well tolerated by chemically sensitive people. Use water-based

TIP

Ask friends and family to air toys and books out of boxes before giving as presents. Then a child can play and use them straightaway on opening.

If your child goes to a children's party and is on a special diet, find out from the hosts what food is to be served in advance. Ask if you can make a special dish – for everyone to eat, not just your child – or send special food for your child in advance – in party format, of course!

TIP

The Custom Bake Company makes special occasion cakes and dishes to your own specification of ingredients by mail order (address on page 168).

felt-tip pens (as a bonus, stains from these can usually be washed out!). Watch out for any soft doughs, face paints or similar toys your child uses – these very very rarely cause sensitivity, but it might just happen if your child uses them a great deal.

Support for the Carer

The most neglected person in an allergic or sensitive child's life is often the one who has prime responsibility for managing and caring for the child – the carer. If this is you, make sure that you do not neglect your own needs in the middle of juggling the child's and other family members' needs.

Make sure you take time off for yourself, even if it means leaving partner or other family members to cope without you. They *will* cope. Deal with your anxiety and guilt – you will feel guilty for having an ill child. You will also feel very guilty at times when something you do or could have prevented, or something you test, makes him or her ill for a time, but it is not your fault. Your child will have to make his or her own way in the world – your task is to launch them out as well as you are able and to let them make their way. You cannot protect nor save them from hurt and pain.

You cannot resolve all tensions and competition between siblings – they have to learn that life is unequal and unfair and that you are not responsible for everything. Go easy on yourself, do the best that you can, and ask for help and support – no-one expects you to be perfect, nor to cope alone.

Support groups of people in similar situations can be enormous help. There are often local support groups around the country, attached to national charities or independent allergy support groups. There is also a support group for carers of hyperactive children. Contacts for these are given in CHARITIES and SUPPORT GROUPS.

Cleaning Products

This section covers products used for domestic and general cleaning, and products such as disinfectants, insect repellents and insect killers. For DIY products, >BUILDING AND DECORATING MATERIALS.

What Causes Problems?

Certain chemicals in cleaning products often cause sensitivity and allergy. Chlorine, ammonia and phenol are released from common bleaches, disinfectants and cleaners and can cause reactions if inhaled or touched. Fragrances and perfumes are added to virtually all cleaning products, either to add a pleasant fragrance, or as a masking chemical to block strong odours. Many products contain organic solvents, either used directly as cleaning agents, as in stain removers or dry cleaning fluid, or as solvents to carry other chemicals, as in polishes. Natural chemicals are not automatically safer. Some people are sensitive to chemicals, such as pine oil, coconut oil, lemon oil, acetic acid (vinegar) and lavender oil, which are used in some cleaners. Nor are 'green' or environmentally safer products necessarily less likely to cause reactions. Most contain perfumes and some contain troublesome natural chemicals.

For more information on chemical sensitivity, >CHEMICALS.

What to Use

Use as few cleaning products as possible, and only when you really need to. Most situations or mishaps can be dealt with effectively by rapid intervention with hot water. You can meet virtually all cleaning needs with a cupboard containing just salt, sodium bicarbonate, washing soda and Borax. A low-allergen washing powder, detergent and vinegar (if you can tolerate them) are also handy.

Salt, sodium bicarbonate, washing soda and Borax give off virtually no fumes and are not known to cause chemical sensitivity. Washing soda and Borax are strong chemicals and will cause irritation even to a non-allergic person's skin and airways if not handled with care, so be prudent, but they should not trigger sensitivity reactions.

Some brands of cleaning products are tolerated well by people with allergies and sensitivity. Sensitivity is very idiosyncratic, so they may not suit *you*, but those named below are very often trouble-free. Try them with care at first. If one does not suit you, try another brand. The brands which are consistently reported to be a good choice are The Allergy Shop range, available by post; Amway products, available from local agents; Boots for Sensitive Skin range, available from Boots the Chemist; and Clearspring products by Faith in Nature, available from health food shops or by post. (For addresses, >pages 339–40.)

It is not a good idea to carry out home tests, such as the Sniff Test or Patch Test (>CHEMICALS for details), with cleaning products. Many cleaners contain powerful chemicals, even if they do not cause sensitivity. If you apply them straight on to your skin or inhale them directly, they may cause irritation and other symptoms. In normal use, they should cause no such problems. Your best course is to use products according to the directions; protect your hands, do not inhale them directly and always rinse thoroughly after use.

Chemicals at Work or School

Your reactions may be caused by cleaning products used at your workplace or school. You could ask the management or people responsible for the cleaning to use products which you tolerate better. If necessary, give them a packet or bottle to try.

Cleaning Products

The following products are discussed on the following pages:

- Air Fresheners
- Bath Cleaners
- Bleaches
- Brass Polishes
- Car Cleaners
- Carpet Cleaners
- Deodorisers
- De-scalers
- Disinfectants
- Dishwashing Products
- Drain Cleaners
- Dry Cleaning Fluids
- Fabric Softeners
- Furniture and Floor Polishes
- General Cleaners
- Glass and Tile Cleaners
- Insect Repellents and Killers
- Leather Polishes
- Mould Inhibitors
- Oven Cleaners
- Scouring Powders
- Shoe Cleaners and Waterproofers
- Silver Cleaners
- Stain Removers
- Toilet Cleaners
- Washing Powders and Liquids
- Window Cleaners

Addresses for suppliers are given at the end of the section (see pages 339–40).

Air Fresheners

Do not use solid or spray air fresheners. Some contain chemicals such as limonene (a synthetic lemon scent) to perfume the air; others contain chemicals which block and mask odours. The chemicals are usually complex hydrocarbons and can cause sensitivity. Toilet freshener blocks often contain paradichlorobenzene, which is a troublesome chlorinated hydrocarbon.

Air fresheners really are not necessary. Keep rooms well ventilated and open windows to remove unpleasant odours fast. If you want to remove or kill smells, see **Deodorisers** below.

If you like natural perfumes and are not sensitive to plant terpenes (>PLANTS AND TREES), try using pot pourri, dried herbs or lavender bags as air fresheners.

Bath Cleaners

General cleaners (see page 334) can be used effectively as bath cleaners. See also **De-scalers** (page 331).

Bleaches

Bleaches are of two basic types – chlorine bleaches and oxygen bleaches. Chlorine bleaches are often troublesome and should be avoided; oxygen bleaches are usually well tolerated.

Liquid bleaches and scouring powder bleaches (such as Vim or Ajax) are chlorine bleaches. Avoid using these if you can; they give off free chlorine. If you do ever use them, above all do not do so together with anything containing acid (such as toilet cleaner or de-scalers). Mixing chlorine bleach and acid can bring about a chemical reaction which releases large amounts of chlorine.

Use an oxygen bleach for preference. Oxygen bleaches can cause irritation even to a non-allergic person's skin and airways if handled carelessly, but they should not cause sensitivity. Amway sell an oxygen bleach. They have a network of local agents; contact Amway at the address below to find your nearest agent. Ecover also make an oxygen bleach. This can be ordered via a health food shop or is available by post from The Green Catalogue (address on page 340).

Brass Polishes

Most brass polishes are solvent-based and can cause reactions. Two alternative polishes are:

- *either* dip a piece of lemon in salt and rub it over the brass,
- *or* make a paste of equal parts of vinegar, flour and salt and rub it over the brass

Do not leave either of these on the brass for long as they can be caustic. Rinse off the mixture, dry and buff up the brass with a cloth.

For silver and chrome polishes, see Silver Cleaners, below.

Car Cleaners

Most car-care products are solvent-based and can be troublesome. Either use general cleaners or detergents which you tolerate or try a special range of solvent-free products made by Simoniz. These are available from most car accessory shops such as Halfords.

Carpet Cleaners

To clean a carpet, you can use a steam-cleaning machine with just plain water and no detergent.

If you want to use a detergent, use a washing-up liquid or general cleaner that you tolerate (see below). Mix one part liquid with four parts boiling water. Allow to cool, then whip the mixture with an egg beater until it foams. Sponge it into the carpet and wipe it away thoroughly with a damp cloth.

If you are allergic to house dust mites or to moulds, make sure that the carpet dries very thoroughly. Damp conditions encourage dust mites and moulds.

For killing smells in a carpet, see **Deodorisers**, below.

Deodorisers

Sodium bicarbonate, available from any chemist, is an effective deodoriser. It absorbs smells in rooms, or in enclosed spaces such as cupboards or refrigerators.

To kill smells in a refrigerator, place some sodium bicarbonate in a small glass jar. Pierce the lid and place the jar in the refrigerator. Replace the powder after a couple of months. Fridge Fresh is also a very effective refrigerator deodoriser. It contains activated carbon in an egg-sized, hard plastic container and absorbs smells more effectively than sodium bicarbonate. One container lasts for four months. These are sold in major supermarkets. Fridge Fresh can also be used as a deodoriser in cars.

Another way to reduce smells in a refrigerator or freezer is to wash down the surfaces with a solution of sodium bicarbonate or domestic Borax (one dessertspoonful to a bowl of warm water). Domestic Borax is stocked by or can be ordered from Boots the Chemist.

To remove smells from a carpet, sprinkle sodium bicarbonate generously over it. Leave for a couple of hours, then vacuum or brush vigorously to remove.

To remove smells from a cupboard or room, you can use Fridge Fresh (see above) or place sodium bicarbonate in an open bowl and leave it for a few days, or permanently. Replace every few months.

Persistent smells from a toilet are caused by bacteria and moulds in the bowl and under the rim. Either clean with an oxygen bleach (see **Bleaches**, above) or with a solution of Borax, as above.

To kill smells from a drain, place a tablespoon of washing soda (available from supermarkets) on top of the drain and pour very hot or boiling water down the drain.

To kill dustbin or wastebin smells, sprinkle neat sodium bicarbonate and Borax in the bin. Wash the bins regularly and leave to dry in the open air.

De-scalers

Most de-scalers are based on acids. Kettle de-scalers use much stronger acids than bath de-scalers. Acids do not usually cause sensitivity reactions but they are irritant and strong chemicals and if you use them, do so with care.

A milder choice is to use vinegar if you tolerate it. Wipe on vinegar and leave it to stand, then rinse off.

Ecover's toilet cleaner contains acetic acid, which is vinegar, and can be effective on toilets and on baths, but be careful since it also contains essential natural oils and can cause sensitivity if you react to natural chemicals.

___ **TIP** ___

Protect your hands whenever you use a cleaning product, especially if you have sensitive skin. >HAND PROTECTION for advice on what gloves are available.

Disinfectants

Most domestic disinfectants are based on quaternary ammonium compounds or on phenol (carbolic acid). They also contain fragrances, usually complex hydrocarbons. Disinfectants are unpleasant and troublesome chemicals. Do not use them unless you have a strong need – say, infection or an invalid in the home.

Very hot water, and plenty of it, is the best way to clean up after any baby messes and mishaps. Most kitchen surfaces are effectively disinfected by thorough washing and rinsing with hot water. A solution of Borax or sodium bicarbonate will serve as a mild disinfectant for most purposes, as will oxygen bleach. For toilets, see **Toilet Cleaners** (below). To kill smells around the home, see **Deodorisers** (above).

TIP

Air conditioning systems are often regularly disinfected to protect against bacterial infections such as Legionnaire's Disease. This may affect you at work in the days immediately after the disinfection, while the fumes are blown through the system. Ask the people responsible to give you warning so that you can be prepared, or out of the building.

If you need to use a strong disinfectant, The Allergy Shop make an anti-bacterial concentrate which some people tolerate well. Unscented Dettox (available from supermarkets) is also tolerated well by some people with chemical sensitivity. Try these with care.

Dishwashing Products

The following dishwashing liquids are well tolerated by people with allergy and sensitivity – Boots for Sensitive Skin, available from Boots the Chemist, and Clearspring by Faith in Nature, stocked or to order from a health food shop, or by post from Faith in Nature (address below). Both have very little fragrance, which is the most common cause of sensitivity to other liquids.

If you cannot tolerate these, you could try using Amway's LOC Regular which is a concentrated general cleaner (see **General Cleaners**, below). Alternatively, you could use a shampoo that you tolerate. This is an expensive option, so use with moderation. >**PERSONAL HYGIENE** for advice on shampoos.

You can also use washing soda for washing dishes. Use a dessert-spoonful in a washing-up bowl full of hot water. This is very effective for cutlery and normal plates and glasses; but if you have very dirty dishes, or burnt or greasy pans, you would be best to soak them for at least half an hour in a solution of washing soda before finally washing them. Do *not* use washing soda on aluminium utensils.

TIP

Remember always to rinse washing-up very thoroughly to remove any traces of detergent or washing soda, so that you are not ingesting any when you use your utensils.

Remember to use gloves as hand protection, especially if you have sensitive skin. >HAND PROTECTION for full advice.

For dishwashing machines, you can use washing soda as a detergent. Simply fill the detergent container full of soda and use as normal. You will not need rinse aid. Salt used for softening is no problem and can be used. Faith in Nature make a liquid for dishwashing machines called Clearspring Dishwasher Liquid, which is virtually unperfumed and is well tolerated by people with allergy and sensitivity.

Drain Cleaners

To clean drains and to kill smells, place a tablespoon of washing soda on top of the drain and pour very hot, or boiling, water down the drain.

Dry Cleaning Fluids

Dry cleaning fluids are solvents, usually chlorinated hydrocarbons such as tetrachloroethene. They can cause irritation at high levels to healthy people, as well as sensitivity reactions.

Avoid having clothes and other items dry-cleaned wherever possible. The solvents air off, however, so if you have to have clothes or other items cleaned, air them for a few days or longer in a spare room before using. Do not wear anything that has just been cleaned. Unless you are extremely sensitive, airing off the items will be enough to prevent you reacting. (>also **Stain Removers**, below.)

Fabric Softeners

The main function of a fabric softener is to reduce static electricity on fabrics and thereby make them feel more supple and soft. They are often strongly perfumed and can be very troublesome. Avoid using them, or any laundry agents containing them in combination with a soap powder. Alternatively, try Boots for Sensitive Skin fabric conditioner which is unperfumed and well tolerated. Static electricity on clothes usually arises from tumble-drying, or from synthetic fabrics – so if it bothers you, you could either tumble-dry clothes less, or use natural fibres more.

Furniture and Floor Polish

Spray polishes for polishing while you dust contain solvents, and often strong perfumes. They are best avoided. Damp-dusting (>page 177) is an effective way of removing dust while cleaning.

If you need to polish furniture or wood floors, most wax polishes are solvent-based and perfumed. As an alternative, try true beeswax polish or the Allergy Shop's low-allergen furniture polish.

True beeswax polish is relatively trouble free. The beeswax is held in a solvent, often turpentine, linseed oil or methylated spirits; and while it might bother you as you use it, the solvent disperses very fast and leaves no trace. Polish furniture once or twice a year only. Major supermarkets stock a pure beeswax polish called Lord Sheraton, which is based on natural linseed oil and pine turpentine. Quince Honey Farm, The Healthy House and The Green Catalogue sell a beeswax polish by post. The Healthy House also sell other natural solvent-based polishes. Livos make a range of natural-solvent based polishes, and will supply samples to test.

General Cleaners

Washing soda (available from supermarkets) is an effective general cleaner for all kinds of uses, but do not use on anything made of aluminium. Dissolve a tablespoonful in a bowl of hot water.

You can use washing soda for washing paintwork; for cleaning baths and tile work; for washing floors; for cleaning windows; for washing cars. It is less effective than detergents or dishwashing liquids at cutting grease, so use in combination with one that you tolerate if you need extra grease-cutting power. Washing soda can damage some oven surfaces (see **Oven Cleaners**, below).

Amway make a general cleaner, LOC Regular, a concentrated and powerful detergent which is generally well tolerated. Available via Amway agents (address on page 339).

Livos make a range of low-allergen general cleaners. These are new on the market and we have no reports of how well they are tolerated. Livos will send small samples to try before purchase.

Glass and Tile Cleaners

To clean glass and tiles, you can use a general cleaner such as washing soda or Amway's LOC Regular. If you tolerate vinegar, you can also mix white vinegar half and half with water. Apply lightly to the surface and polish with a soft cotton cloth.

To clean scum and mould from tiles and grouting, sprinkle Borax or sodium bicarbonate on a nailbrush and scrub thoroughly. Borax and sodium bicarbonate inhibit mould growth.

Insect Repellents and Killers

The active ingredients in fly and wasp killers are often powerful toxic agents such as dichlorvos, fenitrothion or lindane. Some use pyrethroids, which are natural toxic agents derived from plants. All of these can cause unpleasant reactions and should be avoided.

If you have a troublesome wasp nest which has to be removed, get professional help from your local authority and see if they can use means such as smoke or water to remove the nest before using chemicals. If you have to kill ants, you can do so by pouring boiling water on the nest.

To repel and deter insects, keep all dustbins and wastebins sealed. Empty and clean regularly. Wipe up food spills. Keep food covered and cupboards closed. To remove insects, use a fly-swat or a fish-slice. Open the windows and chase them out.

Lavender and citronella are natural insect repellents, as are many herbs. If you tolerate plant oils, hang dried lavender and herbs around. You can also dab lavender oil or citronella (available from pharmacies) on cloths and hang them in the kitchen.

Leather Polish

>**Shoe Polishes and Waterproofers**, below.

Mould Inhibitors

Borax and sodium bicarbonate inhibit mould growth, as do bleaches. Wash surfaces in bathrooms, kitchens, fridges or freezers, or mouldy walls with a solution of these to deter moulds. For advice on killing moulds, >MOULDS.

Oven Cleaners

Most oven cleaners are based on caustic soda and are highly corrosive and irritant, even to normal, healthy people.

The best way to keep your oven clean is never to allow grease and spills to become encrusted. Wash it down each time you use it while it is still warm with a solution of sodium bicarbonate in hot water (one tablespoon to 300 ml/½ pint water), or clean with washing-up liquid. Never allow grease to build up. It is hard work, but make it a habit and it will save you using a noxious cleaner.

If the oven is already dirty, sprinkle salt or sodium bicarbonate on to the moistened surfaces when the oven is warm, and allow them to stand for some time. Rinse and wash thoroughly.

Washing soda is a very effective oven cleaner, but it cannot be used on self-cleaning liners or on certain enamels as it will damage the surfaces. Read your cooker's instructions or contact the manufacturers to find out if you can use it.

Scouring Powders

Avoid chlorine bleach scouring powders (see **Bleaches**). You can use sodium bicarbonate or ordinary salt as a scouring powder. Sprinkle a little powder on to the surface and scour thoroughly with a sponge. Use steel wool for resistant spots.

Shoe Polish and Waterproofers

Most shoe polishes are based on solvents and oils and give off strong fumes. Proprietory waterproofers can also cause sensitivity. Silicone liquid polishes are less troublesome and are tolerated by some people.

Livos make a range of natural oil-based products; these are new and we have no reports as to how well they are tolerated. Livos will send samples before purchase.

Lord Sheraton make a Leather Balsam for cleaning and polishing leather. It is made from beeswax with a rich emollient, which is less aggressive than other solvents. Available from major supermarkets.

Saddle Soap is a leather cleaner made from beeswax and glycerol, which is a mild solvent. Glycerol can cause sensitivity in some people, but saddle soap is generally less troublesome than other leather cleaners.

Neatsfoot Oil is an effective old-fashioned means of waterproofing leather. Made from calves' feet, it is available from pharmacies.

Silver Cleaners

Most silver cleaners are solvent-based and give off fumes. To clean tarnished silver, make a solution of one part washing soda and 20 parts water in a washing-up bowl. Put in a piece of aluminium foil. Immerse the silver and leave for about one minute. This causes a chemical reaction (non-hazardous) and the tarnish from the silver is transferred to the foil. Rinse well, dry and buff with a dry cloth.

Chrome can be polished with a solution of sodium bicarbonate.

Stain Removers

Stain removers are of a number of different types. Some are laundry agents, to be used for soaking or washing things. Others are spot removers, to be applied to small areas to remove specific stains.

Laundry agents usually list their ingredients. They often contain enzymes, which can be troublesome, and perfumes. They are best avoided. To remove stains on things you plan to launder, soak them overnight before washing in a solution of ordinary salt in cold water (one tablespoonful to a large bowl). You can also sprinkle a washing powder you tolerate directly on to the stain with a little cold water and leave it to stand for a few hours. Scrub with a nailbrush.

Spot removers are usually solvents, similar to dry cleaning fluids (see above); they are best avoided.

To remove stains, start to work on them immediately they arise. Start with cold water first; hot water loosens grease but can cook, and set in, food stains. For wine stains, pour on salt with a little water. Try also for beetroot and fruit. For non-greasy stains, try a solution of either salt or Borax (one part Borax to eight parts water). Wipe on and allow to dry before laundering. For oily stains (like oil, grease, grass stains), try a mild solvent like glycerol or eucalyptus oil (available from pharmacies). Take care; these are mild chemicals but are known to cause reactions. Rubbing on a pure hand soap, such as Simple Soap or Kay's Soap (>PERSONAL HYGIENE), and leaving to stand for a while can also help dissolve greasy stains.

Toilet Cleaners

Toilet cleaners are usually based on an acid material, sodium hydrogen sulphate, which is an irritant chemical. Ecover make an acetic acid-based cleaner, which is effective, but the acetic acid and its natural perfumes upset some people. The best choice for many people is to use an oxygen bleach (see **Bleaches**, above).

You can also use Borax to sprinkle under the rim and in the bowl.

Washing Powders and Liquids

Sensitivity to washing powders and liquids is very idiosyncratic; one product will affect one person, and not another. The ingredients which most often cause reactions are enzymes, chlorine bleaches, perfumes and a stabiliser ethylene-diamino-tetra acetate (EDTA). Other petro-chemical-based chemicals in laundry agents also cause problems. Avoid enzyme powders and combined conditioner and detergent products.

TIP

If you think you react to your washing powder or liquid, it may be that it is not being rinsed out adequately. If you live in a soft-water area, or if you use low temperature programmes a lot, detergent residues may not be rinsed out and can remain in the laundry when dry. Try running an extra rinse programme on every wash.

Doing hand-washing may expose you to too much of your detergent. You may be inhaling or touching enough to make you react, while using machine-washing and rinsed clothes may be fine. Avoid hand-washing if possible – use a wool or fine materials programme on a machine.

The following products are tolerated well by most people with allergies and sensitivities. Amongst ordinary brands, Persil Original Formula is often well tolerated. Some people tolerate pure soap flakes (such as Lux) well. These can be used in a washing machine by mixing half and half with washing soda. Filetti soap powder (available from some supermarkets or by post) is also well tolerated.

If you are very sensitive, the following products are often tolerable: The Allergy Shop washing liquid, Amway SA8 Plus concentrated powder, Boots for Sensitive Skin laundry products, and Ecover washing powder. One brand may suit you while another may not, so keep trying. Product sources are given below.

If you are exceptionally sensitive and find that nothing suits you, you can use sodium bicarbonate, washing soda or Borax as laundry agents. Use a tablespoonful of powder per washing load. They are effective cleaners for normal use. They do not always remove greasy stains, and you may have to soak these in salt (see **Stain Removers**, above) or use a detergent wash occasionally to remove stains and grease.

TIP

Run the machine empty for a few rinses before trying a new product. This will flush out any residues in the machine and clear it out.

Use less powder or liquid than instructed and do an extra rinse. This will remove residues and may make you able to tolerate a product.

If you find you are still reacting even when you have changed laundry agents, or used sodium bicarbonate, washing soda or Borax for some time, it may be that you are extremely sensitive and are reacting to minute residues of your former laundry agents in your clothes and other items. To see if this is the case, buy a new item of clothing (e.g. a vest or T-shirt), wash it thoroughly in sodium bicarbonate or your new laundry agent several times, dry thoroughly and wear or sleep on it. If a new garment like this gives you no more problems, and you are confident you are not reacting to fibres, then you are reacting to residues of your former detergents in your existing clothing.

Window Cleaners

>**Glass and Tile Cleaners** (above).

Addresses of Suppliers

The following are suppliers of cleaning products:

The Allergy Shop
PO Box 196
Haywards Heath
West Sussex RH16 3YF
Tel: 0444 414290

Amway (UK) Limited
Michigan Drive
Tongwell
Milton Keynes
Buckinghamshire MK15 8HL
Tel: 0908 679888

(Manufacturer; contact for agents)

Boots plc
1 Thane Road West
Nottingham NG2 3AA
Tel: 0602 506111

Ecover
Full Moon
Mouse Lane
Steyning
West Sussex BN44 3DG
Tel: 0903 879077

Faith in Nature
Kay Street
Bury
Lancashire BL9 6BU
Tel: 061 764 2555

Filetti
Swiss Products (UK) Limited
P O Box 27
Liskeard
Cornwall PL14 6XS
Tel: 0752 361321

Fridge Fresh
Brookline Delta
Unit 10
The Robert Eliot Centre
No. 1 Old Nichol Street
London E2 7HR
Tel: 071–739 5655

(Manufacturer; contact for
stockists)

The Green Catalogue
3–4 Badgworth Barns
Notting Hill Way
Weare
Axbridge
Somerset BS26 2JU
Tel: 0934 732469

The Healthy House
Cold Harbour
Ruscombe
Stroud
Gloucestershire GL6 4DA
Tel: 0453 752216

Livos
Tony Robinson
PO Box 103
Warwick CV34 6QZ
Tel: 0926 400821

Lord Sheraton
Lucerne
18 St. George's Square
Stamford
Lincolnshire PE9 2BM
Tel: 0780 66787

(Manufacturer; contact for
stockists)

Quince Honey Farm
North Road
South Molton
North Devon EX36 3AZ
Tel: 0769 572401

Simoniz
Spectra Brands
Treloggan Industrial Estate
Newquay
Cornwall TR7 2SX
Tel: 0637 871171

Clothing

This section falls into two main parts. The first part, 'What to Look For', discusses clothing in general, describing what often causes problems and how to work out what is upsetting you. There is general advice on what to choose, and on how to avoid trouble.

The second part is an alphabetical guide by type of clothing baby clothes, men's clothes, underwear, etc. In each sub-section, there is more detailed advice on how to avoid trouble. Full lists of suppliers are given. If you know you are looking for specific items of clothing, go straight to the sub-section you need.

WHAT TO LOOK FOR

Symptoms

The most common reactions caused by clothing are breathing and nasal symptoms, and sensitive skin, but other symptoms can result. Do not therefore exclude clothing as a possible sensitiser just because your symptoms (such as arthritis or headaches) seem remote.

Clothing can cause allergic or sensitivity reactions not just by contact with it, but also by inhaling fibres from the clothing, or inhaling chemicals used in, or applied to, the materials. Contact with fastenings, trimmings, linings and elastic can also give trouble.

Before You Start

Clothing may appear to be the prime suspect if you have persistent problems whatever you wear, but there are other possible candidates which may be worth checking before you pursue clothing further.

The cause of persistent symptoms could be your laundry agents, or products you use as toiletries, cosmetics or for personal hygiene. If you want to check these first, >CHEMICALS for general guidance, then CLEANING PRODUCTS, COSMETICS, TOILETRIES AND SKINCARE, or PERSONAL HYGIENE.

If you have occasional, rather than continual problems, these could be caused by dry-cleaning fluids. Check to see if wearing dry-cleaned clothes matches the pattern of your symptoms (>CLEANING PRODUCTS for avoidance advice).

Minute spores of moulds cling to clothes unless they are bone dry. If you are unusually sensitive to moulds, these tiny traces can upset you. Make sure that clothes are kept very dry, especially before wearing. Change out of clothes if they become damp or sweaty. >MOULDS for further information.

What Causes Problems?

Clothing can cause reactions by contact with, or inhaling vapours or particles from:

- fibres
- chemical treatments and finishes
- fastenings and trimmings

Wool and synthetic fibres are the most usual causes of allergy and sensitivity to fibres. Allergy to cotton and linen is relatively rare. Silk is more allergenic than cotton and linen, but because few people have any significant exposure to it, the incidence of allergy to silk is low.

Wool and synthetic fibres often cause irritation, even if you are not actually allergic or sensitive to them. They can irritate already sensitive skin and airways, so are often best avoided.

Fabric resins, applied to give easy-care properties, can be a cause of sensitivity to fabrics. They are applied to certain types of pure cotton, to polycotton blends, to viscose and rayon, and to some linen fabrics. They are hardly ever used on wool and never on silk, nor on pure synthetics. Other fabric treatments, such as dyes, mordants, fire-retardant treatments and bleaches, can cause reactions, but they are less common causes.

Clothes that you have to wear for work or school may be the cause of reactions. This can be a difficult area to sort out and find alternatives (>CHILDCARE). Also >**Children's Clothes** (page 354) for details of sources of school uniform clothes in pure cotton.

Leather, suede and fur clothing can be high-risk choices. Tanning agents and dyes used on leather and suede can upset the chemically sensitive, unless the clothes are quite old or well-worn (>**Leather** in MISCELLANEOUS ALLERGENS). Fur clothing can upset people who are sensitive to animal hair (>PETS AND OTHER ANIMALS).

Fastenings and trimmings are relatively easy to identify as a source of trouble. If you suspect these, see page 350 for how to investigate and avoid trouble. Remember that reactions caused by contact and by inhaling do not necessarily occur at the site of the body where contact takes place. Contact reactions also occur frequently after a delay – sometimes a few days after.

How To Detect The Cause Of Reactions

It is not always straightforward to work out whether specific fibres are causing your reactions or whether it is chemical treatments and finishes. The best way to proceed is to test fibres systematically using the information below (page 344) and in FIBRES. You can do this in such a way that chemical treatments and finishes should not interfere with the test. Once you know what fibres you do or do not tolerate, you can investigate chemical treatments and finishes (page 346) if you are still having problems with clothing.

How to Avoid Problems

If you don't need a systematic approach, here is some basic advice. Pure cotton clothes are very often a good choice for people with allergies and chemical sensitivity. Allergy to cotton is rare, and much less common than sensitivity to wool, pure synthetics or blends. Some cotton clothes are treated with chemicals. If you have to wear cotton but are very sensitive to these, there are ways to detect and avoid them (see page 346).

If you are allergic to cotton, but have to wear it because of multiple allergies, there are certain types of cotton clothes which produce much less flock and particles, and can be better tolerated by people allergic to cotton (see page 344). Some people allergic to cotton can tolerate it in a polycotton blend. This may be worth trying. If you cannot wear wool and synthetics, and wear mainly cotton, it can be very difficult to keep warm. For advice on what to do, see page 345.

Silk is often a good choice. It can be invaluable for lightweight warmth, and chemically sensitive people tolerate it well because no resins are used on it. Silk jersey underwear and T-shirts are available now at relatively affordable prices. They can be very useful to protect sensitive skin against irritation from other fibres and as nightwear. Sources are given below.

Choosing Cotton Clothes

If You Are Allergic To Cotton

If you are allergic to cotton but choose to wear it because of mulitiple allergies, or reasons of cost or practicality, certain types of cotton fabric are less troublesome than others.

Cotton causes allergy when you inhale, or come into contact with, the cotton flock – the small particles given off from the fibre. You can avoid cotton flock by wearing only very smooth cotton fabrics, such as cotton jersey, poplins and lawns. Avoid fibrous cotton such as knitted cotton sweaters, fine flocky underwear, or towelling. Some people tolerate cotton corduroy and cotton fleece fabric (tracksuit material) quite well, even though they are a bit flocky.

If you are allergic to cotton but have to wear it

Try smooth fabrics	Avoid flocky fabrics
Cotton jersey	Knitted sweaters
Cotton lawn	Flocky underwear
Cotton poplin	Towelling
Cotton corduroy	Brushed cotton
Cotton fleece-backed	Winceyette

If you are chemically sensitive, see also page 346.

Choosing Fibres

If you would like full information on fibres and how to detect allergy or sensitivity to them, you should go to FIBRES. For a short guide to detection, read on.

There is a relatively cheap and easy way to test at home whether you are allergic or sensitive to specific fibres – the Pillow Test (see page 110). Washing the cloth with sodium bicarbonate and drying thoroughly before use will minimise the possibility of sensitivity to laundry agents, chemicals or moulds interfering with the test.

You will get clearer results from the test if you are able to avoid totally the fibre you are planning to test for at least a day, preferably several days, before you do the test. You can then confirm the results of the Pillow Test by avoiding totally (or as far as is practicable) the fibre or fibres you suspect for a period of a week and then reintroducing it –

How to Keep Warm

If you cannot tolerate wool or synthetics, keeping warm is one of life's real challenges for the allergy sufferer. Here are some useful tips

Wear lots of layers. Layers of thin clothing trap air and keep warmth in. Lots of thin layers of clothing can be surprisingly warm. Wear a vest under a T-shirt under a sweatshirt. You might feel like the Michelin Man but you won't look it! Wear thin socks under thicker ones, or leggings. And don't forget the old string vest.

Cover your head. Fifty per cent of body heat loss is from the head. Wear scarves or knitted hats. Wear a scarf under a hat in really cold weather. Wear a hat or scarf indoors if you need to. Wear a nightcap – they had their uses!

Use silk if you tolerate it. Silk jersey underwear is relatively affordable, and offers lightweight warmth. Larger children can wear smaller women's sizes. It washes well in a machine on a delicate cycle. Wear silk scarves, glove liners, socks and balaclavas.

Sources of Supply for hats, gloves, socks and warm underwear are given in the alphabetical guide on pages 351–68.

TIP

If you have multiple allergies or sensitivities and have to avoid many fibres, you may simply have to choose your safest options and stick to them. Some people with sensitive skin find that they can tolerate a fibre to which they usually react, provided they do not wear it next to the skin. So try wearing a vest or shirt of a different fibre next to your skin under other garments. If this works, you may not have to replace large parts of your wardrobe.

You can also try *rotating* fibres (wearing one specific fibre per day or one per week), to give your system a rest. Don't shun anything – you may react, say, to nylon or wool, but they could be better than any other choice you have. Stay flexible and keep varying your options until you find the one that suits you best.

TIP

Take precautions if you borrow clothes to test them out. Check out what soap powder or conditioner has been used. Sniff for any perfumes that might cling to them.

Take great care if you buy clothes secondhand or from charity shops. Ask about soap powders and conditioners. Look out for dust, cigarette smoke or animal hairs which might cling.

Avoiding your worst culprits may make you able to tolerate them again after a while. You could be able to wear them occasionally or even regularly. Never throw anything away.

Do not have a massive clearout and replace everything at once. You can sometimes tolerate something well for a while, then find it comes to upset you. Take one step at a time.

by wearing or using it again. Monitor any symptoms for the period of avoidance and on reintroduction.

Fabric Treatments and Finishes

If, after you have tested fibres, you find that you are still reacting to clothing without apparent pattern of explanation, then fabric treatments and finishes may be the cause.

Detecting fabric treatments and finishes

Most fabric treatments and finishes wash out well. Unless you are exceptionally sensitive to the chemical traces left, you will not react to a well-washed garment. Wash all clothes well before wearing and only buy clothes that can be washed.

The Iron Test

This is a rough and ready test for fabric finishes. Iron a portion of a garment that you have just washed and dried. Do this with care in case you react strongly. The heat will cause any residual resins to be released from the fabric. Inhale the vapours gently. See if you detect any distasteful smell, or if symptoms arise.

The Iron Test (see page 346) can also give you a guide as to whether it is tiny traces of chemical from a garment that are upsetting you. Try this on any garment you suspect.

Where treatments and finishes are used

The most common causes of reactions to chemical treatments and finishes are fabric resins applied to give easy-care properties (see page 348 for full information). Other causes of reactions include fire retardants (applied to some night and workwear), and certain kinds of dyes, germicides and moth repellents. Some people are sensitive to bleached fabric even though the bleaches are very thoroughly washed out before finishing.

Starches and sizes are often applied to stiffen clothes when new. They are of a variety of chemicals – denim, for instance, often has corn starch applied. Starches and sizes wash out readily, however, and should be well tolerated.

Some fabric treatments are generally not troublesome. 'Mercerisation', for instance, is a process whereby cotton is scoured with caustic soda. The soda is extremely thoroughly washed out, and should not be the cause of sensitivity.

If you are sensitive to fabric resins

If you are exceptionally sensitive to resins, wear wool, pure silk or pure synthetics if possible. You can buy resin-free cotton clothes – usually called 'formaldehyde-free' – for babies, children and adults. Sources are given below.

You can also find certain kinds of cotton clothes that are much less highly treated than others. These are often well tolerated even if you are sensitive to resins. If you are unable to wear wool, silk or synthetics, and want to have a wider choice of cotton clothing, choose relatively untreated cotton clothing as follows:

Try	Avoid	Take care with
Cotton jersey	Cotton poplin	Brushed cotton
Cotton fleece	Cotton drill	Cotton lawns
Cotton corduroy	Denim	Cotton voiles
Cotton towelling	Easy-care	
Knitted cotton sweaters	Permanent Press	
Indian cottons	Sanforised	
Third World cottons		

Fabric Resins

What Are Resins?

A significant proportion of allergic reactions and sensitivity to clothing are caused by resins, applied to give easy-care properties. The resins used are mostly formaldehyde polymers. They make fabrics more resistant to shrinking, creasing, and going out of shape. They improve dye absorption and restrict fading. The feel of clothes, and the way they hang, can also be improved. Formaldehyde resins are used for stain and grease resistance, waterproofing, and permanent pleating and pressing.

Resins and additives other than formaldehyde resins can also be applied (such as acrylates to reduce creasing and silicates to improve the feel of fabric). Catalysts can also remain in the fabric but are removed when the garment is first washed. These are not generally known as major causes of reactions.

Wash New Clothes

Resins wash out readily, but not all fabrics or clothes are washed during manufacture, and new clothes can have very high levels of fumes. You can reduce the level to tolerable amounts by washing new clothes before wearing them. If you add a dessertspoonful of sodium bicarbonate to the water, this also helps to neutralise the resins. You may have to wash new clothes several times before you can wear them, but, for virtually everyone, this is sufficient to avoid any major problems. Unless you are extremely sensitive, washing clothes well will make resins tolerable.

Which Clothes Are Treated?

Fabric resins are not applied to silk, nor to pure synthetics. They are rarely applied to wool or to linen. Virtually all cotton, viscose and polycotton fabrics are treated with formaldehyde resins.

Some sensitive people learn to develop the ability to judge whether a fabric is highly treated or not. There is often a distinctive, sweet, aromatic smell to the fabric which a sniff (gentle, just in case!) can detect. Some people can tell by the feel of the fabric; some say that their skin prickles when they hold it. Another test is to place one drop of water with an eye-dropper on the fabric. If it holds in place without being absorbed, then there is a finish to the fabric.

Generally speaking, the more glazed, stiff and shiny the fabric, the more likely it is to have high levels of resins. If clothes are labelled, 'Easy Care', 'Permanent Press', 'Sanforised' or any variant of these, then they will be treated heavily. Cotton poplin, stiff cotton drill and denim are often treated and may be best avoided.

Conversely, cotton jersey (including cotton loopback), cotton fleece, towelling, knitted cotton sweaters and cotton corduroy are much less treated and are often no problem once washed. Brushed cotton is also sometimes untreated. Some cotton lawns and voiles are treated; others are not. Indian and Third World cotton fabrics are less likely to be treated heavily, and thus are often acceptable to people who are sensitive to most other fabrics.

TIP

Watch out for shirt collars on men's cotton shirts. These are sometimes much more highly treated than the shirt itself. Look for shirts with softer collars.

If You Are Sensitive to Bleached Fabric

Try wearing unbleached cotton and linen clothes if you are sensitive to bleached fabric. Sources of these are given below. Sources of unbleached fabric for making clothes are given in **FABRICS**. Unbleached cotton fabric is more flocky than ordinary cotton and can upset you if you are very sensitive to cotton.

If You Are Sensitive to Other Chemicals

If you are generally chemically sensitive, it is better to avoid chemical treatments, such as fire retardants, moth repellents and germicides, as far as possible. Cotton winceyette is often treated and is best avoided.

Dyes rarely cause allergy or sensitivity but a group known to cause problems are mostly chemicals known as the Disperse azo dyes. These are rarely used on cotton, viscose, rayon or wool, but commonly on synthetics. Colour is unfortunately no guide to the chemicals in question. (>also **CROSS-REACTION** for information on Paraphenylenediamine (PPDA), a chemical with many uses which cross-reacts with azo dyes.)

Dyes in nylon stockings and tights are known to cause reactions. You can get dye-free nylons and wearing these may help you to work out if dyes rather than fibres are causing your symptoms. (see **Socks, Stockings and Tights**, page 361.)

Avoid overprinted fabrics, or T-shirts with placement prints if you are very sensitive. The dyes or fabric inks used in these can be troublesome.

Some mordants are known to sensitise. These are metallic salts used to fasten a dye to a fabric. Chromates (salts of chromium) are known to produce reactions. They are a common cause of occupational dermatitis, having wide industrial uses (>MISCELLANEOUS ALLERGENS). If you know you react to chromates, these may be behind unexplained reactions to clothing.

Workwear, such as overalls or uniforms, is often treated with fire retardants, germicides or other protective chemicals. These may be the source of problems.

Fastenings, Trimmings, Linings and Elastic

Finally, trouble with clothing can result from reactions to fastenings, trimmings, linings and elastic. Mostly the problem is obvious, through a contact reaction with a metal fastening or with lace trim, or an elastic strap or waistband, for instance. Look out, however, for garment linings, which are often synthetics or viscose. The thread used to sew seams in clothes can also be bothersome.

If a garment lining causes discomfort, cut it out and see if the trouble goes away. Cut off lace and trims if necessary. Elastic or sewing thread next to the skin can be a severe problem, where the sensitivity is often exacerbated by sweat and friction. To avoid problems with elastic or sewing thread, try any of the following:

- Look for underclothes or nightwear with cased elastic bands which will protect the skin
- Wear underwear inside out so that fabric is next to the skin
- Wear a thin silk vest under bras or close-fitting underwear
- Place cotton handkerchieves or silk scarves under the elastic to protect the skin
- Dust sodium bicarbonate or magnesium carbonate gently on the areas of friction to relieve the reaction
- Swab those areas with Boots Cream of Magnesia liquid to calm symptoms
- Avoid cotton clothes containing Lycra or Elastane

Silk clothes and underwear can be useful because they are often sewn with silk thread.

Look out for waddings, paddings and shoulder pads. Remove them if you have to. Be careful with cotton interlinings, which can be treated with formaldehyde resin to strengthen them. Watch out for pocket linings and zips. To protect against metal fastenings or buttons, use any of the protection methods suggested for elastic and thread above.

TIP

If you cannot work out what is causing a contact skin reaction, bear in mind that contact reactions to things like fastenings and trimmings do not necessarily occur at the site where the offending object makes contact. Contact reactions can occur at other parts of the body. They can also occur with a delayed reaction – sometimes a few days later. You may have to experiment carefully with clothing to establish a pattern.

A–Z OF CLOTHING

The following is an index of clothing, listed alphabetically by category, providing detailed advice, plus sources of unusual and hard-to-find products. The sources given are mainly for pure cotton, silk and linen clothes, and clothes with low levels of chemical treatment. Wool most synthetics, viscose and synthetic blend clothes are widely available and sources for these are not given, except for nylon clothes, since these are now hard to find.

TIP

When reading brochures from any of the suggested suppliers, check the materials of each garment carefully. Some firms selling pure untreated cotton, for instance, also sell polycotton or other materials. Read brochures carefully and check with the supplier yourself if you need to.

The addresses of all manufacturers and suppliers of the clothes mentioned are on pages 369–74.

Baby Clothes

Here's some advice on finding clothes, especially untreated pure cotton clothes, for babies and toddlers.

Avoid cotton winceyette if you or your baby are very sensitive. Winceyette clothes, especially sleepwear, are often treated with fabric finishes. If you buy cotton poplin or denim clothes, wash them very well before using. If you or your baby are very sensitive to resins, avoid them altogether. Look for clothes made of :

- cotton jersey
- cotton tracksuit fleece
- cotton plush velveteen jersey
- 100 per cent cotton corduroy
- brushed cotton

High Street Names

It is relatively easy to find 100 per cent cotton jersey vests, underwear and sleepsuits for newborns and up to 12-month size (80–90 cm). Boots, Mothercare and Woolworths, in particular, are good sources, but check labels to make sure that all cuffs and trimmings are of cotton. Marks and Spencer usually have a selection of pure cotton babywear, but these are more highly treated and not always well tolerated. Next sell a very good range of soft 100 per cent cotton jersey rompers and nightwear for babies. They often have cotton fleece all-in-ones which are much warmer than sleepsuits for winter babies. Most of their baby clothes have very little fabric finishes applied, unlike Next adult clothing in cotton jersey which is often highly treated. Next sell by mail order as well as in their High Street shops.

One brand name to look out for in the High Street shops is Fix, who make virtually all their range in 100 per cent pure cotton. Their clothes are not treated with formaldehyde and are not chlorine-bleached. Another name to look for is Stummer who make pure cotton velveteen rompers and outfits; these are warmer than cotton jersey for tiny babies. Honeybee make a good range of sleepsuits, sweat shirts, polo neck jumpers and T-shirts.

Outerwear

Tracking down outerwear or snowsuits that are not of man-made fibre or of polycotton mixes is virtually impossible. It is occasionally possible to find corduroy snowsuits, anoraks and leggings with brushed cotton linings. These still have polyester wadding, but since these are enclosed by 100 per cent cotton, they cause less problems. Heskia produce a range of such outerwear. Their clothes are sold by John Lewis and House of Fraser stores.

Footwear, Socks and Tights

Cotton corduroy boots and padders in 100% cotton are made by many firms and are easy to find. Pex make 100 per cent cotton socks in newborn and baby sizes. These are widely available in children's shops

Table 10: **Suppliers of Baby Clothes**

SUPPLIERS	Formaldehyde-free cotton	Chlorine bleach-free cotton	Cotton jersey	Cotton fleece	Cotton velveteen	Cotton socks & tights	Cotton outerwear	Silk and other bleached clothes	Wool and wool bleached clothes
Blooming Marvellous			●	●					
Clothkits			●	●					
Cot 'n' Kids	●	●	●						
Cotswold Clothing Company				●					
Cotton On	●	●	●			●			
Fix	●	●	●						
Freemans			●						
The Green Catalogue		●	●						
Heskia							●		
Honeybee			●	●					
Kid's Stuff			●						
Littlewoods			●						
Manhattan Kids			●						
Mothercare Home Shopping			●						
MUS			●	●					
Next Directory			●	●			●		
Pex						●			
Schmidt Natural Clothing	●	●	●			●		●	●
Stummer					●				
You and Yours			●						

and large supermarkets. Hundred per cent cotton tights in baby sizes are sold by mail order by Cotton On and by Schmidt Natural Clothing.

Sources of Clothing

Table 10 gives the names of suppliers, mostly mail order, of relatively problem-free clothes for babies. Addresses are on pages 369–74.

Cotton On's range is specifically designed and chosen for babies with eczema and skin conditions. Their clothes are formaldehyde-free, chlorine bleach-free and do not use other well-known irritants. Cot'n Kids, Fix and Schmidt Natural Clothing also sell formaldehyde-free and chlorine-free clothing. The Green Catalogue sell unbleached cotton underwear. Schmidt Natural Clothing sell silk, silk blend, wool and wool blend clothing.

The large mail-order catalogues companies (such as Littlewoods, Freemans, You and Yours, Grattan) also often sell a selection of cotton jersey sleepsuits and underwear.

Children's Clothes

If your child is chemically sensitive, or has irritable eczema or asthma, avoid synthetics and wool. Pure cotton is generally better tolerated, although some unlucky children are sensitive to it, particularly flocky or knitted cotton. When choosing cottons, take care with fabric finishes and:

- wash poplin or denim very well before using to remove any finishes. If very sensitive, avoid altogether
- avoid winceyette, especially sleepwear

Look for clothes made of:

- cotton jersey
- cotton tracksuit fleece
- 100 per cent cotton corduroy
- brushed cotton

Wash everything very well before wearing at all.

The most difficult clothes to find for children in pure cotton are:

- school uniform
- knitwear
- socks and tights
- hats and scarves

- outerwear and waterproofs

School Uniform and Knitwear

Cotton On sell by post a range of school uniform clothes (trousers, shorts, shirts, jumpers, socks) in pure cotton, as well as a range of plain tracksuit tops and bottoms. These are formaldehyde and chlorine bleach-free. Cotton school cardigans and jumpers are available from Sheila Stewart. Angela Knitwear make school uniform, novelty and striped jumpers for children in pure cotton.

Socks and Tights

Pex manufacture 100 per cent cotton socks for children. They are widely available. Cotton On (details above) sell pure cotton socks for children, and 100 per cent cotton tights for babies and children. Some of their socks are 98 per cent cotton, 2 per cent synthetic fibre, but no reports of reactions have been received. Schmidt Natural Clothing sell pure cotton socks and tights for children by mail order.

Hats and Scarves

Cotton On also sell warm, knitted cotton hats and scarves.

Outerwear and Waterproofs

It is virtually impossible to find warm, waterproof outerwear for children that does not contain some synthetics. One solution is to buy a waxed cotton jacket, and let it hang until the fumes from the new waxing have given off; these are then usually tolerated well, even by the chemically sensitive. Re-wax rarely. Another solution to achieve warmth is to make a coat or jacket liner out of cotton blankets (>BEDDING for sources) and wear it under a waxed coat or corduroy jacket.

The Cotswold Clothing Company make dry wax waterproof rainwear of pure cotton, with a brushed cotton lining. They also have a range of padded pure cotton corduroy and brushed cotton jackets. Next Directory sell soft cotton anoraks with polyester wadding. Joan Hollings makes Liberty cotton wadded jackets and waistcoats. Annie Jo Retail make pure cotton needlecord and poplin padded jackets. The wadding in each case is polyester, but encased so should not cause trouble. You can also try PVC raincoats. If rinsed through with water, and left to air for some time, the new plastic smell goes, and they can be tolerated reasonably well.

Sources of Clothing

Table 11 gives sources for children's clothing, mostly mail order. Once again, check all details in catalogues and, if necessary, by telephone. For formaldehyde-free and chlorine bleach-free clothes, see Cotton On, and Schmidt Natural Clothing. Schmidt also make silk and silk blend underwear for children. The Green Catalogue sells unbleached cotton underwear for childen.

Coats and Outerwear

If you are allergic to wool, and, in addition, are sensitive to a wide range of synthetic fibres or fabrics, it can be virtually impossible to find warm, windproof and waterproof outerwear, with tolerable linings. There are no reliable solutions, or sources of clothing, but here are some suggestions on how to cope.

It is not difficult to find warm jackets with 100 per cent cotton outers, 100 per cent cotton linings, with polyester wadding or quilting for warmth. The exceptionally sensitive will be bothered by fumes from the wadding. For most people, however, even if chemically sensitive, the wadding is enclosed sufficiently to reduce the level of fumes; airing the jacket before wearing, and washing it if possible, should be enough to avoid discomfort.

If you tolerate silk and want to make your own jacket, a source for silk wadding is given in FABRICS, as well as sources for untreated fabrics.

Look for corduroy jackets or coats. Although not waterproof, corduroy is often better tolerated than cotton poplin, because it is less treated with fabric finishes. Waxed 100 per cent cotton jackets with cotton linings are also on sale everywhere. While these can cause problems when new, the fumes from the wax do wear off; and the jackets can be tolerated quite well by chemically sensitive people. Waxed coats are surprisingly warm in cold weather. Re-wax only rarely; get someone to do it for you if you can.

In camping and mountaineering shops, you can find anoraks and jackets in proprietary 100 per cent cotton fabrics which are weatherproof and waterproof. Some chemically sensitive people can tolerate these, but there are no makes which emerge as more acceptable than others. You can waterproof fabrics yourself by applying a solution of Alum, alkaline salts, in water. You can buy this at any chemist. This also acts as a fire retardant. Unfortunately, the solution often leaves

Table 11: **Suppliers of Children's Clothing**

SUPPLIERS	Formaldehyde-free cotton	Chlorine bleach-free cotton	Cotton jersey	Cotton fleece	Cotton corduroy	Cotton lawn	Brushed cotton	Cotton school uniform	Knitted cotton sweaters	Cotton socks & tights	Cotton hats and scarves	Cotton outerwear & waterproofs	Silk & silk blend underwear
Angela Knitwear								●	●				
Angela Master						●							
Annie Jo Retail					●							●	
Blooming Marvellous			●	●	●		●						
Cloth Kits			●	●	●								
Cotswold Clothing Co.			●	●	●		●					●	
Cotton On	●	●	●					●	●	●	●		
Freemans			●			●	●						
The Green Catalogue		●	●										
Joan Hollings						●							
Kids' Stuff			●										
Littlewoods			●		●		●						
Manhattan Kids			●	●									
MUS			●	●									
Next Directory			●		●	●						●	
Pex										●			
Sara-Jane Brown								●	●				
Schmidt Natural Clothing	●	●	●									●	●
Sheila Stewart									●	●			
You and Yours			●			●	●						

white streaks on the garment, so only use if you do not object to this. Avoid proprietary waterproofing compounds unless you can find out from the manufacturer what is in them. PVC rainwear gives off its fumes quite rapidly and can be well tolerated if rinsed in water and then left to air for some time.

Cut out linings if they upset you but the outer shell does not. For advice on how to keep warm, see page 345.

Maternity Wear

Mothercare usually have within their range a selection of cotton jersey maternity clothes. They also sell cotton jersey nightwear and a 100 per cent cotton maternity bra. Mothercare sell by post as well as in their High Street shops. Mum's The Word at Dorothy Perkins usually have a selection of cotton jersey T-shirts and corduroy clothes.

By mail order, Blooming Marvellous have a wide choice of 100 per cent cotton maternity clothes, including cotton jersey, fleece and corduroy. Heinz Baby Club sell by post a 100 per cent cotton maternity bra.

Men's Clothes

Leisurewear for men in pure cotton is generally easy to find, but more formal clothes for men can be problematical, particularly if you have to wear suits or tailored clothes for work. If you are sensitive to wool, or are chemically sensitive and cannot tolerate fabric finishes, or dry cleaning fluids, then you may have to dress more casually than you would wish in pure cotton clothes that can be washed. Cotton corduroy can be useful for tailored suits and jackets.

Tailored Cotton Clothing

Next Directory usually sell a wide range of pure cotton tailored clothes, available by post. Pure cotton poplin shirts are widely available in High Street shops. If you are very chemically sensitive, the fabric finishes on even a well-washed shirt will affect you; some people also find finishes on shirt collars a problem. Look for shirts with softer feeling collars as you may be able to tolerate these better. Seymour's Shirts will make pure cotton shirts with soft collars on request.

Untreated Cotton Clothing

Cotton On and Schmidt Natural Clothing sell by post pure cotton casual clothes for men which have not been treated with formaldehyde, nor bleached with chlorine bleach. Natural Facts sell by mail order pure cotton clothes made from organically grown cotton, and free of bleaches, dyes, and formaldehyde. The Green Catalogue, Next Directory, Friends of the Earth and Greenpeace sell unbleached, undyed cotton clothes free of formaldehyde; some of these are made from organic cotton.

Silk Clothing

Alternatively, you may find silk shirts more tolerable. Patra sell men's silk shirts, and silk jersey T-shirts at reasonable prices, by mail order. James Meade and Complete Essentials also sell silk shirts by post. Orvis sell silk jersey polo necks by mail order. These, like the silk T-shirts from Patra, can be very useful as a means of keeping warm if you cannot wear synthetics or wool. Orvis also sell silk and cotton blend knitted sweaters which are reasonably priced and exceptionally warm.

Linen Clothing

Look for men's fashions in linen as an alternative fibre. Next Directory and Complete Essentials commonly stock linen and linen/cotton blend men's clothes in their summer range.

Sources of Clothing

Table 12 gives mail order suppliers of men's clothes.
   >**Nylon Clothes** (below) for sources of nylon shirts and pyjamas. For cotton, linen and silk underwear and nightwear, >**Underwear and Nightwear** (below). For cotton and silk socks, see **Socks, Stockings and Tights**, (below).

Nylon Clothes

Most people with allergies find that they can tolerate cotton, linen and silk reasonably well and are better off avoiding synthetics. Some people, however, are very sensitive to natural fibres and find they are

Table 12: **Suppliers of Men's Clothes**

SUPPLIERS	Formaldehyde-free cotton	Chlorine bleach-free cotton	Organic cotton	Cotton jersey	Cotton fleece	Cotton corduroy	Cotton shirts	Soft collar cotton shirts	Cotton casual clothes	Cotton tailored clothes	Cotton sweaters	Cotton outerwear	Cotton workwear	Silk & cotton sweaters	Silk polos & T-shirts	Silk shirts	Linen clothes
Angela Knitwear											●						
Bridgedale											●						
Complete Essentials			●			●	●		●	●						●	●
Cotton On	●	●	●						●								
Cotton Traders			●				●		●		●	●					
Edinburgh Woollen Mill											●						
Empire Stores				●		●			●			●					
Freemans				●	●				●			●					
Friends of the Earth	●	●	●	●	●				●								
Grattan				●		●			●			●					
Great Universal Stores				●		●			●			●					
The Green Catalogue	●	●	●	●					●								
Greenpeace	●	●	●	●	●				●								
James Meade						●										●	
Kay & Co				●		●			●			●					
Littlewoods				●		●			●			●					
Natural Fact	●	●	●	●					●								
Next Directory	●	●	●	●	●	●	●		●	●	●	●				●	●
Orvis				●		●	●		●		●			●	●	●	
Patra														●	●		
Racing Green				●		●	●		●		●	●					●
Rainbow Leisure				●					●	●							
Sander & Kay				●		●			●			●	●				
Schmidt Natural Clothing	●	●	●	●					●								
Seymour's Shirts							●	●								●	
Woody				●		●	●		●			●					
You and Yours				●		●			●				●				

more comfortable in nylon and purely synthetic fibres. It is now quite difficult to find sources of nylon clothing, although polyester, acrylics, viscose and polycotton blends are very easy to obtain.

Celic sells a range of nylon clothing (men's and women's nightwear, men's nylon shirts) by mail order. Seymour's Shirts sell men's nylon shirts by mail order. See **Socks, Stockings and Tights** (below) for information on nylon stockings and tights.

Socks, Stockings and Tights

Nylon Stockings and Tights

For women, if you find you react to nylon stockings and tights, it is natural to assume at first that it is the fibre itself which is the cause. For many women, this is indeed so. Some women, however, are sensitive to the dyes in stockings and tights; certain dyes (particularly Disperse azo dyes) are known irritants. The colour itself of the hosiery is not necessarily a guide, since a mixture of colours (principally red, yellow and blue) is used to make up flesh-colour. Black and navy colours, however, use acid dyes and are probably less irritant than browns, which use Disperse dyes. So try black and navy before flesh and brown colours.

Aristoc make a range of stockings, tights and knee highs in natural colour which contain no dyes at all. This is called the 'JUST' range. If you tolerate these well, then you will know that you react to dyes, not to the synthetic fibre itself.

If, however, you are sensitive to synthetic fibres, do not give up ordinary tights or stockings, before you try wearing knee highs. They do not touch the sweaty areas at the back of the knees, or at the top of the thighs, and therefore can often be tolerated. Disguised with a long skirt or trousers, they look just like longer stockings or tights.

Silk and Cotton Hosiery

If you cannot wear wool, or synthetic fibres, silk or cotton hosiery may be your only solution.

Pure cotton socks are sold by mail order by Cotton On, The Green Catalogue, Natural Fibres, Sander and Kay, and Schmidt Natural Clothing. The Green Catalogue sell 100 per cent cotton tights for women. Cotton On sell 85 per cent cotton tights for women, which are often well tolerated.

For men's socks, look in High Street shops or specialist men's outfitters for the brand names Wolsey (who include thin mercerised cotton socks in their range), and John Brown of Australia, who make a thicker walking or sports sock. For women, Sock Shop stock a range of thin cotton socks.

Sources of Supply

Mail order suppliers of cotton and silk socks, stockings and tights are shown in Table 13.

Table 13: **Suppliers of Socks, Stockings and Tights**

SUPPLIERS	Dye-free nylons	Cotton socks	Cotton tights	Cotton stockings	Silk socks	Silk stockings
Aristoc	●					
Cotton On		●	●			
Funn Stockings				●		●
Green Catalogue		●	●			
Natural Fibres		●		●		●
Orvis					●	
Patra					●	
Sander and Kay		●			●	
Schmidt Natural Clothing		●	●			
Survival Aids					●	

Underwear and Nightwear

Cotton Underwear and Nightwear

Pure cotton underwear is relatively easy to find in High Street shops. Cotton jersey vests and pants are commonly sold by all the major clothing chains, as are warmer knitted cotton winter underwear. Flocky knitted cotton underwear can sometimes irritate sensitive skin where cotton jersey (also called cotton interlock) does not. If you are very sensitive, stick to cotton jersey. You may need to beware of trimmings, lace and elastic upsetting you. Follow the guidelines in **What to Look For** (page 350) if you have problems with fastenings, trimmings and elastic.

Nightwear can be harder to track down. Some chemically sensitive people react to cotton poplin, cotton lawn and winceyette, because of fabric treatments. Again, cotton jersey can be safer. Most High Street chains usually have a selection of cotton jersey nightwear for women and children. Marks and Spencer commonly stock 100 per cent cotton poplin men's pyjamas. Mail order sources for cotton jersey nightwear are given below. Information on a source of untreated linen nightwear is given at the end of the section.

Finding 100 per cent cotton bras can also be tricky. Specialist underwear shops or departments usually stock light cotton jersey sports bras which are practicable if you need only light support. Playtex make a 100 per cent cotton support bra, the 'Whisper' bra. Natural Fibres supply 100 per cent cotton bras by post, with a size range up to 115 cm (46 inches). David Nieper also supply 100 per cent cotton bras by post. Schmidt Natural Clothing sell a silk and cotton blend bra top. Maternity bras are commonly available in pure cotton. Even if not pregnant, you may find them useful, since they are designed for proper support (see **Maternity Wear**, above).

Nice Irma's sell Indian cotton dressing gowns. Women's slips and petticoats in cotton are sold by post by David Nieper.

Silk Underwear and Nightwear

Silk underwear is extremely useful to people with multiple sensitivities who cannot tolerate wool, cotton or synthetics. It is invaluable as a light layer of warmth and can be used as pyjamas. It can also be very helpful to people who are sensitive to elastic, seams and fastenings, as silk underwear can be worn as a thin layer under other clothes or underwear to insulate or protect sensitive areas. Silk underwear is often sewn with silk thread – a help to people who react to synthetic thread.

There are three basic materials used in silk underwear. One is a smooth knitted jersey fabric which lacks stretch, but which is very silky and smooth next to the skin. The second is a slightly brushed knitted fabric, more like a traditional knitted vest fabric; only women's underwear is available in this type of silk. The third is a more satiny fabric, woven not knitted. Underwear of this fabric is usually more exotic than practical.

In silk jersey underwear (often called ski underwear), you can obtain by mail order a wide range of underwear including vests, leggings, long johns, camisoles, briefs and boxer shorts, women's slips and petticoats and T-shirts. Conoley & Johnson, Myerscough-Jones and Woods of Morecambe sell by mail order women's silk underwear made from slightly brushed knitted fabric. Schmidt Natural Clothing sells silk blend underwear, including a silk/cotton bra top.

Silk nightwear, for men and women, including dressing gowns, is available from Orvis and Patra. David Nieper sell women's satin nightwear and lingerie.

Linen Nightwear

Irish Looms make nightshirts for men and women from totally untreated, unbleached, pure linen. Contact them for stockists.

Sources of Supply

Table 14 gives details of suppliers.

Women's Clothes

Pure cotton clothing for women has become much more widely available over the last few years, as have silk and linen clothes at more reasonable prices. This section first gives advice on finding relatively safe sources of cotton clothing. Details of silk and linen clothing follow at the end of the section.

Cotton Clothing

Some items of clothing can be hard to find in pure cotton, such as cotton swimwear, pure cotton tracksuits, or unusual or stylish fashion clothes. The sources provided are chosen therefore because they sell unusual clothes, as well as being better tolerated by people with allergies and sensitivities.

Of the High Street suppliers, Benetton pure cotton clothes are generally well tolerated, once they have been washed – especially their corduroy, cotton jersey and tracksuit fabric clothes. They are a very useful source for warm winter clothing if you can tolerate nothing but cotton. Mixed reports are received of Marks and Spencer and Laura Ashley cotton clothes, in cotton poplin and drill in particular. Some people tolerate these very well; others find they do not. Proceed with caution!

Table 14: **Suppliers of Underwear and Nightwear**

SUPPLIERS	Men's and Women's	Men's only	Women's only	Formaldehyde-free cotton	Chlorine bleach-free cotton	Cotton jersey underwear	Knitted cotton underwear	Cotton bras	Cotton slips & petticoats	Cotton dressing gowns	Cotton lawn nightgowns	Cotton jersey nightwear	Men's cotton pyjamas	Silk jersey underwear	Women's knitted silk underwear	Silk nightwear	Silk dressing gowns	Silk-cotton bra	Satin underwear	Linen nightgowns
Conoley and Johnson	●					●	●								●					
Cotton On	●			●	●	●						●								
David Nieper			●													●		●		
The Green Catalogue	●			●	●	●														
Irish Looms																				●
Myerscough-Jones	●					●	●								●					
Natural Fibres			●				●													
Nice Irma's	●								●											
Nightingales			●								●									
Nightshift			●									●								
Orvis	●													●		●	●			
Patra	●													●		●	●			
Piklik			●									●								
Playtex			●					●												
Sander & Kay	●													●						
Schmidt Natural Clothing	●			●	●	●						●							●	
Survival Aids	●												●							
Tuttabankam			●								●									
Woods of Morecambe	●					●	●						●		●					

While Next's clothes for children are relatively trouble-free, some of their women's cotton jersey fashions have higher levels of fabric finishes and cause more problems, even after washing. Again, handle with care! Next now sell a range of formaldehyde-free organic clothes.

Look out for soft cotton Indian or Third World fashions, which are usually relatively untreated. Cotton voiles and cotton lawns are also often better tolerated than stiffer cotton drill or poplin.

With all cotton clothing, follow the guidelines in **What to Look For** (page 341) for washing and drying before wearing.

Sources of Supply

Mail order suppliers of cotton clothing for women, are given in Table 15. The mail order catalogues, such as Littlewoods or Grattans, are good sources of cheap pure cotton clothes. Cotton On, Schmidt Natural Clothing, Friends of the Earth, Green Catalogue, Greenpeace, and Natural Fact and Next Directory, are sources of formaldehyde-free and chlorine bleach-free clothes. Friends of the Earth, Greenpeace, Green Catalogue, and Natural Fact and Next Directory, also sell clothes made of organically grown cotton.

For maternity wear, see **Maternity Wear** (page 358).

Silk Clothing

In the High Street, Monsoon has a wide range of silk clothing for women. Next and Wallis also sell silk fashions for women.

By mail order, the supplier with the widest choice of silk clothes at reasonable prices is Patra. For women, their range includes raincoats and suits, as well as blouses. They have silk/cotton blend clothes, and a range of silk jersey T-shirts. One of Gillie's make silk bikinis to order, as well as a range of co-ordinates and dresses. Table 15 gives names of further suppliers of silk clothes.

Linen Clothing

Linen is a natural fibre (sometimes called flax) which is expensive and not very practical in everyday life because it creases easily. It often has fabric finishes when new to prevent creasing, but once washed, loses its finish and some people with allergies and sensitivities tolerate it well. Table 15 gives names of suppliers of linen clothing.

>FABRICS for a source of untreated, unbleached pure linen for dress-making.

Table 15: **Suppliers of Women's Clothing**

SUPPLIERS	Formaldehyde-free cotton	Chlorine bleach-free cotton	Organic cotton	Cotton jersey	Cotton fleece	Cotton corduroy	Cotton voile	Cotton lawn	Indian & Third World cotton	Brushed cotton	Cotton poplin	Cotton outerwear	Cotton swimwear	Knitted cotton sweaters	Silk clothes	Silk swimwear	Linen clothes
Angela Gore				●				●		●							
Angela Knitwear														●			
Bridgedale														●			
Clothkits				●	●	●				●							
Colores										●							
Complete Essentials				●						●				●	●		●
Cotton On	●	●	●														
Cotton Traders				●						●	●						
Edinburgh Woollen Mill														●			
Editions				●			●			●				●	●		
Empire Stores				●	●					●	●			●			
Freemans				●	●					●	●			●			
Friends of the Earth	●	●	●	●					●								
Grattan				●	●					●	●			●			
Great Universal Stores				●	●					●	●			●			
The Green Catalogue	●	●	●	●	●												
Greenpeace	●	●	●	●													
Joan Hollings								●			●						
Kaleidoscope				●						●							
James Meade										●						●	
Kay & Co				●	●					●	●			●			
Littlewoods				●	●					●	●			●			

continued

Table 15: **(continued)**

SUPPLIERS	Formaldehyde-free cotton	Chlorine bleach-free cotton	Organic cotton	Cotton jersey	Cotton fleece	Cotton corduroy	Cotton voile	Cotton lawn	Indian & Third World cotton	Brushed cotton	Cotton poplin	Cotton outerwear	Cotton Swimwear	Knitted cotton sweaters	Silk clothes	Silk swimwear	Linen clothes
Natural Fact	•	•	•	•	•	•											
Natural Fibres				•													
Next Directory	•	•	•	•	•	•					•	•		•	•		•
Nightingales										•	•						
One of Gillie's			•								•		•	•	•		
Orvis											•		•				•
Oxfam Trading									•								
Panache Mail Order									•								
Patra															•		
Paul Costelloe																	•
Penny Plain									•					•			
Racing Green				•	•						•	•	•	•			•
Rainbow Leisure				•										•			
Schmidt Natural Clothing	•	•	•	•													
Selective Marketplace				•			•										
Seymour's Shirts											•				•		
The Silk Road															•		
Traidcraft									•								
Woody				•							•			•			
Workshop						•					•				•		•
You and Yours				•		•					•	•		•			
Zigzag											•						

Addresses of Suppliers

Angela Gore Ltd
Slogarie House
By Castle Douglas DG7 2NL
Tel: 06445 611

Angela Knitwear
Ferndale
Manor Road
Writhlington
Radstock BA3 3LZ
Tel: 0761 433637

Angela Master
2 Shrubbery Grove
Royston
Hertfordshire SG8 9LJ
Tel: 0763 247277

Annie Jo Retail
5 Swan Walk
Thame
Oxford OX9 3HN
Tel: 084421 5431

Aristoc
North Street
Langley Mill
Nottinghamshire NG16 4BT
Tel: 0773 716177

(Manufacturer; contact for
stockists)

Blooming Marvellous
PO Box 12F
Chessington
Surrey KT9 2LB
Tel: 081–391 0338

Bridgedale
First Rate
La Ramee
St Peter Port
Guernsey
Channel Islands
Tel: 0481 710981

Celic Ltd
PO Box 7
Ashburnham Road
Bedford MK40 1DL
Tel: 0234 354811

Clothkits
PO Box 2500
Lewes
East Sussex BN7 3ZB
Tel: 0345 900200

Colures
19 The Oval
Bath
Avon BA2 2HB
Tel: 0225 314115

Complete Essentials
139 Clapham Road
London SW99 1EE
Tel: 0345 900400

Conoley and Johnson
PO Box 309
Leicester
Leicestershire LE5 5NW
Tel: 0533 733622

Cot'n Kids
PO Box 133C
Esher
Surrey KT10 0DH
Tel: 0344 873247

The Cotswold Clothing
Company
The Ridge House
Duns Tew
Oxfordshire OX5 4JL
Tel: 0869 40791

Cotton On
29 North Clifton Street
Lytham
Lancs FY8 5HW
Tel: 0253 736611

Cotton Traders
Kaleidoscope
Admail 50
Leicester LE5 5DL
Tel: 0274 571611

David Nieper
PO Box 14
Somercotes
Derby DE55 4QW
Tel: 0773 836000

Edinburgh Woollen Mill
Trading by Post Ltd
FREEPOST
Waverley Mills
Langholm
Dumfriesshire DG13 0BR
Tel: 03873 80092

Editions
139 Clapham Road
London SW99 0HR
Tel: 0345 900300

Empire Stores
Freepost
Bradford BD99 4YB
Tel: 0924 370144

Fix of Sweden Ltd
95a High Street
Blaina
Gwent NP3 3BN
Tel: 0495 291648

(Manufacturer; contact for
stockists)

Freemans plc
139 Clapham Road
London SW99 0HR
Tel: 071–735 7644

Friends of the Earth
56–58 Alma Street
Luton
Bedfordshire LU1 2YZ
Tel: 0582 482297

Funn Stockings
PO Box 102
Steyning
West Sussex BN44 3DY
Tel: 0903 892841

(Manufacturer; contact for
stockists)

Grattan
Freepost
Bradford
West Yorkshire BD99 2FP
Tel: 0800 333444

Great Universal Stores
Freepost
Royal Avenue
Widnes WA8 7BR
Tel: 0800 838785

The Green Catalogue
3–4 Badgworth Barns
Notting Hill Way
Weare
Axbridge
Somerset BS26 2JU
Tel: 0934 732469

Greenpeace UK
Canonbury Villas
London N1 2PN
Tel: 071–354 5100

Heinz Baby Club
Vinces Road
Diss
Norfolk IP22 3HH
Tel: 0379 651981

Heskia
279 Dover House Road
London SW15 5BP
Tel: 081–788 7747

(Manufacturer; contact for
stockists)

Honeybee
Unit 1B
Tomlins Lane
Gillingham
Dorset SP8 4BH
Tel: 0747 824479

(Manufacturer; contact for
stockists)

Irish Looms Ltd
St Ellen Industrial Estate
Shaw's Bridge
Belfast BT8 8LG
Tel: 0232 491225

James Meade
48 Charlton Road
Andover
Hampshire SP10 3JL
Tel: 0264 333222

Joan Hollings
Leycam
Great Sampford
Saffron Walden
Essex CB10 2RL
Tel: 0799 86 461

Kaleidoscope
Admail 50
Leicester LE5 5DL
Tel: 0274 571611

Kay & Co Ltd
Freepost
Worcester WR1 1BR
Tel: 0905 27141

Kids' Stuff
Tennant House
London Road
Macclesfield
Cheshire SK11 0LW
Tel: 0626 511888

Littlewoods Warehouses Ltd
Staley Avenue
Crosby
Liverpool L70 2TT
Tel: 051–949 1111

Manhattan Kids
Green Lane
Spennymoor
Co Durham DL16 6JF
Tel: 0800 521530

Mothercare Home Shopping
PO Box 145
Watford WD2 5SH
Tel: 0923 210210

MUS
23 Addison Park Mansions
Richmond Way
London W14 0GA
Tel: 071–603 6792

Myerscough-Jones
8 Lonsdale Avenue
Leigh
Lancashire WN7 3UE
Tel: 0942 674836

Natural Fact
30–40 Elcho Street
London SW11 4AU
Tel: 071–228 9652

Natural Fibres
2 Springfield Lane
Smeeton Westerby
Leicester
Tel: 0533 792280

Next Directory
PO Box 299
Leicester LE5 5GH
Tel: 0345 100500

Nice Irma's
Ground Floor
Spring House
Spring Place
London NW5 3BH
Tel: 071–284 3836

Nightingales Ltd
Meadowcroft Mill
Off Bury Road
Rochdale
Lancashire OL11 4AU
Tel: 0706 620919

Nightshift
Little Cambourne Farmhouse
Goudhurst
Kent TN17 1LR
Tel: 0580 211997

One of Gillie's
Llantrithyd
Cowbridge
Glamorgan CF7 7UB
Tel: 0446 781357

The Orvis Co
The Mill
Nether Wallop
Stockbridge
Hampshire SO20 8ES
Tel: 0264 781212

Oxfam Trading
Murdock Road
Bicester
Oxon OX6 7RF
Tel: 0869 245011

Panache Mail Order
16–18 Dock Street
London E1 8JP
Tel: 071–481 8769

Patra
1–5 Nant Road
London NW2 2AL
Tel: 081–209 1112

Paul Costelloe
Moygashel
Dungannon
Co Tyrone
Northern Ireland BT71 7PB
Tel: 086 87 22291

(Manufacturer; contact for
stockists)

Penny Plain
10 Marlborough Crescent
Newcastle-upon-Tyne NE1 4EE
Tel: 091–232 1124

Pex
Palma Group PLC
577 Ayleston Road
Leicester LE2 8TD
Tel: 0533 833461

(Manufacturer; contact for
stockists)

Piklik
30 Buckingham Palace Road
London SW1 0RE
Tel: 071–931 9941

Playtex Ltd
Industrial Estate
Port Glasgow
Renfrewshire PA14 5UY
Tel: 0475 41631
(Manufacturer; contact for
stockists)

Racing Green
Spring Mill
Earby
Colne
Lancashire BB8 6RN
Tel: 0282 443332

Rainbow Leisure
92A Elm Grove
Hayling Island
Hants PO11 9EH
Tel: 0705 469382

Sander and Kay
101–113 Scrubs Lane
London NW10 6QU
Tel: 081–969 3553

Sara-Jane Brown
Bank House
Longden
Shrewsbury
Shropshire SY5 8ES
Tel: 0743 860319

Schmidt Natural Clothing
155 Tuffley Lane
Gloucester
Gloucestershire GL4 0NZ
Tel: 0452 416016

Selective Marketplace
Bolton Road West
Loughborough
Leicestershire LE11 0XL
Tel: 0509 235235

Seymour's Shirts
S Seymour & Co Ltd
136 Sunbridge Road
Bradford BD1 2QG
Tel: 0274 726520

Sheila Stewart
97 Danes Drive
Scotstown
Glasgow G14 9EW
Tel: 041–959 7030

The Silk Road
20 Fountainhall Road
Edinburgh EH9 2NN
Tel: 031–667 3470

Stimmer
5–6 The Ivories
Northampton Street
Islington
London N1 2HY
Tel: 071–226 7246
(Manufacturer; contact for
stockists)

Survival Aids Ltd
Morland
Penrith
Cumbria CA10 3AZ
Tel: 09314 444

Traidcraft
Kingsway
Gateshead NE11 ONE
Tel: 091–491 0855

Tuttabankem
Loddington Hall
Loddington
Leicester LE7 9X2
Tel: 057 286 332

Woods of Morecambe
42 Queen Street
Morecambe
Lancs LA4 5EL
Tel: 0524 412101

Woody
Hawkshead Countrywear
Main StreetHawkshead Village
Cumbria LA22 0NT
Tel: 05394 34000

Workshop
2 Lawrence Street
Cheyne Walk
London SW3 5NB
Tel: 071–351/6108/3478

You and Yours
Anchor House
Ingleby Road
Bradford
West Yorkshire BD99 2XG
Tel: 0274 577411

Zigzag Designer Knitwear
Riverford Mill
Stewarton
Ayrshire KA3 5DH
Tel: 0560 85187

Cosmetics, Toiletries and Skincare

This section covers products and toiletries used on skin, body and hair for cosmetic, grooming and beauty purposes.

For emollients and moisturisers used for medical purposes, >MEDICAL HELP. For basic daily care and personal hygiene products, >PERSONAL HYGIENE. For babycare products, >BABYCARE.

Basic Advice

Cosmetics, toiletries and skincare products cause reactions by contact and by inhaling. They are common causes of sensitive skin, asthma and itchy eyes. They can also cause nasal symptoms, headaches, and wider symptoms such as joint and muscle aches and mental symptoms (>SYMPTOMS).

A wide range of chemical ingredients in grooming and beauty products cause sensitivity and allergy, the most common being perfumes and preservatives. Natural plant extracts or oils are no less allergenic than synthetic chemicals and are not automatically safer.

Hypoallergenic (low-allergen) products exclude the most allergenic substances. This does not mean that they are totally safe, but the major sensitisers are absent and most people tolerate them well.

Sensitivity to skincare products is highly idiosyncratic. You may not be able to tolerate one brand of products, but could tolerate another brand, or selected products within a range, quite well. If you react to a hypoallergenic product, do not therefore assume that you will react to any low-allergen product or brand. Try another with care and see how you go.

If you want to know how medical treatments can help you cope, >MEDICAL HELP. >CHEMICALS for full information on chemical sensitivity.

If you know that you are sensitive to cosmetic and skincare products, your best advice for avoidance is to:

● Use unperfumed products where possible

- Try low-allergen products (details below) until you find some that suit you
- Use as few products on your skin, hair and body as you feel able to. Reducing the load will help your system cope
- Use perfume, cologne or aftershave as seldom as possible

If you suspect that you are sensitive to cosmetic and skincare products and want to find out,

Either
- Switch to low-allergen products and see if you see any improvement

or
- Reduce the amount that you use or cut out certain products

or
- Stop using products altogether for one week. Use low- allergen soap and shampoo only (>PERSONAL HYGIENE), then reintroduce products one by one, at intervals of at least a day and preferably one a week. Use either your previous products, or low-allergen brands. Monitor any symptoms carefully.

Caution
You may feel worse before you get better when you stop using things you have used regularly. This is a form of withdrawal and new symptoms can result (>SYMPTOMS).

You can also use the Sniff Test and the Patch Test (see pages 88) to test a small amount of product to see if it upsets you. If you want more detailed advice about sensitivity to cosmetics, toiletries and skincare products, >page 378.

TIP

> Avoid using *fragrance-free* products if you are very sensitive to perfume. These are legally allowed to contain one perfume, usually for the purpose of masking the smells of other ingredients. Use *unperfumed* products in preference – these cannot contain any perfume at all.

High Street Brands

The following are hypoallergenic brands of skin, body and haircare products which are widely available in High Street shops. These brands are well tolerated by many people with allergies and hypersensitivity. Simple produce hair, skin and body products but no make-up products. Clinique and RoC include suncare products and a wide choice of skin products in their ranges. Contact the manufacturers directly if you want to know more about their products.

Almay
225 Bath Road
Slough
Bucks SL1 4AU
Tel: 0753 523971

Boots No 7 Pure Care
Boots plc
1 Thane Road West
Nottingham NG2 3AA
Tel: 0602 506111

Clinique Laboratories
54 Grosvenor Street
London W1X 0EU
Tel: 071–499 9305

RoC
Laboratoires RoC UK
13 Grosvenor Crescent
London SW1X 7EE
Tel: 071–823 9223

Sensiq
17 Cavendish Square
London W1M 0HE
Tel: 071–409 1413

Simple
Smith and Nephew
Allum Rock Road
Allum Rock
Birmingham B8 3DZ
Tel: 021–327 4750

Mail Order Suppliers

The following are specialist mail order suppliers of skin, body and hair products. Allerayde and The Allergy Shop have chosen their products especially for people with allergies and can give you advice on which to choose. The others sell products which people with allergies have reported to be relatively trouble free. Crimpers sell hair products only.

The Allergy Shop and Cosmetics to Go sell a small number of products which have absolutely no preservatives. They need to be kept in the fridge to prevent mould and bacteria growth and have a limited life.

Allerayde
147 Victoria Centre
Nottingham
Notts NG1 3QF
Tel: 0602 240983

The Allergy Shop
PO Box 196
Haywards Heath
West Sussex RH16 3YF
Tel: 0444 414290

Blackmore's Laboratories
Natural Health Products
Unit 7
Poyle Tech Centre
Willow Road
Poyle
Slough
Bucks SL3 0PD
Tel: 0753 683815

Cosmetics to Go
24 High Street
Poole
Dorset BH15 1AB
Tel: 0800 373366

Crimpers
63–67 Heath Street
Hampstead
London NW3 6UG
Tel: 071–794 8625

Faith Products
Unit 5
Kay Street
Bury
Lancs BL9 6BU
Tel: 061–764 2555

Honeycomb Cosmetics
Old Acres Farm
Stour Provost
Gillingham
Dorset SP8 5LT
Tel: 0747 85373

Natural Beauty
Western Avenue
Bridgend Industrial Estate
Mid Glamorgan CF31 3RT
Tel: 0656 766566

Read on if you would like more detailed information on cosmetics and skincare, such as:

- What causes problems
- How to detect allergy or sensitivity
- How to avoid trouble

What Causes Problems?

A wide range of chemical ingredients in cosmetics and skincare products can cause allergy or sensitivity. To know more about what chemical sensitivity is and likely symptoms, >CHEMICALS.

The most common causes are:

- Perfumes and fragrances
- Preservatives
- Hair dyes
- Lanolin

Perfumes and fragrances most frequently cause sensitivity to cosmetics, toiletries and skincare products. Perfumes, aftershaves and colognes are themselves common sensitisers. If you react to any products (for instance, soap, hair gels, bath lotions, hairspray or make-up), the most likely cause will be perfume added to disguise the smell of ingredients. Natural oils used as fragrances (such as cinnamic alcohol or musk ambrette) are known sensitisers and allergens. Musk ambrette, commonly used in aftershaves, is a known photoallergen, causing reactions under certain conditions of sunlight (>**FURTHER READING**) Look for unperfumed products wherever possible. This move alone may solve any problems you have with toiletries.

Preservatives are also known to sensitise, especially chemicals known as the parabens. Preservatives are necessary to give any product shelf-life. Without them, products would grow mould and bacteria within a few days. For people with sensitive skin, some preservatives are more likely to cause reactions than others when used on already inflamed skin, but are virtually hypoallergenic when used on areas not already sensitised. Therefore they continue to be used in many hypoallergenic products, although it is known that they can sensitise.

It is virtually impossible to avoid preservatives if you use grooming and beauty products. To avoid problems with preservatives, do not apply products directly to areas of highly inflamed skin unless you absolutely have to.

The Allergy Shop and Cosmetics To Go (addresses above) sell a small selection of preservative-free products.

TIP

If you know you are sensitive to a specific chemical, you can identify products which do not contain it by using the National Eczema Society's database of ingredients (address in **CHARITIES**).

Among hair products, permanent hair dyes are the commonest cause of allergy. They often contain a highly allergenic chemical, PPDA. You should always follow the advice on the packet of these dyes to patch-test behind the ear or on the forearm 24–48 hours before using. If a hairdresser is to apply the dye for you, make sure that you patch-test 24–48 hours before the appointment. Semi-permanent dyes and temporary rinses are also known to cause reactions. Henna, a vegetable dye, is not reported to cause allergic eczema or dermatitis, but can cause sneezing, nasal symptoms and asthma.

If you bleach your hair, ammonium persulphate is added to hydrogen peroxide to speed up the process. Ammonium persulphate is highly irritant and has been reported to cause immediate reactions such as facial swelling, asthma and hives. Irritant eczema can also result if the solution is left on too long.

Permanent wave solutions are known to cause reactions, but the cause is most usually the perfume used to disguise the unpleasant smell of the ingredients. The ingredients of the waving solution and neutralisers themselves can sometimes irritate and cause allergy. Alkaline solutions (for home and salon use, with ammonium thioglycolate as the waving solution) are reported to cause reactions less often than acid solutions (using glyceryl thioglycolate – salon use only) or sulfite wave (using sodium sulfite – home use only).

Lanolin is a natural fatty substance obtained from the fleece of sheep. It is a complex material, the chemical composition of which varies greatly in purity; and the reaction of people with allergy or sensitivity varies correspondingly to different brands or preparations. It is commonly found in cosmetic products such as cleansers, ointments, hand creams, soaps, lipsticks and hair products. People sensitive to lanolin can sometimes tolerate one lanolin preparation but not another. Some cosmetic brands and moisturisers are either lanolin-free or use new purified lanolin which is often better tolerated. To avoid problems, use hypoallergenic brands, try different brands to find one that suits, and write to the manufacturer if necessary to find lanolin-free products in their range.

Other ingredients known to cause sensitivity and allergy include resins in nail polishes, some dyes used in blushers and lipsticks, and propylene glycol which acts as a solvent and preservative, and keeps products moist. It is also an ingredient in lubricating jelly (>SEX AND CONTRACEPTION).

How to Detect Allergy and Sensitivity

The most reliable way to detect if cosmetics and skincare products are causing you problems is to *stop using them altogether* for at least one week and see if any improvement results. During that period, use only the minimum of basic personal hygiene products (>PERSONAL HYGIENE). Put the things you regularly use away in a box or cupboard so that you do not inhale the ingredients.

You may feel worse and have a few new symptoms (for instance, headaches, muscle aches, sometimes nausea) for the first few days when you stop using products. This is withdrawal as the chemicals clear from your body. Some people do not notice any withdrawal symptoms at all, while others can feel quite ill for a few days.

Monitor any symptoms for the week that you do not use products, allowing for withdrawal. If you experience improvement, either continue not using the products or reintroduce them one at a time, not more than one a day, preferably one per week, and see if any change in symptoms results.

If total abstinence is too radical a step for you, then you can try either not using one product for a week and then reintroducing it; or switching to a hypoallergenic alternative and trying it for a while. These are often more tolerable approaches and less disruptive, but they can give you misleading results and some people find that they end up taking more time and effort than a short, sharp programme.

TIP

Before trying any new product, use the Sniff Test (page 88) or the Patch Test (page 88) to see if the product upsets you.

Rather than buying a product before patch-testing, ask the shop assistant to apply a sample for you from a product or apply a patch from samples on display.

You can also write to manufacturers or suppliers to ask for samples to test.

Avoiding Trouble

If you are exceptionally sensitive, you may not be able to wear even low-allergen products (details on page 375). You may have to avoid toiletries and cosmetics altogether. It can be very difficult to have to give up something that is a source of self-esteem or pleasure, and can be a hard decision. On the other hand, total abstinence may be your only route to being well.

If you know you react to skincare products, have done all you can to avoid things yourself, yet are still having problems, the source may well be other people's products. You can react to these by inhaling them, or by contact with them. This can be a real problem at work, or in public places where people gather – such as pubs, shops, cinemas and clubs. If you feel ill after a sports activity, it may well be because of other people's bodycare products.

Eczema or asthma in babies and children can often be caused by products that parents or siblings wear, or those worn by a childminder, babysitter or relative caring for them, classmates at school, or teachers. Teenagers' problems could perhaps be caused by a boyfriend's or girlfriend's toiletries.

Dealing with other people's products is a tricky area. Within the family, you may have to negotiate and agree that everyone wears products that the person with allergies or sensitivity can tolerate, at least within the home. With a childminder or relative carer, you may have to agree on products they can wear. At work or school, you may be able to negotiate so that people close to you or your child use less of the things that upset you, or use products that are tolerable.

If your work involves considerable exposure to things that upset you, it may not be possible for you to continue with it (>MEDICAL HELP). Most situations will be beyond your control and you will have to find ways of minimising your exposure.

TIP

If you go to the barber's or hairdresser's, go at a time when the place is relatively empty and free of substances first thing in the morning, or early in the week. Take your own products if necessary. Or get a hairdresser to come to your home.

At a cinema, theatre or concert, sit at the end of a row or at the back or front, so that you are not totally surrounded by other people. Arrive as late as you can.

Ask people coming to your home not to wear perfumes, after-shave, hair gels or sprays or other perfumed products.

Carry a handkerchief or scarf with you. Place over your nose and breathe through it if you have to go into places where perfume and cosmetic smells are intense.

In pubs, clubs or at parties try to move near a door, windows or fan ventilation so that you are breathing cleaner air.

Fabrics

If you want to know what materials you react to, you are best advised to start with FIBRES where basic advice on materials, and on detecting allergy and sensitivity, is given.

This section focuses on finding tolerable fabrics for people who are chemically sensitive and have to avoid synthetic fibres and chemical treatments. It gives information on what to look for, and sources of hard-to-find materials.

There follows advice on choosing fabrics for:

- Furnishing
- Dressmaking
- Household linens and general use

Furnishing Fabrics

If you are exceptionally sensitive to synthetic fibres, you may have to avoid using them in curtains, furnishings and upholstery. Your choices then come down to pure cotton, wool, linen or silk. Pure cotton is for most people the best choice, for reasons of cost, practicality and the fact that it is usually washable. However, pure cotton furnishing fabrics are commonly treated with three types of chemical finishes which can cause sensitivity:

- Formaldehyde resins
- Fire retardant treatments
- Stain resistant finishes

Dyes and other fabric treatments rarely cause reactions.

Formaldehyde resins protect the fabric against stains, grease, water and creasing. They restrict dyes fading, and improve the feel and body of the fabric. Formaldehyde is a common sensitiser and irritant.

Most major manufacturers of pure cotton furnishing fabrics in the UK apply fire retardant finishes to most or all their fabrics. Fire retardant treatments are of two basic kinds. The first, more common, are proprietary chemicals applied to cotton fabrics at the final stage of production. Two of the most widely used in the UK, Pyrovatex and Proban, release formaldehyde and have been known sometimes to cause irritation and reactions. The second kind of fire retardant treatment is to apply a thin backing layer of a rubber-like chemical.

Stain resistant treatments are not so widely applied to cotton fabrics. The fabric is usually labelled with a proprietary name, or is called 'stain-resistant'.

TIP

If you are not sure whether you react to fabric finishes on a piece of fabric, you can use the Iron Test to help you find out (see page 346). You can do this on a sample of fabric before you buy it to see if you react.

If you want to find out whether Pyrovatex, Proban, other chemicals or back coating have been applied to any fabric you want to buy, ring the fabric manufacturers to find out. They are invariably courteous and helpful.

Pure wool fabrics are not treated with formaldehyde resins, nor with fire retardant chemicals since they meet fire safety regulations without treatment. They are sometimes treated with stain protection chemicals. Wool furnishing fabric may therefore be a good option for the chemically sensitive, if you are confident you do not react to wool.

TIP

If you are very sensitive to fabric treatments and synthetics, and are allergic to cotton and wool, wooden shutters or roller blinds of wood, rushes or paper may be an alternative to curtains.

Wooden shutters without varnish or paint finish are made by:

The London Shutter Company
St. Martin's Stables
Windsor Road
Ascot
Berkshire SL5 7AF
Tel: 0344 28385

Blinds of wood, rush and paper are sold by Habitat.

Fabric roller blinds are sprayed with stiffening chemicals which can cause reactions. Avoid blinds or only use after airing off for a while.

Using Untreated Fabrics

It is possible to obtain untreated pure cotton furnishing fabrics. These are mostly fabrics from India where chemical treatments are less applied. Sources for these are given below. Some of these fabrics are washable. There is no problem at all about using these untreated fabrics for curtains, soft furnishings or bedding under fire safety regulations. You can also use them for upholstered furniture, but you need to take care to comply with the fire safety regulations.

New upholstery

For new upholstery, untreated pure cotton furnishing fabric does not pass a fire safety test known as the match test; but it can be used to upholster furniture, provided that the furniture on which it is used contains a fire-resistant interliner. This interliner can be of pure cotton fabric but it has to be treated to meet the regulations.

The fire-retardant chemicals used on interliner fabrics, are known to be less irritant than Pyrovatex or Proban. Some manufacturers of cotton interliner use water soluble phosphate salts which do not cause sensitivity but can irritate. Others use proprietary chemicals which bind and adhere to the fabric. None of these chemicals is 100 per cent free of reports of reactions, but reports are very rare. The interliner cotton fabric is covered by a layer of upholstery fabric and hence is:

- Not directly in contact with your skin
- Less freely inhaled

Most chemically sensitive people will have no problems with this combination.

For new upholstered furniture, therefore, the best solution to meet fire safety regulations for the chemically sensitive is to use either:

- Wool fabrics since they meet regulations without treatment
- Untreated pure cotton fabric with a fire-resistant interliner underneath

Re-upholstering Old Furniture

The fire safety regulations for fabric fire resistance do not apply to the sale or re-upholstery of furniture made before 1950. You can therefore buy older (pre-1950) or antique furniture covered in totally untreated materials, re-upholster yourself or have such furniture re-upholstered in untreated materials of your choice.

Contact the Association of Master Upholsterers for specialists in

upholstery who may be able to help (address on page 387). >FURNI-
TURE for further advice on upholstering furniture.

Sources of Supply

Table 16 gives sources of supply of relatively safe pure cotton furnishing fabrics. The companies listed will send samples and will supply by
mail order.

Dressmaking Fabrics

Information is given in Table 16 on sources of supply of untreated cotton fabrics, untreated linen, and of silk fabrics and wadding for dressmaking. >CLOTHING for full advice on how to choose safer alternatives
in fibres for clothing. Suppliers given in Table 16 will send samples
and supply by mail order.

Cotton corduroy and pure cotton jersey for dressmaking are available in many High Street fabric shops. Wash before sewing to remove
any fabric treatments.

The Silk Association of Great Britain can provide further addresses
of suppliers of silk fabrics and yarns (address on page 388).

Household Linens and General Use

Limericks Linens sell by mail order a range of fabrics for making up
sheets or household linens. They can supply by the metre:

- Unbleached cottons and sheeting
- Terry towelling
- Irish linen
- Hessian
- Linen tea towelling

Limericks also sell for household use:

- Cotton dishcloths
- Cotton stockinette
- Linen window cleaners
- Calico ironing board covers
- Butter muslin
- Cheesecloth

MacCulloch and Wallis and Russell and Chapple (addresses on page
388) sell untreated calico and butter muslin.

We cannot track down any supplier of silk sheeting fabric. Contact

Table 16: **Sources of Supply for Fabrics**

SUPPLIERS	Untreated Indian cottons for furnishing	Furnishing silks	Untreated cotton calico	Dressmaking silks	Untreated linen	Indian cottons for dress-making	Butter muslin	Silk wadding	Household fabrics
Allans				●					
Conran Shop	●								
Irish Looms					●				
P N Jones Trading	●	●		●		●			
Limericks Linens			●				●		●
MacCulloch and Wallis			●	●			●		
Ian Mankin	●								
Nice Irma's	●								
Parisienne Fabrics				●					
Pongees				●					
Russell and Chapple			●				●		
Silks for Handspinners								●	

TIP

Wash all fabrics before handling or making up to remove fabric treatments as much as possible.

---

any of the silk suppliers in Table 16 or the Silk Association of Great Britain for details of wide-width silks.

Addresses of Suppliers

Allans of Duke Street
56–8 Duke Street
London W1M 6HS
Tel: 071–629 3781

Association of Master Upholsterers
Unit One, Clyde Road Works
Clyde Road, Wallington
Surrey SM6 8PZ
Tel: 081–773 8069

The Conran Shop
Michelin House
81 Fulham Road
London SW3 6RD
Tel: 071–589 7401

Ian Mankin
109 Regents Park Road
London NW1 8UR
Tel: 071–722 0997

Irish Looms Ltd
St Ellen Industrial Estate
Shaw's Bridge
Belfast BT8 8LG
Tel: 0232 491225

Limericks Linens
Hayle
Cornwall TR27 6BR
Tel: 0736 756054

MacCulloch and Wallis
25–6 Dering Street
London W1R 0BH
Tel: 071–629 0311

Nice Irma's
Ground Floor
Spring House
Spring Place
London NW5 3BH
Tel: 071–284 3836

Parisienne Fabrics
4 Worsbrough Hall
Worsbrough
South Yorkshire S70 5LN
Tel: 0226 299358

P N Jones Trading
18 Holly Grove
Peckham Rye
London SE15 5DG
Tel: 071–639 2113

Pongees
184–186 Old Street
London EC1V 9BP
Tel: 071–253 0428

Russell and Chapple
23 Monmouth Street
London WC2H 9DE
Tel: 071–836 7521

The Silk Association of Great
Britain
c/o Rheinbergs
Morley Road
Tonbridge
Kent TN9 1RN
Tel: 0732 361357

Silks for Handspinners
The Mill
Tregoyd Mill
Three Cocks
Brecon
Powys LD3 0SW
Tel: 0497 847421

Face Masks

Face masks come in three basic kinds:

- dust masks
- activated carbon masks
- respirators

which give varying degrees of protection against inhaled particles and chemical fumes.

You can use face masks to protect you in situations where you are unavoidably exposed to things which upset you – doing dusty tasks, vacuuming or household cleaning, doing DIY or car maintenance, at work, riding a bike, or even when driving a car (>TRAVEL).

Dust Masks

Dust masks are the simplest of all masks. They do not protect against chemical vapours, but will protect to some extent against irritant dusts and particles. The most common type, found in DIY shops, has a pure cotton gauze filter pad held in place across the nose by a light aluminium face-piece. Another type, also found in DIY shops, made of a cotton/synthetic blend, is a moulded white mask.

No guarantee is given of the size or type of particle which these masks keep out. Dust masks are not helpful in protecting against most chemical vapours, but they do offer some (but not total) protection against dusts, and against allergens such as house dust mites, moulds and animal allergens.

They are cheaper than other masks (£1–2 at 1992 prices) and unless you are very highly sensitive to inhalant allergens, such as house dust mites, they will offer you sufficient protection to allow you to do most tasks.

These masks are widely available at DIY stores or by post from Safety Equipment Centre (address on page 391). Safety Equipment Centre has a small-order charge for orders less than £25.

Activated Carbon Masks

Activated carbon masks come in various designs but all combine a fibre layer or web which will trap particles, and activated charcoal which absorbs a wide range of gases and vapours. They are designed to fit well around the nose, mouth and cheekbones to seal the areas where air can enter. They will protect against both small particles and chemical vapours.

One of the most effective is made by 3M. It is made of a dense synthetic fibre web which traps particles effectively, and activated charcoal filter media within the fibre web. It is one of the most effective, and light and relatively comfortable to wear. It will not protect 100 per cent against chemicals and particles, and if you are extremely sensitive to synthetic fibres, you may react to the fibres of the mask, but reactions of this kind are rare and most people find it useful. The mask will need replacing every six months, or more often if you use it intensively. The 3M mask costs around £5–6 at 1992 prices and is available by post from Allerayde or The British Lung Foundation. A similar mask by Pirelli is available from Safety Equipment Centre. (Addresses on page 391.)

TIP

One solution, if you react to contact with the materials of a face mask, is to line the inside of the mask with a pure cotton handkerchief or cotton muslin nappy, or with a silk scarf if you are sensitive to cotton. This helps protect skin in contact.

More expensive versions of charcoal filter masks are made by Respro. One version, the Respro Bandit (£10–12), is a 100 per cent cotton scarf with a nose clip, which incorporates a charcoal filter, laminated into the scarf. It is chemically treated to be fully washable; if you are exceptionally sensitive, you may react to the treatment. Wash it before use to try and avoid problems. The scarf looks more attractive than a nose and face mask, however, and may be more comfortable.

Respro also make the City Pollution Mask at £20 with a replaceable charcoal filter, which has a stretchable fitting to fit comfortably around the face. This fitting is made of neoprene, with a lycra lining, which again may upset you if you are exceptionally sensitive to synthetic rubber and elastomers.

Both Respro products are available from The Green Catalogue and Renaissance Design (addresses below).

Respirators

If you want to go further, you can obtain respirators which are designed for working with toxic fumes in construction and manufacturing industries. These have replaceable charcoal filters designed to take out a wide range of chemicals, and you can choose the filter medium which suits you best. The Safety Equipment Centre have a full range. The Sussex 300 is one of the cheapest and simplest. The face piece is made of low-allergen rubber – less likely to cause reactions than other types of rubber, although it still may upset you. The Sussex 300 costs about £12, and its cartridges are £2–3 each, before postage and packing. If you work with chemicals each day, a respirator of this kind could be valuable, as long as you are able to tolerate the face-piece.

Sources of Supply

Allerayde
147 Victoria Centre
Nottingham NG1 3QF
Tel: 0602 240893

British Lung Foundation
8 Peterborough Mews
London SW6 3BL
Tel: 071–371 7704

The Green Catalogue
Badgworth Barns
Notting Hill Way
Weare
Axbridge
Somerset BS26 2JU
Tel: 0934 732469

Renaissance Designs
28 South Island Place
London SW9 0DX
Tel: 071–587 3663

Safety Equipment Centre
11–15 Bridge Street
Huddersfield
West Yorkshire HD4 6EL
Tel: 0484 537730

First Aid and Home Medicine

You can deal effectively with most domestic mishaps and ailments, and ease allergic reactions, with a medicine cupboard that contains:

- sodium bicarbonate
- salt
- cream of magnesia liquid
- paracetamol
- cotton wool, lint, plasters and bandages
- an icepack
- a hot water bottle
- boiled, cooled water

There are a few more things you can add if you want to (or borrow from the kitchen cupboard), but basically that's all you need!

Here is advice on what you can use without causing sensitivity reactions (if used with care) in the following situations:

- allergy turn-off
- antiseptics
- athlete's foot and other fungal infections
- bandages and dressings
- blocked noses
- boils and infections
- bruising and sprains
- burns and scalds
- catarrh
- cuts and grazes
- cystitis
- diarrhoea
- earache
- eyewash
- fever
- head colds
- head lice
- indigestion relief
- inflammation of joints
- insect repellent
- insect stings
- laxatives
- mouthwash
- nappy rash
- painkillers
- period pains and PMT
- piles
- rashes and itchy skin
- shock
- sinusitis
- spots and pimples
- sore throats and coughs
- sunburn
- toothache
- wind

>CHEMICALS if you want to know more about what specific chemicals to avoid and why.

If you are on a low-salt diet, be careful throughout and consult your doctor about taking sodium and other salts by mouth.

Allergy Turn-Off

You can relieve the effects of a strong reaction by taking alkali salts. This works for food intolerance and chemical sensitivity, as well as for allergy. In a reaction, the environment in the body becomes acid; alkali salts neutralise the reaction and can relieve its effects, or even stop them dead. The simplest way to take these is to dissolve a teaspoon of sodium bicarbonate in a glass of water and drink it.

Some people find that sodium bicarbonate on its own does not suit them as well as other mixtures of alkali salts. You could also try the following mixtures; ask your pharmacist to mix them for you:

- *Sodium and potassium salts*
  Mix two parts sodium bicarbonate to one part potassium bicarbonate. Dissolve one teaspoonful in a glass of water.

- *Tri-salts*
  Mix three parts sodium bicarbonate to two parts potassium bicarbonate and one part calcium carbonate. Dissolve one teaspoonful in a glass of water.

The salts mixtures can be laxative. Do not take more than three times a day, and preferably only once a day. Consult your doctor if you are on a low-salt diet before using.

Vitamin C also helps relieve reactions. Take a teaspoon in a glass of water. You can also add a teaspoon of vitamin C to a glass of any of the alkali salts mixtures above. Ask your pharmacist for pure vitamin C powder (ascorbic acid).

Some people find that taking a salts mixture regularly each day helps to deter and control reactions. This could be worth trying as a controlling measure.

You can obtain sodium bicarbonate and vitamin C powder by post from:

Green Farm Foodwatch
Burwash Common
East Sussex TN19 7LX
Tel: 0435 882482

If you have an attack of nettle rash (hives or urticaria), or other local skin reactions, bathing the area in an alkaline solution will help relieve the discomfort. Use Boots Cream of Magnesia Liquid; Boots own brand does not contain flavourings, or bathe the skin with a solution of alkali salts.

TIP

To help control reactions, avoid extremes of heat and cold, or sudden big swings in temperature, as these can trigger reactions. Also avoid getting too hungry, as this can trigger reactions. Avoid swings, or excessive highs or lows, in blood sugar levels.

Antiseptics

The best way to disinfect a cut or wound is to bathe it in a sterile solution of salt (saline). The easiest way to do this is to take a cup of boiled, cooled water and dissolve a teaspoon of salt in it, then wash the wound gently with a clean or sterile dressing. This is a very effective antiseptic.

For convenience, you can buy from a pharmacy sterile saline solution in sachets (Normasol or Steripod). These are handy for first aid kits, for workplace or school, or for travelling.

TIP

Be careful to use water (for solutions or for drinking) which you tolerate well. You can be sensitive to tapwater, and this may make you react when you use it for medicinal purposes. Use filtered, mineral or distilled water if you are not sure, and >WATER AND WATER FILTERS for full advice.

Boric acid, dissolved in boiled, cooled water, can be used as a stronger antiseptic. It should not be used on young children, nor on broken skin. You should consult your doctor or pharmacist before using it.

Calendula, a homeopathic ointment or tincture, is antiseptic. Some allergy sufferers tolerate it well. Patch Test (>CHEMICALS) or use with care, to see if you tolerate it.

If you have a persistent infection or sepsis in a cut or wound, you should always consult a doctor.

Athlete's Foot and Other Fungal Infections

Bathing the site of athlete's foot or other fungal infections in a solution of potassium permanganate will help cure it. Ask your pharmacist for advice on dosage.

You can react allergically to the fungus itself, and this can aggravate the symptoms. Removing the infection as above will relieve this.

Bandages and Dressings

Use pure cotton wool balls, cotton buds and dressings wherever possible if you are chemically sensitive, or have sensitive skin. Many brands of cotton wool are not 100 per cent pure cotton, but a cotton/viscose blend.

Use absorbent pure cotton lint for a padded dressing for a cut or wound. Secure with low allergen (hypoallergenic) dressing tape; Micropore or Dermicel tape are usually well tolerated.

Use pure cotton gauze bandages when you need a bandage. Avoid elasticated bandages unless you know you do not react to elastic or rubber.

For simple plasters, Boots Clear Washproof Plasters are well tolerated by people with sensitive skin, or allergies. Micropore, Elastoplast and Band Aid also make low-allergen (hypoallergenic) plasters.

Blocked Noses, Sinusitis, Catarrh and Head Colds

The symptoms of blocked noses, sinusitis, catarrh and head colds can all be relieved by a simple steam inhalation. Fill a bowl or jug with very hot water (not boiling to avoid scalds). Place a towel over your head and breathe in steadily over the bowl for a few minutes. This should loosen and ease the blocked passages.

Saline nose drops dilute the secretions of the nasal passages and help relieve nasal symptoms. Use a sterile saline solution (as described in **Antiseptics**, above, boiled, cooled water plus a teaspoonful of salt, or buy Normasol or Steripod sachets); place a few drops in each nostril.

Ice cubes held on sore and inflamed sinuses can bring relief.

Use a menthol or plant oil inhalation (such as Karvol) only if you are not chemically sensitive and not sensitive to plant terpenes

(>PLANTS AND TREES for further information). Add a spoonful or a capsule to hot, but not boiling, water and inhale the vapour.

Boils and Infections

For boils, or infected spots or scabs, a dressing of magnesium sulphate paste will help to bring out and ease the infection. First wash the area with cooled boiled water and cotton wool. Apply a covering layer of paste, and cover with a pure cotton dressing secured with low-allergy adhesive tape (Micropore or Dermicel).

A hot water bottle held on the site of infection, once covered with dressing, can also speed recovery by increasing blood flow to the infected area. See a doctor if infection persists.

TIP

If you are sensitive to rubber or plastics, use an old-fashioned ceramic hot water bottle. Search in attics, or junk shops, or see page 180 for manufacturer.

Bruising and Sprains

Apply an ice pack to bruises and sprains to reduce swelling. If you are sensitive to soft plastics, place ice cubes in a plastic bag and wrap it in a cloth or pillowcase to mask it. You could also use a bag of frozen vegetables wrapped in a cloth or pillowcase.

Witch Hazel is a natural plant extract that is astringent and eases bruising and swelling. It can cause sensitivity reactions, but if you tolerate it, it is very useful. Sniff it gently in the pharmacy before buying; if you feel unwell on inhaling, or strongly dislike the smell, do not use it. Apply liberally to a cloth and hold it to the site of bruises and sprains.

Burns and Scalds

Cool the area of the burn or scald to relieve pain. Keep the burned area in cold water or hold it under a cold running tap until the pain stops, or for at least 10 minutes. Do not prick or burst any blisters, or apply any ointment or lotion.

If the burn or scald is serious, seek emergency medical help. If the burn or scald is superficial, but rubs against clothing, cover it with a dressing of pure cotton lint and secure it with a cotton bandage. Do not use fluffy cotton wool.

Cuts and Grazes

Clean cuts and grazes and disinfect following the advice in **Antiseptics** (page 394). Leave open to the air unless it is a large or deep wound. Use plasters or dressings, if necessary, following the advice in **Bandages and Dressings** (page 395).

Cystitis

Drinking alkali salts can ease the symptoms of cystitis. Dissolve a teaspoon of sodium bicarbonate in a glass of water and drink it. Consult your doctor if you are on a low-salt diet.

Diarrhoea

Taking arrowroot will stop diarrhoea very effectively. You can buy this as a powder at a pharmacy and make a paste by adding water. Consult your pharmacist to get the right dosage.

If you need rehydration salts after severe diarrhoea, do not take any of the proprietary ready-mixed products which can cause reactions. Rehydration salts are a mixture of sodium and potassium salts, and glucose in the right ratio; ask a pharmacist to mix these for you.

Earache

If you tolerate olive oil, warm a teaspoonful of it. Drop it into the ear, then close the earhole with pure cotton wool.

An alternative to this is sodium bicarbonate BPC, which is available in an eardrop solution.

Eyewash

For sore and itchy eyes, use a sterile saline solution to ease the itchiness. Either make a solution yourself, as in **Antiseptics** (page 394) or buy Normasol or Steripod in sachets from a pharmacist. Bathe the eyes with the solution in an eyebath, or put a few drops into the eye with a dropper.

Fever

Aspirin sensitivity is common, so avoid it. Use paracetamol BP to reduce fever. It is well tolerated by people with allergies and sensitivities, and reduces high fever effectively. Most allergics tolerate ordinary Paracetamol BP tablets well.

If you are very sensitive, you may perhaps react to powders used in tabletting the paracetamol. Your doctor can prescribe for you pure paracetamol powder which has no other constituents. It is bitter and does not dissolve well, so is difficult to take; but it may suit you better.

If your baby or child reacts to the paracetamol liquids made for children, the cause may be colourings or flavourings. High fever in an infant or young child can be dangerous; take your doctor's advice about alternatives to liquid paracetamol for babies and children.

Head Colds

See **Blocked Noses** (page 395) and **Fever** (above) and **Sore Throats and Coughs** (page 401).

Head Lice

Most proprietary treatments for head lice use very strong and troublesome chemicals. To prevent head lice infestation, shampoo hair frequently with hot water and brush regularly. This can damage young insects before they become established and prevent them laying eggs.

There is no natural remedy for head lice. Some treatments are made up in a water-based (aqueous) solution. These are better tolerated than those made up with alcohol.

Indigestion Relief

For indigestion, dissolve a teaspoon of sodium bicarbonate in a glass of water and drink. Take not more than three times a day, and not for prolonged periods. Consult your doctor if you are on a low-salt diet.

Persistent indigestion may be a symptom of food intolerance or allergy (>FOOD AND DRINK).

You can also take Boots Cream of Magnesia liquid for indigestion relief.

Inflammation of Joints

For an inflamed joint, you can apply a Kaolin poultice. Ask your pharmacist for instructions. You can also apply an ice pack, or a hot water bottle or hot cloths to ease joint inflammation. Do this gently at first.

Insect Repellent

Unless you are sensitive to plant terpenes, try using lavender oil, dabbed on heels, ankles, throat, and inner elbows to deter insects. Citronella can also be effective, but again take care if you are sensitive to plant oils.

Insect Stings

Bee stings are relieved by alkali solutions; wasp stings by acid solutions. Therefore, apply a solution of sodium bicarbonate to bee stings; apply vinegar or lemon juice to wasp stings, unless you react to these; in which case, you should use a weak solution of boric acid.

For emergency treatment if anaphylactic shock results from insect stings, >EMERGENCY TREATMENT.

If your skin reacts badly to mosquito and other insect bites, dab on Boots Cream of Magnesia Liquid and allow to dry. This will soothe and reduce swelling.

Laxatives

Taking Boots Cream of Magnesia Liquid by mouth is an effective mild laxative. Use Epsom Salts if you need a stronger laxative. Dissolve one teaspoonful in a glass of water and drink.

Mouthwash

You can use sodium bicarbonate (one teaspoonful in a glass of water) as a mouthwash. It kills smells very effectively.

Nappy Rash

For avoiding and relieving nappy rash, >BABYCARE.

Nettle Rash

>**Rashes and Itchy Skin** (right).

Painkillers

For painkillers (analgesics), use paracetamol. For information on which form to use, see **Fever** (page 398). Paracetamol is a powerful pain-reliever and will be adequate for home medication.

Period Pains and PMT

Use paracetamol as a painkiller; see **Fever** (page 398). If you suffer from low muscle cramps at the time of your period, try placing a hot water bottle on your lower abdomen to relieve pain.

Some women have found that Evening Primrose Oil helps relieve pre-menstrual and menstrual problems. Some react, however, to the gelatine of Evening Primrose Oil capsules. If this affects you, try taking the oil either by mouth in drops, or rub the oil gently into the fine skin of the inner elbow. It is absorbed readily into the bloodstream by the latter method. You may not be able to take as large a dose that way but you may tolerate the oil better. It is still possible to react to the oil itself, so take care.

Some women find that keeping blood sugar levels even and avoiding excessive highs and lows helps a great deal with hormonal problems. Eat something, even a small bite, every two or three hours and don't go long between meals at pre-menstrual or menstrual times.

Piles

External piles can be relieved by sitting on, or applying an ice pack. You can also apply a solution of Witch Hazel but it stings mightily. Piles can be a symptom of food intolerance or allergy (>FOOD AND DRINK).

Rashes and Itchy Skin

If you have eczema, or dermatitis, take your doctor's advice about emollients and moisturisers (>also MEDICAL HELP). The National Eczema Society (>CHARITIES for address) is an invaluable source of counselling and advice.

For nettle rashes, other fleeting rashes, sunburn, insect bite swellings, chicken pox and itchy skin, dab the affected area with Boots Cream of Magnesia Liquid and allow to dry. It is wonderfully soothing.

Urtica Urens, a homeopathic tincture or ointment, can also relieve nettle rash and other rashes. Some allergics tolerate it well, but use with care.

Shock

For how to deal with anaphylactic shock, >EMERGENCY INFORMATION.

Sinusitis

See **Blocked Nose** (above).

Sore Throats and Coughs

A steam inhalation will soothe sore throats and ease coughs; see **Blocked Nose** (page 395). Leaving a just-boiled kettle to steam gently in a room can ease severe coughing, especially at night.

If you tolerate lemons and a sweetener such as honey or sugar, squeeze fresh lemon juice, dilute with hot water and add honey or sugar to taste.

Unless you are chemically sensitive, a spoonful of Glycerin (from your pharmacy) will soothe coughs. If you are chemically sensitive, do not use it.

Spots and Pimples

Maintain scrupulous cleanliness to keep spots, blackheads and pimples at bay. Wash with a soap that you tolerate (>PERSONAL HYGIENE) and plenty of water. Dab dry with a towel.

You can use Rosewater and Witch Hazel as a cleanser, or Witch

Hazel solution on its own as an astringent. Your pharmacist will make these up for you. You can be sensitive to these; sniff both before using to see whether they affect you, and use with care. Witch Hazel may sting a little on use. Do not use it on skin with any deep cuts, where it will sting badly.

Sunburn

Apply Boots Cream of Magnesia Liquid liberally on skin and allow to dry. Very soothing! Apply an ice pack to very hot, angry areas.

Toothache

Apply oil of cloves directly to the tooth. Sniff it first, or take care, as you can be sensitive to the natural oils in cloves. (>PLANTS AND TREES).

Wind

Take a few drops of peppermint oil in a glass of water to relieve severe wind. Again the oil can cause sensitivity, so take care to sniff and use prudently.

Furniture

What Causes Problems?

If you are allergic to house dust mites, or to moulds, these are the most likely causes of reactions to older furniture. Both house dust mites and moulds thrive in damp, dark, warm places. If pets sleep or rest on furniture, the cause may be allergens that they have left behind. Try the avoidance measures for all of these, especially airing, cleaning and vacuuming, to see if this helps. (>HOUSE DUST MITES, MOULDS and PETS AND OTHER ANIMALS.)

You may be allergic or sensitive to the materials used to make the furniture – feathers and horsehair in upholstery are common allergens, especially in older furniture. (>FIBRES and MISCELLANEOUS ALLERGENS for more information.)

Chemicals are also a common cause if you are chemically sensitive. People are often sensitive to fumes from synthetic foams and fillings, to synthetic fibres and fabrics, and to chemical treatments on fabrics, although all of these are much less troublesome on older furniture which has aired off. Most veneered furniture is based on chipboard, also used in fitted kitchens and bedroom furniture. It gives off free formaldehyde for some time after manufacture. If you are exceptionally sensitive, it may bother you even for years if you have a lot of chipboard furniture in your home. Office furniture and surfaces in shops are often made of coated chipboard. Melamine veneers and sheets give off fumes initially but usually air off fast. Adhesives on veneered furniture can also be troublesome at first, but well tolerated in the long term.

Solid wood furniture rarely gives problems. Some people react to resinous woods, such as pine or cedar, but these are rarely a problem once they are polished or varnished. If you think you react to wood, it is extremely rare. It is more likely that you are sensitive to the actual varnish or polish that has been used on the wood (>PLANTS AND TREES).

Reactions to metal furniture are also extremely rare. Some people are sensitive to the enamel paints used on metal surfaces, but these are usually only a problem when new, or if the furniture becomes warm for any reason.

Glass and marble furniture, mirrors, stone, slate and ceramic tiles or surfaces do not cause reactions.

How to Avoid Problems

If you are allergic to house dust mites and moulds, you are best advised, apart from taking the usual precautions of airing, drying and vacuuming, to avoid upholstered furniture as much as you can, especially in beds. Avoid padded or upholstered headboards and bed-bases. A simple slatted bed or divan base in wood or metal allows ventilation, evaporation of damp and easy cleaning. For living room furniture, keep padded and upholstered furniture to a minimum. Choose chairs or sofas with easily removable cushions, or seats which can be aired or vacuumed, or even washed. Avoid flocky fabrics which harbour dust and moulds.

If you are chemically sensitive, you are best advised to avoid new veneered furniture and fitted furniture based on chipboard, as much as you can. If you have old veneered furniture or fittings, which have been there for several years, then they are probably fine and you may be better to leave them be, rather than replace them with something which may not be an improvement. Use solid wood or metal furniture, if you can (see below for further advice). >also BUILDING AND DECORATING MATERIALS for advice and alternatives to chipboard.

Some chemically sensitive people tolerate aired-off or washed synthetic foams, fibres and fabrics quite well. Again, if you have had furniture for some time, it may no longer give off vapours and is best left in place. If you are extremely sensitive, or if you need to replace a piece of furniture, avoid synthetic materials if possible. If you do buy them, leave them to air off fumes out of the way for some time before bringing into use.

Pure cotton, although more expensive, is often a good choice for upholstered furniture for chemically sensitive people, although you need to be careful to avoid cotton fabrics and materials which have been treated with fabric finishes and protective chemicals. You can use pure cotton wadding for upholstering fillings and cushions. This is invariably treated for fire retardancy with boric acid, which does not give off vapours and does not cause sensitivity, although it can cause irritation if you handle the powder itself. In enclosed upholstered wadding, it causes no sensitivity problems. For cushions, you can also use kapok (>FIBRES).

Untreated cotton fabrics for upholstery use are available, but they need to be combined with a pure cotton interliner which meets fire safety regulations. It is possible to do this in a combination which min-imises exposure to chemicals and meets the fire safety regulations. >FABRICS for full details of what to do, and where to obtain materials. See below for information on furniture makers. For information on mattresses, >BEDDING.

One way to use totally untreated materials and meet the fire safety regulations is to re-upholster furniture made before 1950, to which the regulations do not apply. You can legally buy older (pre-1950) or antique furniture in totally untreated materials, or you can re-uphol-ster yourself, or have it re-upholstered in untreated materials of your choice.

Your first problem in doing this is to obtain the materials. Sources of fabrics are given in **Fabrics** (page 387). John Cotton manufacture cotton wadding and will give names of stockists. Your second problem is to persuade an upholsterer to do the work if you do not do it your-self. Many are reluctant to use untreated materials on old furniture, even though it is legal, because they may be liable in case of accident. It is legal, however, and you can persist in persuading them. Contact the Association of Master Upholsterers for specialists in upholstery who may be able to help (address on page 407).

Some people react to even tiny traces of varnishes and sealing pol-ishes used on solid wood furniture. Furniture that is not new is usually little problem. Furniture made before the 1940s is usually trouble free, since many varnishes, lacquers and polishes used then were water-based, so buy or use older furniture for preference.

If you are exceptionally sensitive to varnish fumes, or need to buy or have made a new piece of furniture, you could use water-based var-nishes rather than solvent-based ones. These are well tolerated, but do not give full protection against splashes, spills or marks, and are thus not really satisfactory in everyday use. There are alternative compro-mise solutions which are satisfactory; full details of these are given in BUILDING AND DECORATING MATERIALS. If you have furniture made spe-cially, ask the maker to use a varnish of your choice. If you buy new wooden furniture, allow it to air off varnish before use.

French polish, shellac and Japanese lacquer are solvent-based and can cause sensitivity when being applied, and shortly after, while vapours are being released. Do not use these if possible. If you do use them, ventilate well afterwards and leave the piece of furniture to air before use. If using adhesives in upholstery or repairs to furniture, >BUILDING AND DECORATING MATERIALS for products to use.

If you are sensitive to resinous woods, like pine and cedar, look for furniture of less troublesome wood, such as beech, ash or oak. It may help to apply several coats of varnish to pine or cedar furniture to cut down fumes. Varnish the inside of drawers and cupboards and shelves as well. >BUILDING AND DECORATING MATERIALS for varnishes to use.

If you are sensitive to enamel paints on metal furniture, sniff carefully before buying. Wash down surfaces with a solution of one dessertspoonful of domestic Borax in a bowl of warm water. Allow to air before use and keep away from sources of heat.

Use glass and marble furniture, and mirrors, stone, slate or ceramic tiles and surfaces if you can.

Sources of Supply

Simple slatted beds of solid wood and metal are readily available. Mail order companies, such as Freemans, Littlewoods and Grattans, sell metal frame beds by post (addresses below). Habitat and IKAEA do not sell by post but have a choice of wooden, metal, glass and even marble furniture at reasonable prices. Contact them for details of local branches.

If you want to have upholstered furniture made for you, Multiyork will make chairs, stools and sofas upholstered in cotton wadding, on a beech frame. They will use a totally untreated cotton cover fabric if you supply it (>FABRICS for sources) over a pure cotton barrier interliner fabric to meet fire safety regulations. They have branches around the country or will take postal orders.

Alternatively, contact the Association of Master Upholsterers for local specialist upholsterers.

Treske will make solid wood furniture in any wood of your choice, with a varnish of your choice.

TIP

Directors' chairs made of cotton canvas and varnished wood, are often well tolerated and comfortable. You can also use them to carry with you if you go on holiday, on a visit or if you have problems at work. They are widely available at Habitat, DIY stores and department stores. Also try folding chairs of wood and metal.

Addresses of Suppliers

Association of Master
Upholsterers
Unit One
Clyde Road Works
Clyde Road
Wallington
Surrey SM6 8PZ
Tel: 081–773 8069

Freemans plc
139 Clapham Road
London SW99 0HR
Tel: 071–735 7644

Grattan
Freepost
Bradford
West Yorkshire BD99 2FP
Tel: 0800 333444

Habitat Design Limited
Hiphercroft Road
Wallingford
Oxfordshire OX10 9EU
Tel: 0491 350000

IKAEA Limited
Drury Way
North Circular Road North
London NW10 0JQ
Tel: 081–451 5566

John Cotton (Mirfield) Limited
Nunbrook Mills
Mirfield
West Yorkshire WF14 0EH
Tel: 0924 496571

Littlewoods Warehouses
Limited
Staley Avenue
Crosby
Liverpool L70 2TT
Tel: 051–949 1111

Multiyork
Stephenson House
Stephenson Way
Thetford
Norfolk IP24 3RD
Tel: 0842 764761

Treske
Station Works
Thirsk
North Yorkshire YO7 4NY
Tel: 0845 522770

Hand Protection

Protect Your Hands Where Necessary

It can be important to protect your hands against substances which upset you, especially if you have severe eczema or dermatitis on them. Wear gloves to protect your hands as much as you can when handling anything that upsets you. Wear cotton, silk or waterproof protective gloves as appropriate. A choice of gloves of various materials, and addresses of suppliers, are given below.

Always wear protective gloves to do washing-up, when doing DIY, or when handling any strong chemicals such as cleaning products or adhesives. Try to get children to wear gloves, if using play materials that upset them.

Use gloves in any other situation where you are particularly sensitive. Some people react to handling food, such as milk, the juice of fruit or vegetables, or eggs; if this applies to you, then wear gloves to prepare food. Some people react to handling laundry or clothes, or even paper and newspapers, or the steering wheel of their car. Again wear gloves.

Wear fine gloves (choices given below) if you need to. Remember, if eye surgeons can do micro-surgery in gloves, you can certainly brush your dog, chop carrots, or do the gardening in gloves.

If You Are Sensitive To Gloves

Some people find that they are sensitive to contact with protective gloves made of rubber (latex) or synthetics. You can buy protective gloves made of a choice of materials (such as vinyl, latex and polyethene). It is a good idea, if you react to one particular material, to try gloves of another type to see if you tolerate that material better. Sometimes it is the lining material that can cause reactions, so try unlined gloves as well.

Boots the Chemist stock a selection of waterproof protective gloves in several materials. Their Sensitive Skin glove is made for people who react to latex. If you tolerate latex, but react to synthetics, they make a pure latex glove without lining. They also have gloves of other materials which are well labelled. Try each kind if you need to.

TIP

New rubber or protective gloves often smell strongly at first and give off fumes. Wash thoroughly inside and out and leave them to air for a while before use, until the fumes disappear.

Thin protective gloves for delicate manoeuvres are also sold by Boots the Chemist. These are made of polyethene. As an alternative, Mates gloves are sold in most chemists and some supermarkets. They have a choice of materials – Handi-mates are made of vinyl, Medi-mates are made of latex. They make types of other materials as well: contact them for brand names and details if you need them.

For thicker protection, try cotton calico gloves or thick leather or suede gloves. These are both sold in most garden centres.

If you still cannot find a protective material that suits, wear a thin liner glove of cotton or silk inside protective gloves.

Cotton and Silk Gloves

Pure cotton gloves are sold by Boots the Chemist (called Minette gloves, available in bleached or unbleached cotton). Seton cotton gloves are available from most chemists. The Healthy House sell cotton gloves by post. The smaller sizes of all of these will fit larger children. Lohmanns sell cotton stockinette gloves for dermatological use. Scratch mitts for babies are available in pure cotton from Boots and Mothercare. Mothercare have a postal service (address below).

Fine silk liner gloves are available by post from Orvis, Patra, Sander and Kay and Survival Aids. These are finer than cotton gloves and are useful if you are allergic to cotton. Some makes have a synthetic cuff but you can turn this up so that it does not touch your skin.

TIP

If your hands are irritated when doing washing-up, it can help to use tepid rather than hot water, as well as to wear gloves. Also try using a low-allergen washing-up liquid (>CLEANING PRODUCTS) in case inhaling fragrances or other chemicals upsets you.

Addresses of Suppliers

Boots plc
1 Thane Road West
Nottingham NG2 3AA
Tel: 0602 506111

The Healthy House
Cold Harbour
Ruscombe
Stroud
Gloucestershire GL6 4DA
Tel: 0453 752216

Lohmanns
Credsee House
Oxford Road
Stone
Aylesbury
Buckinghamshire HP17 8PL
Tel: 0296 747272

Mates Healthcare
Ansell House
119 Ewell Road
Surbiton
Surrey KT6 6AY
Tel: 081–541 0133

(Manufacturer; contact for
stockists)

Mothercare Home Shopping
PO Box 145
Watford WD2 5SH
Tel: 0923 210210

The Orvis Co Inc
The Mill
Nether Wallop
Stockbridge
Hampshire SO20 8ES
Tel: 0264 781212

Patra Selections
1–5 Nant Road
London NW2 2AL
Tel: 081–209 1112

Sander and Kay plc
Mail Order House
101–113 Scrubs Lane
London NW10 6QU
Tel: 081–969 3553

Seton Healthcare Group Ltd
Tubiton House
Oldham OL1 3HS
Tel: 061–652 2222

Survival Aids Ltd
Morland
Penrith
Cumbria CA10 3AZ
Tel: 09314 444

Personal Hygiene

In this section, you will find advice on substitutes if you find you react to things you use regularly for your personal hygiene.

The causes of reactions are commonly:

- Fragrances and perfumes
- Preservatives
- Lanolin
- Chemicals used as active ingredients, or in formulation

For more information, >CHEMICALS, COSMETICS and TOILETRIES AND SKINCARE.

The topics covered here are:

- Contact lenses
- Denture cleaning
- Deodorants
- Depilatories
- Hand cleansers
- Incontinence protection
- Sanitary protection
- Shampoos
- Shaving
- Soaps
- Tissues
- Toilet paper
- Toothpaste

For first aid and the home medicine cupboard, >FIRST AID AND HOME MEDICINE. For contraception, >SEX AND CONTRACEPTION.

Contact Lenses

The chemically sensitive should be careful with the hygiene solutions they use on their lenses.

Soft Lenses

Soft contact lenses need particular care. The material of the lens acts like a sponge and takes up fluid from the eye, and from cleansing and soaking solutions. A significant proportion of the volume of the finished lens can in fact be fluid and any chemical in the solutions used on the lenses will be absorbed into the lens itself, and be held in contact with the eye.

Older preservative-based soft lens cleansing systems use a wide range of chemicals as germ-killing agents. All are liable to cause irritation and symptoms in the average soft lens-user, not just in the chemically sensitive. You should look for a preservative-free system.

Some modern preservative-free cleansing systems use hydrogen peroxide as the germ-killing agent in an aqueous solution. If used properly, these peroxide systems cause no problems at all to the chemically sensitive. The soft lens is soaked in the peroxide solution overnight. In the morning, the lens needs to be rinsed to remove the peroxide which will cause smarting, but no harm, if it is left on the lens. A neutralising agent is therefore used in the morning to remove the peroxide.

There are three leading brands of peroxide system in the UK: 10/10, Oxysept and Perform. They differ in the neutralising agent used in the second step of the system. In 10/10, the neutraliser contains sodium pyruvate; this is a chemical produced naturally in the body as a by-product of metabolism and is well tolerated. The neutraliser in Oxysept is an enzyme called catalase; in practice, few problems arise with this. In Perform, the neutraliser is sodium thiosulphate. This is a less powerful agent than sodium pyruvate or catalase. Follow the manufacturer's instructions carefully and it should prove acceptable.

Some other modern preservative-free systems use as their germ-killing agent chemicals which release free chlorine in the process. These type of systems do not require a neutralising agent; they are cheaper to buy and less time-consuming to use. In theory, the chlorine released should disperse during soaking overnight and not cause problems in the morning. In practice, most people do not have problems with this type of system but even some people who are not chemically sensitive find that they get irritation from the minute traces of chlorine left on the lens.

On balance, the more expensive and less convenient peroxide plus neutralising agent systems, such as 10/10 and Oxysept, are a better choice for the chemically sensitive.

For some people, protein builds up on soft lenses over a period of wearing the lenses. This needs to be cleaned and removed by a protein-removing agent. One brand of tablet, Amiclair, is relatively free of problems and should be better tolerated by the chemically sensitive. The Amiclair tablets can be used by dissolving them in distilled water or a saline solution.

Alternatively, opticians have found that Ultrazyme tablets work well used in combination with the Oxysept peroxide system; the Ultrazyme tablets can be dropped into the overnight soaking solution and left to work overnight. Some people who have reacted to Amiclair tablets used on their own have been able to tolerate Ultrazyme if used in combination with Oxysept in this way.

If you need to use wetting drops for your lenses, try Clerz sold in single dose sachets. This is a preservative-free system and is well tolerated. If you use a surfactant cleaner before using a peroxide solution, use Mirasept with the 10/10 system. This is generally trouble-free.

You can ask any pharmacist or optician to obtain those systems for you if you cannot readily find them in shops.

Hard Lenses

Hard lenses do not absorb fluid in the way that soft lenses do. Even in gas-permeable lenses, only a tiny amount of fluid is taken up by the lens. Preservative-based systems can therefore be used on hard lenses without trouble by the chemically sensitive, since the agent can be thoroughly rinsed off before wearing.

The rinsing solution used is a sterile saline solution sold in ozone-friendly aerosol cans. Some brands of saline are buffered with chemicals that maintain the pH of the solution; these can cause problems. Make sure you are using an unbuffered saline solution – there are half a dozen brands readily available. Ask your optician or pharmacist to check for you if you are not sure which to use.

If you use a surfactant cleaner for your hard lenses, these will be thoroughly removed by overnight soaking and rinsing in saline.

Denture Cleaning

See **Toothpaste** (below).

Deodorants

Mum Unperfumed Roll-on Deodorant is tolerated reasonably well by people with chemical sensitivity. On sale in major chemists, or contact the manufacturers:

> Mum
> The Bristol-Myers Company Ltd
> Swakeleys House
> Milton Road
> Ickenham
> Uxbridge UB10 8NS
> Tel: 0895 639911

Alternatively, make a weak solution of sodium bicarbonate (one tea-spoon to 600 ml/1 pint water) and wash yourself under your arms with this.

Depilatories

Shave with an electric razor without soap if possible, rather than use a depilatory or wax agent.

Hand Cleansers

Some sensitive people find that they can use a cooking oil (one which they tolerate or to which they are not allergic) to clean off substances like paint, thick grease, oil and stubborn dirt. Massage the oil into the hands until the substance dissolves, then rinse the oil away.

Incontinence Protection

If you cannot tolerate incontinence pads, try re-usable towels. The Green Catalogue sell re-usable sanitary towels with a waterproof back-ing. They are made of unbleached cotton, with an absorbent felt of vis-cose and polyester. Some people may not tolerate these, but they might be worth trying. Contact:

> The Green Catalogue
> 3–4 Badgworth Barns
> Notting Hill Way
> Weave
> Axbridge
> Somerset BS26 2JU
> Tel: 0934 732748

The Green Catalogue also sell disposable sanitary towels in non-chlo-rine bleached pulp if you are sensitive to chlorine.

If you can tolerate neither of these, try using a pure cotton muslin nappy (usually sold for babies). Fold the nappy and wear it with a pair of plastic waterproof pants over it, if you tolerate the plastic. If you do not tolerate the waterproof pants, try using a pair of thick cotton pants with a thin strip of plastic cut from a plastic bag placed between them and the folded nappy. Pin the nappy to the pants if you wish. Boots and Mothercare sell muslin nappies, usually non-chlorine bleached.

If you want to disinfect them after use and kill smells, make a solution of Borax in a bucket. Put one dessertspoonful of Borax in a bucket of warm water. Soak for up to a day, rinse and launder, preferably on a hot programme. Boots stock, or will order, domestic Borax.

Sanitary Protection

Tampons are made of a blend of cotton and viscose. Some brands are treated with glycerol which is a mild solvent. Sanitary towels are made of wood pulp, with a lining of some type of plastic to provide waterproofing. Most brands are bleached with chlorine, although it is now possible to find unbleached and non-chlorine bleached products. Most will contain formaldehyde to provide wet strength, and some brands are perfumed.

If you are chemically sensitive, it is probably better to avoid tampons unless you absolutely have to use them. The vagina, being a mucosal area of the body, absorbs chemicals very readily. You are more likely to react to a tampon than to a sanitary towel. Boots own brand are not treated with glycerol and may be a better choice if you have to wear tampons.

Some brands of sanitary towels are better tolerated than others by chemically sensitive women. Try using Simplicity towels to see if they suit you, or Boots own brand towels.

The Green Catalogue (address above) sell disposable sanitary towels in non-chlorine-bleached pulp, and 100 per cent cotton non-chlorine-bleached tampons. They also sell re-usable sanitary towels in unbleached cotton with absorbent felt of viscose and polyester and a waterproof backing. These may not be tolerated by some women but could be worth a try.

If you can use none of these, try using a pure cotton muslin nappy, usually sold for babies. These are usually non-chlorine bleached. Fold the nappy, and pin it to your pants if necessary. Cut the nappy in half or smaller if it is too bulky. Boots and Mothercare sell these.

For details on how to disinfect and launder, >**Incontinence Protection** (above).

Some other women successfully use vaginal sponges if they have a light flow. Buy a tiny natural sponge – sold usually for applying cosmetics – and place high in the vagina. Remove and rinse several times a day. Rinse it thoroughly and keep very clean between periods.

Another option is to use a contraceptive cap to collect the blood. You will need your doctor to fit a cap for you. Insert the cap without spermicide and empty it frequently. This works well if you have a light flow, unless you are sensitive to the latex of the cap (>MISCELLANEOUS ALLERGENS).

Shampoos

The following shampoos are tolerated well by people with allergies and sensitivities:

> Crimpers Shampoo
> 63–67 Heath Street
> Hampstead
> London NW3 6UG
> Tel: 071–794 8625

> Simple Shampoo
> Smith and Nephew
> Allum Rock Road
> Allum Rock
> Birmingham B8 3DZ
> Tel: 021–327 4750

> (Available in most chemist's)

Shaving

For shaving, use an electric razor which will not require soap or lather. For a wet shave, Simple, Gillette and Wilkinson make shaving foams or gels for sensitive skins. If you want to use soap, choose one of the soaps given below. For aftershave, use Witch Hazel, available from pharmacies, which is an astringent.

Soaps

Use soap sparingly. You only really need it to remove grease or severe dirt.

Two soaps that are tolerated well by people with sensitive skins and other allergies are Kays Vegetable Oil Soap (available in Superdrug and most supermarkets), and Simple Soap by Simple (available in most chemist's). Most supermarkets also sell their own brand of 'pure' soap or 'simple' soap. These are worth trying. Beware of fragrance-free soaps and look for unperfumed (>page 376). Health food stores sell pure olive oil soap. Wash E45 is tolerated well by some sensitive people; ask your pharmacist.

Tissues

To avoid formaldehyde and bleaches, use handkerchieves rather than tissues.

Toilet Paper

Toilet paper will contain formaldehyde for wet strength. Some brands will be chlorine-bleached. Some toilet papers are perfumed; avoid these.

Try different brands to see if one suits you better than others. Sniff before buying. If the smell is unpleasant or you get symptoms, try another. Air the rolls before using if you can. Keep supplies out of the toilet, in a cupboard or outhouse, until you need them, to keep down the fumes.

Try using non-chlorine-bleached or unbleached toilet paper. Some people tolerate these better; others find they make little difference. If you find you cannot use toilet paper, use pure cotton handkerchieves instead. To disinfect and kill smells, >**Incontinence Protection** (above).

Toothpaste

Flavourings (such as menthol or thymol) and active ingredients in toothpastes can cause reactions. Herbal toothpastes can equally give you trouble. Here are two alternative toothpowders:

- Mix one part salt with two parts sodium bicarbonate. Apply to brush with a little water and use as usual.
- Use sodium bicarbonate on its own in exactly the same way.

If you have young children and want to give them fluoride, you can give it to them in the form of drops made up with distilled water. These are available from dentists or chemists.

For cleaning dentures, mix up the salt and sodium bicarbonate powder as above, and clean the dentures thoroughly with a brush. You can use sodium bicarbonate on its own just as well if you prefer.

Sex and Contraception

Before You Start

Genital and urinary symptoms are commonly caused by infections. Make sure that you have eliminated these as possible causes before considering allergy or sensitivity. Consult your doctor.

If allergy or sensitivity is the cause, genital and urinary symptoms are not always caused by sexual activity and contraception. Symptoms such as itchy discharge, cystitis, rashes, irritation and hives around the genitals, can also result from sensitivity to foods, and to chemicals that you use elsewhere, not just from sexual contact. So if you are sensitive to these, or you find that the advice in this section does not help, it may be worth investigating foods and chemicals further (>FOOD AND DRINK and CHEMICALS).

Candidiasis and thrush can also cause genital and urinary symptoms in men and women. An overgrowth of a fungal organism which grows naturally in the body, candidiasis often accompanies allergy and sensitivity. For more information on candidiasis, >FOOD AND DRINK and SYMPTOMS.

What Causes Problems?

Any symptom can result from reaction to things used in connection with sex and contraception, including the classic symptoms of allergy, such as asthma and rhinitis, and the symptoms of chemical sensitivity (>SYMPTOMS). Most commonly, however, localised symptoms result, on the genitals, anus and surrounding skin and tissues, plus urinary symptoms and, for women, inflammation or pain in the pelvic region. Dermatitis can also be connected to sexual activity, especially around the mouth, neck, lower face and upper thighs.

There are three main categories of causes. The first, and most common, is chemicals used by you or your partner as toiletries, personal hygiene, or cosmetics; as laundry agents; or on products such as sanitary towels, tampons or incontinence protection. You may be sensitive to things that you use, or that your partner has used. They may be things that you tolerate well unless you have contact in an intimate area. Sweat and friction increase the likelihood of reaction – they make the skin and tissues more permeable and more likely to absorb chemicals. So, for instance, a soap powder or deodorant that normally does not bother you, may make you react when you have intimate contact.

Drugs or ointments that you are taking to treat these symptoms, or some other condition, can also cause genito-urinary symptoms. Take medical advice on whether to discontinue these.

For advice on how to cope with all these chemicals, >page 420.

The second cause, less common, is contraceptives, lubricants and sexual aids. If you use barrier contraceptives, such as a condom, a cap or diaphragm, these are made usually of pure latex and you can be allergic to it. Most condoms often contain a spermicide lubricant and you can be sensitive to this. Spermicides, used in conjunction with barrier methods of contraception, are based on phenols and alcohols and these can cause reactions.

Some women can become sensitive to the coil or IUD (intra-uterine device). These are made either of plastic, or of plastic plus copper. Some contain slow-release contraceptive chemicals such as progestogen. Although the specific cause of sensitivity is not really understood, women with a tendency to allergy and sensitivity sometimes do not tolerate the coil well.

Nor is the Pill well tolerated by many women with allergies and sensitivity. It often exacerbates food and chemical sensitivity. The reasons for this are not understood.

Lubricating jelly (such as KY) can be the cause of reactions. This is used invariably for internal gynaecological examinations, for smear tests, and on ante-natal checks, so women may be exposed to this, even if not using it for sexual intercourse.

Sexual aids, such as vibrators or other objects inserted into the vagina or rectum, or held to the penis, have been known to cause reactions.

For advice on how to cope with contraception, lubricants and aids, >page 422.

The final category is of reaction to human semen, mucus, saliva, and skin. It is possible to be allergic or sensitive to another person. It is extremely rare, and the other causes above are much more likely, but it does sometimes happen.

For advice on how to cope with sensitivity to human allergens, >page 423.

TIP

If you practise oral or anal sex, symptoms in these areas of the body may result. You may confuse the causes of these with some other cause. Stop for a while to see if things improve.

How to Deal With Reactions to Sex and Contraception

Start with Chemicals

If you suspect toiletries, cosmetics, or personal hygiene products as a cause of reactions following sexual activity, your best course of action is to use nothing in the genital area and to use the absolute minimum on the rest of your body and hair. In particular, stop using any douches, deodorants, perfume, talcum or home medicines on the genitals. Do this for a while and see if things improve. To use the absolute minimum on the rest of your body, stop using toiletries, cosmetics, aftershave and perfume, and >PERSONAL HYGIENE for suggestions for soap, toothpaste and shampoo.

Wash your genitals, upper thighs, and neck, face and hands after sexual intercourse. Wash your face, neck and hands and any other part of the body that needs it after kissing and petting. Use filtered or bottled water (>WATER AND WATER FILTERS) if you are sensitive to water.

TIP

Bathing the genitals in salt water can help relieve symptoms. Drinking alkali salts can also help reduce or stop reactions, and relieve cystitis. >FIRST AID AND HOME MEDICINE for information on how to take alkali salts.

If this does not improve things greatly, the next step is for your partner to follow suit. (If your partner is happy to co-operate, you can do this from the outset.) If you have no regular sexual partner, the only thing you may be able to achieve is for him or her to wash or shower before you touch, but that can be difficult to organise.

The third step is to change to laundry agents (for clothes and bedding) which are much less likely to cause sensitivity, and for you and your partner both to use these if possible. >CLEANING PRODUCTS for choices. It helps to wash underwear just in plain water, or water plus sodium bicarbonate, and to wear loose-fitting pure cotton underwear. Women often benefit from avoiding wearing tights.

If you suspect sanitary protection, stop using tampons and use sanitary towels instead. If these still upset you, use muslin nappies or cloths. >PERSONAL HYGIENE on how to use. You could also stop using lavatory paper for a while to see if it helps. >PERSONAL HYGIENE for alternatives. >also PERSONAL HYGIENE for advice on incontinence protection.

Try Different Methods of Contraception and Protection

If you are highly sensitive to many things, it can be difficult to find an acceptable and effective method of contraception, or protection against HIV and AIDS. For contraception, the Pill and the coil do not seem to suit many women with allergy and sensitivity and are probably best avoided unless you have very strong reasons to choose them.

If you are allergic to latex, you should avoid using condoms, cap, or diaphragm made of pure latex. To work out whether you are allergic to latex, >MISCELLANEOUS ALLERGENS. There are no alternatives to pure latex caps and diaphragms. Durex make a condom with the alluring name of Allergy made of non-allergenic latex. It also has a water-based lubricant, Sensitol, which does not contain spermicide. Try this to see if it suits you better. This may be your best option for protection against HIV and AIDS. It can be ordered through pharmacists, or contact Durex for stockists.

Durex
The London Rubber Company
North Circular Road
London E4 8QA
Tel: 081–527 2377

Spermicides are often risky to people who are chemically sensitive. Try the Sniff Test and Patch Test (>CHEMICALS for how to carry out) to see if they cause you to react – but with the caveat that you may be more sensitive to them on intimate contact than you are under test conditions. Most brands are of similar composition, so trying different ones will not help greatly. If you are sensitive to spermicides, stop using them, plus vaginal sponges and condoms containing them. Try the Durex Allergy condom, described above, which has no spermicide lubricant.

You are left, if you are sensitive to many things, with virtually no choice in contraception except natural methods. The most effective method of natural contraception is called the sympto-thermal method, combining the mucus method (also known as the ovulation or Billings method) with measuring temperature changes and other changes in bodily symptoms. Used correctly, the sympto-thermal method has a failure rate equivalent to a cap or diaphragm used with spermicide, a condom, or a coil, according to the Family Planning Service. Most women are fertile for only about seven days each month around ovulation. Learning to monitor the signs can help you identify the times when unprotected sexual intercourse will not result in pregnancy. The mucus produced by the cervix has characteristic changes on days prior to and just after ovulation. Body temperature also has identifiable changes around the time of ovulation. Other symptoms, such as abdominal pain, bloated tummy and breasts, and an increase in libido often accompany ovulation. During the few days each month when the woman is fertile, you can either abstain from intercourse, or use a method of contraception which you can tolerate in small amounts.

The drawbacks of this method are that it requires a lot of attention and monitoring, and that it is probably only possible for people who have a regular and co-operative partner, or who are in a stable relationship. Furthermore, for women who have an extremely irregular cycle, or do not menstruate, it can be impossible to detect the bodily changes.

A good family planning clinic or experienced doctor will be able to help you work out what to do. Two books which are helpful are listed under FURTHER READING.

Reactions to Lubricants and Sexual Aids

If you are using lubricating jelly, stop for a while to see if it improves your symptoms. Ask for internal examinations and smear tests to be done without jelly. The most common jelly used is KY Jelly which contains propylene glycol, known to cause reactions. Or try using an alternative lubricant, Replens, available from pharmacies. Some people tolerate this if they have become sensitive to KY. Use the Sniff Test or Patch Test (>CHEMICALS) to see if you react.

If you are using sexual aids of any kind, stop for a while to see if your symptoms improve, and stop using them permanently if they are the cause of reactions.

If you are allergic to pets and animals, or to house dust mites, you may get reactions if you make love on a surface where pets often sleep or rest, or which are full of dust mites – such as a carpet, rug, sofa, car seat or bedcover. Cover surfaces with a clean cloth or towel, or try somewhere else.

Reactions to Human Semen, Mucus, Saliva and Skin

It is extremely rare to react to another person's semen, mucus, saliva or skin but it does happen. Only consider these as possible causes if you have eliminated others as above already.

If you think you are sensitive to your partner's semen or mucus, use a condom for sexual intercourse to protect against direct contact. Use Durex Allergy condoms as above if you are sensitive to latex and spermicide. To be extra careful, do not touch sexual organs with hands, and wash hands, body and face thoroughly after intercourse. See if things improve.

It is very rare to be sensitive to someone else's saliva or skin. If you think you are, make sure your partner has been absolutely scrupulous about using no toiletries, cosmetics, perfumes, etc., on skin, and that you both are using low hazard laundry agents. Use no toothpaste, mouthwash, home medicine or anything else that might pass from the mouth. Check whether you react to tapwater (>WATER AND WATER FILTERS).

If you do react to skin, the parts that are most commonly affected are the mouth, face, neck and upper body. Bathe these parts (or others if they require it) in either a solution of alkali salts, or in Cream of Magnesia (>FIRST AID AND HOME MEDICINE) before and after sexual contact. Bathe your partner as well to help protect you.

One last thing that you can try to help you tolerate a partner's semen, mucus, saliva, or skin, is for her or him to avoid foods to which you react. If you are very highly sensitive to a food, you may just be reacting to minute traces of it in your partner's body fluids and skin. This is only likely to be the case if you are exceptionally allergic or sensitive. A tiny number of people find that it can help them if their sexual partner avoids the foods that upset them particularly badly. It can be worth trying if nothing else helps you.

Ask for Help and Support

Sexual difficulties caused by your allergies and sensitivity can erode your self-confidence, destroy your ability to meet and relate to new people, and can eat away at an existing relationship. Sex is often an area of great loneliness and private grief for people with allergies and sensitivity. Little support or counselling is ever offered.

If you are a young person just starting out and need help to cope, you must not feel that you are left alone. Many schools or student organisations can put you in contact with groups that offer sexual counselling, and they will quickly be able to understand the special problems that allergies and sensitivity bring. Family planning clinics and GPs can also refer you to people who will help you. Ask for the help and support you need.

If you are in an existing relationship, and tensions result over sexual abstinence, ways of making love or methods of contraception, contact your local branch of Relate who can provide sexual and relationship counselling.

Travel

If you react and develop symptoms when you travel, by car or by public transport, the most likely cause will be exhaust fumes, or chemical vapours from materials used in the vehicles. Other causes can be tobacco smoke fumes if smoking is allowed in the vehicle, or cleaning products, air fresheners, or disinfectants used in the vehicle. See below for specific avoidance measures. For more information on sensitivity to chemicals, >CHEMICALS.

It is also common, if you are highly allergic to moulds or house dust mites, that these cause you problems in vehicles. Moulds and house dust mites thrive in damp, poorly ventilated places; and cars, buses and trains (even if kept in garages or depots) are rarely dry or aired enough to keep them at bay. (If you feel ill when you first get into a car, or a bus or train just out of a depot, but improve as the vehicle warms up, then the cause is most likely moulds.)

There is little you can do to control moulds or dust mites in cars, beyond vacuuming with a filtered vacuum cleaner and keeping the car as aired and dry as you can. Some car filters will help reduce the level of allergen particles inside a car (>page 430). For more information generally on controlling moulds and dust mites, >MOULDS and HOUSE DUST MITES.

If you are very allergic to pets and animals, you may react when you travel in a vehicle in which pets travel regularly, even if they are not actually present. >PETS AND OTHER ANIMALS for more information on avoidance measures.

If you are allergic to pollens, travelling by car or public transport in the pollen season can make things worse. >POLLENS for advice on how to avoid problems at peak pollen seasons. See page 430 for advice on car filters which can help with reducing pollen levels inside a car.

The rest of this section deals with the following topics:

- Choosing a car
- How to drive to minimise problems
- Car maintenance and cleaning
- Public transport
- Avoidance measures for pedestrians

Choosing a Car

Buying Secondhand

If you are allergic to moulds or house dust mites, you should take care if buying a car secondhand. If a car appears very dusty and damp, or smells fusty, it will probably have house dust mites and moulds. You may be better buying a new car or one of more recent date. (See below for advice on age of car to buy if you are also chemically sensitive.)

If you are allergic to pets and animals, and buying a secondhand car, check with the owner whether any animals (or people in close contact with them) have travelled regularly in the car, even if the owner does not have pets. (Even traces from clothes, or from the rear of a car can upset the very sensitive.) Look for traces of pet hair, often difficult to remove.

If you are sensitive to tobacco smoke residues, check when buying a car secondhand whether anyone has ever smoked in the car. A good tip is to look in all of the ashtrays – these are virtually impossible to clear of smells and ash. You will be able to detect any traces of smokers from the ashtrays even if the owner or dealer cannot say whether the car has been exposed to smoke. When you travel by taxi, ask for a non-smoking taxi.

If you are very sensitive to chemical cleaners and air fresheners, sniff the car carefully to see if any strong agents have been used. Fumes from air fresheners – often stuck to the dashboard, in or under the glove compartment – take a very long time to wear off: avoid a car which has had these recently, if you can. If you buy privately, rather than from a dealer, it is often easier to find out what has or has not been applied to the car. This applies also to recent repairs, rust-proofing or service treatments as well. >**Car Maintenance** (below).

Which Type of Car?

If you are very chemically sensitive, you are best advised not to buy, use or travel in a brand new car. These usually give off high levels of chemical fumes and vapours from new foam, plastics and materials, particularly for the first six months. Many chemically sensitive people will be fine in a new car after six months. Some who are much more sensitive find they can only travel comfortably in a car which is at least two or three years old.

If you are thinking of buying a car, test-drive models and makes of different ages, or travel in friends' or family's cars, to see which age of car suits you best. If you ever have to hire a car, ask for one which is of an age that you tolerate well.

Some models and makes of car have fascia, seats and fittings made of materials which are better-tolerated by some people. The Volvo 340 range and the Volkswagen Polo, for instance, seem to be made of different materials; some people feel better in these, although others notice no difference. The Citroen 2CV and Dyane range have very little plastic fascia, and also cause fewer problems. Some people tolerate leather seats better than those of synthetic materials. Again, test-drive or try out different models or makes to see if one suits you better.

If you are extremely sensitive to exhaust fumes, you could look for a car with a re-circulating air system. A system of this kind does not filter the air, but it provides a cleaner environment than a conventional ventilation and heating system. A conventional system has an air intake direct from outside, entering through vents. Closing these vents and switching off any fan stops most air entering, but then means that you have no ventilation and cannot use the heating. In a re-circulating air system, the system by-passes the normal air intake, and re-circulates air inside the car. This means that you are not taking in fumes continually from outside, and that you can have ventilation and heating operating.

Re-circulating air systems are standard on many larger, more expensive cars, such as the larger Volvos, Mercedes, or Audis. They are installed as standard on Vauxhall Astras from 1991 ('J') registration; you have to select the system by switching it on. A garage can instal a re-circulating air system on any car, but it can be costly and you might be better to change car to one on which it is fitted as standard, or else use a car filter in combination with a conventional ventilation system (see below and page 430).

Some models of car have air intake filters. These have been shown to be extremely effective against pollens, particles and chemical fumes in controlled tests. How these work and fuller information is given on page 000. Air intake filters are installed as standard on Vauxhall Astras since 1991 ('J') registration. They are also installed as standard on all new models of the BMW 300, 500, and 700, the Lancia Thema, and the Mercedes Roadster SI and SB class. Filters are available as options on the Volkswagen Golf and Passat. Currently optional on the Audi 80 and 100, they will soon be installed as standard.

How to Drive

If you are sensitive to vehicle exhaust fumes, you can adapt the way you drive in order to help yourself. Keep windows closed as much as you can. Unless you have a car with a re-circulating air system (see page 427), do not use heating and fan unless you have to, and keep vents closed unless you really need ventilation. A sun-roof can be useful for ventilation – it draws air in and out of the car, directly away from your face.

___TIP___

> If the car gets too cold, or too hot, or condensation develops, use the ventilation and heating system in short intense bursts, then close it down again. Shut off if you have to wait in heavy traffic.

Hang back from the vehicle ahead – especially in busy or stationary traffic – do not stop close to someone else's exhaust, allowing fumes to be drawn directly into your car. Leave as much space as you can. Select a route, or a time, to drive that avoids traffic queues, or sitting stationary at junctions.

When filling your vehicle with fuel, keep windows and vents closed so that fumes from the pumps do not get into the vehicle. If you can find one, go to a service station where someone will serve you, rather than to a self-service garage.

Avoid car journeys in very hot weather if you are very sensitive to vehicle exhausts, or chemical vapours from materials. Materials in cars heat up and give off more vapour in hot weather. It is also impossible to keep windows closed. Only do essential journeys when it is extremely hot, and travel at a cooler time of day if you can. Go earlier to or later from work if possible.

___TIP___

> If you are extremely sensitive, try wearing a face mask (>FACE MASKS) or use a car filter (see page 430). If you cannot afford a filter, hanging damp cloths over air vents will reduce the amount of residual vapours which pass through.

Car Maintenance and Cleaning

Many chemicals used for car servicing, maintenance and cleaning are very troublesome; and there are virtually no good substitutes to suggest for engine maintenance, rust-proofing or repainting. If you are very chemically sensitive, it is probably wise not to do your own car servicing and maintenance.

If you have repairs, rust-proofing or service work done to your car, involving chemicals which upset you, get the garage to keep the car for a few hours, overnight or a day or two extra to allow the fumes to disperse.

For cleaning, Simoniz have a range of solvent-free car cleaners, available from car accessory shops. To clean the inside of a car thoroughly, vacuum, or steam clean if something drastic is needed. Do not use car fresheners. >CLEANING PRODUCTS for more advice. For windscreen wash, fill bottles just with water. Ask garages not to use any detergents in windscreen wash bottles, and not to use any detergents or polishes if they are servicing or repairing your car.

Public Transport

If you travel by public transport, it can be difficult to avoid things which upset you. Buses, trains and coaches can be very dusty and mouldy. Strong cleaners and disinfectants are commonly used. Fumes from tobacco smoke disperse, even into non-smoking areas. Doors and windows are frequently open, allowing traffic exhaust fumes to enter.

If you are allergic to pollens, travelling by InterCity train or air can be an advantage for a long journey, being air-conditioned.

If you are extremely sensitive to anything, and do not mind people staring, wear a face mask (>FACE MASKS). Alternatively, clasp a dampened handkerchief firmly over your nose – it does not stop all fumes, but is of some help.

Some tips which are helpful are to avoid smoking areas, or sit as far from them as you can. On trains or buses, sit away from engines or power units, or from doors which can allow fumes in. Trams are being reintroduced in some British cities – these are electrically powered and often better to travel on, if you have the choice. Spend as little time as you can in underground transport systems.

Advice for Pedestrians

If you have to walk in traffic, choose a route through parallel back streets or pedestrian areas if possible, which avoids having to walk on busy streets. Do not cross the road by walking between stationary vehicles. Hang back from the edge of the road, and cross quickly, at pedestrian crossings or lights if traffic is heavy. Wear a face mask, if

you can cope with the stares (>FACE MASKS), or carry a damp handkerchief to clasp over your nose.

If you have a baby who is chemically sensitive, do not push a
buggy between vehicles with exhausts at the baby's nose level. Cross
at crossings or lights, or where the traffic is light. Choose a pram or
buggy in which the baby sits relatively high up.

Car Filters

There are two basic types of car filters:

- Air intake filters
- Portable interior filters

Air Intake Filters

Air intake filters work by fitting thick fabric or electrostatic filters over the air intake to the ventilation and heating system of a
car, to prevent or reduce particles, such as pollens or fumes, entering the car. Air intake filters permit you to continue to run ventilation and heating systems as normal while the filter is operating.
For full effectiveness, keep windows closed. One make – the
Micronair – is fitted during manufacture as standard to certain
models of car, and is available as optional on others (see page
000). It cannot be fitted after manufacture. Another make – the
Icleen – can be fitted on cars of any make or age.

The Micronair is made of non-woven fabric with an electrostatic charge. The charge attracts particles, and the thick fabric web
prevents larger particles passing. The filter has been shown on
controlled tests to be 100 per cent effective against pollens and
larger particles, 70 per cent effective against virtually all smaller
particles, and 50 per cent effective against the tiniest of particles.
The filter medium loses its charge after one year and needs
replacing. This can be done by main dealers as part of a yearly
service, or separately. The cost of replacement (including parts
and labour) would be between £19 and £25 at 1992 prices,
depending on the dealer.

The Icleen filter is made from a thinner fabric web than the
Micronair, without electrostatic charge. No test information is
available on performance, but reports from users say it makes a
noticeable difference, especially in heavy traffic. The filter is simple to fit – a competent DIYer or any garage can do it – and needs
changing every six months. A pack of two filters costs £43 (at

1992); available from SBP Limited (address below). A garage would charge about £15–20 to instal or change the filter.

Portable Interior Filters

Portable interior filters are powered by plugging into the car cigarette lighter. They draw the air inside the car through a filter medium inside them – either fabric, activated charcoal or an electrostatic surface which attracts particles – or some combination of these. For full effectiveness, keep windows closed.

The benefits of this type of filter compared to the air intake filters are that they are portable, and you can use them in any car or vehicle in which you travel. They also filter the air inside the car – so they can take out particles such as moulds, dust mites, pet hairs, and fumes from plastics, foams and materials in the car. Their main disadvantage is that unless you have a car with a re-circulating air system (see page 427), they are much less effective when you use the ventilating or heating system because of fumes entering from outside. They are best used without operating air vents or heating.

One model – the NSA 600A Auto Air System – has only just been introduced in the UK and there are no reports from users of its effectiveness. It has an electrostatic filter, fabric filters and a thin activated carbon filter to absorb chemical vapours. It has an optional fragrancer which you should not use if you are chemically sensitive. It is close to 30 cm (1 foot) high and has a Velcro mounting to hold it to a surface. Its price is quoted at £110 (at 1992): replacement filters will be required regularly, depending on how much you drive. Contact NSA for names of distributors; ask for a trial period (address below).

Another portable car filter is available for import direct from the United States. The Foust #160A Air Purifier is a free-standing cylinder resting horizontally on a small bracket, about 40 cm (16 inches) in length and 23 cm (9 inches) in height. Made of metal, it contains filter media of activated carbon, alumina with potassium permanganate and a particle filter. If you think you might be sensitive to any filter media, you can obtain test samples in advance of buying a filter and Foust will supply cartridges with different types of filter mix to your needs. The Foust purifier is very effective against chemical fumes. It can be noisy, and get in the way if you have a full car load of people.

The purifier costs $242 (£127 at $1.90 exchange rate). Replacement charcoal, needed every six to twelve months, costs $18 (£10 at $1.90 exchange rate). The Test Kit costs $19 (£10 at

£1.90 conversion). To these prices, you will need to add shipping charges, plus duty and VAT, to be paid when the parcel arrives in this country. Duty at 4.25 per cent and VAT at 17.5 per cent will mean adding £28 to the filter, £2.20 to the cartridge, and £2.60 to the Test Kit. Shipping charges are quoted separately by Foust at time of order.

E. L. Foust will take credit card orders by telephone (address and telephone below).

Sources of Supply

E. L. Foust Co. Inc.
Box 105
Elmhurst
IL 60126
USA
Tel: 010–1–708 834 4952

Icleen
SBP Ltd
Nash House
204A High Street South
Dunstable
Beds LU6 3HS
Tel: 0582 660491

NSA (UK) Ltd
NSA House
1 Reform Road
Maidenhead
Berkshire SL6 8BY
Tel: 0628 776055

(Contact for distributors)

Vacuum Cleaners

For people who are allergic to inhaled particles which collect in dust – such as house dust mites, moulds, animal and pet debris, or fibres such as cotton or wool – using a filtration vacuum cleaner can make an enormous difference. For more information on detecting and avoiding allergens, >relevant sections.

Conventional vacuum cleaners, even the most efficient, blow a share of dust and particles back into the room. Tests have shown that they actually increase the level of airborne particles in a room which explains why so many people with allergies feel worse during and after vacuuming.

Filtration vacuum cleaners, often called 'allergy vacuum cleaners', use a special filter which takes out virtually all particles of major allergens. Tests by *Which?*, by *Good Housekeeping* and other independent bodies, have shown that the two market leaders, Medivac and Nilfisk, both filter out over 99.9 per cent of particles down to 0.3 micron (three-hundredths of a millimetre) in diameter. So virtually no dust is blown around while using the machine, and allergens can be removed from sites where they have collected, such as beds, carpets, curtains or furniture, without dispersing them into the air.

These cleaners are expensive compared to other vacuum cleaners (see below) but people who use them say they would not be without them. Not only do they make cleaning possible in the environment of the highly sensitive with minimum dispersal of dust, but they reduce progressively the level of old or dead allergens collected in furniture, furnishings and bedding.

Most people who have such a machine report that their effect accumulates as time goes on and that they clear out the environment progressively. More than any other product designed to help people with allergies, these cleaners receive shining endorsement from their users. If you can possibly find the money, they are one item really worth buying.

There are two market leaders whose performance is measurably superior to other makes – Medivac and Nilfisk. There are some differences between them, notably price, the Medivac being more expensive (at over £300 at 1992 prices) than the Nilfisk (around £270). They are both canister models on wheels. The Nilfisk is lighter than the

Medivac, but it is made of plastic rather than metal, and if you are sensitive to plastics, the Medivac is preferable. Medivac and Nilfisk both provide efficient service and spares backup.

At the time of writing, Medivac is introducing a new lightweight model at a considerably reduced price. It has similar filters and performance characteristics to the original model, according to the manufacturer, but is not made of stainless steel. It is called the Medivac Lighterweight cleaner. We have no user reports to date, but if Medivac's claims are correct, it should be the most competitive filter cleaner available for people who do not have to have a metal version.

TIP

If you need such a product because of chronic illness, you are not required to pay VAT. Vacuum cleaners can be supplied exempt of VAT if you sign a simple declaration form which the supplier will provide.

Remember to change bags and clean fabric filters regularly. If changing bags or cleaning filters upsets you, enlist someone to do it for you.

The Medivac is available from The Healthy House or direct from Medivac. The Nilfisk is available from Allerayde or direct from Nilfisk. All these suppliers offer a trial period. Other suppliers of allergy vacuum cleaners are BVC, AEG, Miele, Rainbow and Vorwerk. Addresses and telephone numbers below.

The Rainbow machine is worthy of particular mention since users report that they find it more effective than the Medivac or Nilfisk. Dusts and dirt are removed by passing through water and there are therefore no bags to change, or filters to clean. The main drawback is price – it's about £900 (at 1992 prices).

If you absolutely cannot afford to buy such a cleaner, another option is to try exhaust filters, available from Allerayde. These are made of fabric which you tape over the exhaust of any conventional cylinder cleaner, and most hard cased upright cleaners. The fabric is thick synthetic wadding, but has not been reported to cause any reactions. These filters are not as effective as the filtration cleaners. Tests have shown that they are slightly less efficient at trapping particles, and they let out through slightly larger particles. But they still trap over 99 per cent of particles over 0.5 micron in size, which covers most important allergens.

The filters cost £20 for three filters, at 1992 prices, and last about 24 hours of vacuum use. For most people, this would mean replacing them every 12 weeks or so. This is a cheaper solution than buying a filtration cleaner over the long term, unless you use a vacuum cleaner very heavily. Drawbacks are, however, that you are exposed to dusts on changing filters and that it can be fiddly to fix the filters on properly. Again, enlist someone's help to do it for you if you need to avoid dusts.

TIP

Using exhaust filters may be a help if you go away for some time – on holiday or on a prolonged visit.

They may also help to use for a trial period while you decide whether thorough vacuuming will be of benefit to you long term.

Hoover sell High Filtration dust bags for their Turbopower and Turbomaster upright cleaners, which are claimed to reduce the amount of dust passing. A *Which?* survey in 1991 found that 'these gave only a small improvement over their other bags and that they still let through an unsatisfactory quantity of dust'.

TIP

Contact a local allergy support group, or a local group of a national charity, to see if they have members willing to lend you an allergy vacuum cleaner to try for a while (>CHARITIES and SUP-PORT GROUPS).

Addresses of Suppliers

AEG
217 Bath Road
Slough
Berkshire SL1 4AW
Tel: 0753 872101

Allerayde
147 Victoria Centre
Nottingham NG1 3QF
Tel: 0602 240983

BVC
Harbour Road
Gosport
Hants PO12 1BJ
Tel: 0705 584281

The Healthy House
Cold Harbour
Ruscombe
Stroud
Gloucestershire GL6 4DA
Tel: 0453 752216

Medivac
Taylormaid Products Ltd
Bollin House
Riverside Works
Manchester Road
Wilmslow
Cheshire SK9 1BJ
Tel: 0625 539401

Miele
Fairacres
Marcham Road
Abingdon
Oxford OX14 1TW
Tel: 0235 554455

Nilfisk
Newmarket Road
Bury St Edmunds
Suffolk IP33 3SR
Tel: 0284 763163 or Freefone
0800 252296

Rainbow Homecare Ltd
5 London Road
Bicester
Oxfordshire OX6 7BU
Tel: 0869 253105

Vorwerk
Philip Davies
Toutley Road
Wokingham
Berkshire RG11 5QN
Tel: 0734 794753

Water and Water Filters

Some chemically sensitive people find they are sensitive to water that they drink or use in daily life, due to minute traces of chemicals and metals. For some people, it is enough to take care with water that they use for drinking and cooking. Other people, if they are highly sensitive, are affected by washing with, or touching tapwater; some even by inhaling steam or vapours from standing or running water – a flushing lavatory, for instance. Sensitivity of this degree is rare, however, and for most people, it will be sufficient to avoid ingesting the water that upsets them.

Any of the symptoms of chemical sensitivity can result from ingesting, inhaling, or contact with, water. >SYMPTOMS for full details.

This section covers the substances that cause reactions to water, how to detect sensitivity to water, and what you can do to avoid problems. There is detailed information on different types of water treatment equipment and advice on what to buy.

What Causes Reactions to Tapwater?

Low levels of chemicals known to cause chemical sensitivity are found in tapwater, as well as metals known or suspected of causing harm. Water quality regulations permit levels of chemicals which, it is argued, are not harmful to health. Chemically sensitive people are, however, affected by *very low levels* of chemicals, and those present in tapwater are often sufficient to cause them reactions.

The contents of tapwater vary considerably across the country, and even within water company regions. This is partly because the level of industrial or agricultural contaminants differs according to the nature of the local economy. It is also because of local differences in the age and quality of water treatment plants, and mains and pipes. If you live in an area with relatively new treatment plants and pipes, or with little industry, or with low fertiliser use in farming, then your tapwater will contain lower levels of chemicals than that of other places.

Furthermore, some tapwater supplies come from groundwater, drawn direct from springs or boreholes. This often differs little from bottled waters in purity and needs little disinfection and filtration before supply. One third of water in England and Wales is supplied from groundwater, and if this applies to you, you may have few problems with your water apart from chemicals used for disinfection (see **Chlorine** below).

Water that is drawn from other sources (lakes, rivers and reservoirs) is subject to more pollution and needs greater purification, especially water from lowland rivers and reservoirs.

The chemicals found in tapwater which are particularly associated with chemical sensitivity are:

- chlorine
- nitrates
- polycyclic aromatic hydrocarbons
- trihalomethanes
- organic solvents

Aluminium, found naturally or added to purify water in some areas, is linked to some health problems, and lead, found sometimes in lead pipes within the home, is a known health hazard. If you are concerned about lead within your home, ask a plumber to check your system and replace pipes if you need to.

Traces of other heavy metals are also found in tapwater – metals such as copper, zinc and cadmium. Metals do not cause specific sensitivity reactions, but it is thought that absorbing them can depress the immune system, deplete vitamin and mineral levels, and thereby reduce your ability to cope generally with chemical load.

Chlorine

Chlorine is added to water supplies to kill bacteria and viruses. It has a strong taste and a distinctive smell like chlorine bleach. It is a common cause of chemical sensitivity, and responsible for most people's reactions to tapwater.

Nitrates

Nitrate levels in water in some parts of the country have been rising, probably due to the use of nitrogen fertilisers in agriculture. Nitrate levels are highest in East Anglia.

Polycyclic Aromatic Hydrocarbons

Polycylic aromatic hydrocarbons (PAHs) are chemicals which are released into water supplies in some parts of the country from the lining of water mains themselves. Up to the mid-1970s, coal-tar pitch was used to coat the inside of some water mains. If this lining breaks down, PAHs can be released into the water. Coal-tar related chemicals are known to cause sensitivity reactions. Moreover, there are concerns that PAHs, known to cause cancer in animals, may potentially do so in humans.

Trihalomethanes

Trihalomethanes (THMs) are chlorinated hydrocarbons, such as chloroform, which can form in water supplies, from chemical reactions caused by chlorine. These can cause sensitivity.

Organic Solvents

Trichloroethene, also called trichloroethylene, and tetrachloroethylene are organic solvents known to cause sensitivity. They are found in water supplies, probably released from industry and commerce. The chemicals are used as dry-cleaning fluids, and as degreasing and cleaning chemicals in industry.

Get Information from Your Water Company

Water companies are investigating alternatives to disinfection by chlorine, such as using ozone. In addition, a number of them are installing filtration processes, especially activated carbon filters, in order to remove chemical contaminants. You can find out from your local water company what processes they are actually using. They will also be able to tell you if your water comes from a groundwater source.

Water companies are also legally obliged to supply you, free of charge, with a drinking water quality report – an analysis of substances your water contains. These analyses are not complete, however. They only check for a limited range of chemicals. Ask for this, together with a list of the maximum permitted levels of substances under the Water Supply (Water Quality) Regulation, if you want to know something of what is in your water and whether the levels of selected chemicals are high or low.

Bottled Water

Some people who are sensitive to tapwater use bottled water as an alternative, but bottled waters are not always free of problems. Bottled waters are drawn from groundwater sources – springs or boreholes – and some of these can be polluted with chemicals from the environment. If you are exceptionally sensitive, these will trouble you. Some bottled waters are consistently better tolerated than others (see page 441).

Bottled waters have a higher bacteria count than tapwater which has been disinfected. If you use them for babies, or for children or adults vulnerable to infection, you should boil them for five minutes before using, and keep refrigerated once boiled and cooled.

Mineral waters have high alkali salt contents. If you are on a low-sodium diet, you should take medical advice before using them. Spring waters do not generally have high salt levels.

How to Detect Sensitivity to Water

If you suspect you are sensitive to your tapwater, try the following method of detection:

Avoid using unfiltered tapwater for four days, as far as you possibly can.

For drinking and cooking, use bottled water (see page 441 for best choices) or filtered tapwater. (Borrow a jug filter if you can.) Remember to use your chosen water for hot drinks such as tea or coffee. Use it for boiling vegetables, pasta or rice, for washing vegetables before use, or for making soups, casseroles, or other cooking. Use it for cleaning your teeth, or for any water that you swallow.

Stick to the same water if you can throughout the four days, and avoid drinking any made-up or processed drinks – such as fruit juices, canned or bottled drinks, draught beers, lager and cider. These will have been made with tapwater from somewhere. (Most fruit juices are reconstituted with tapwater from concentrated fruit pulp.) Avoid likewise processed foods made up with water – canned soups, fruit or soya milk, for instance. Do not use hot drinks vending machines. Take your own hot drinks or soups to work or school if you need to.

Limit your exposure to water generally. If you can make the effort, use filtered water as much as you can for any use. Bathe and wash hair as little as possible. Avoid showers and baths. It is better simply to do a bodywash at the basin during the four-day test. Get someone else to do the washing-up so that you do not touch or inhale the water. If you have to use water a lot at work, do the avoidance test over a weekend, days off or holiday. Avoid going swimming.

Bottled Water

Many people with chemical sensitivity find that they can tolerate bottled water better than tapwater. But some bottled waters can upset people, even with minute levels of contamination of chemicals. Particular brands of bottled water are consistently better tolerated by chemically sensitive people and, if you are thinking of switching to bottled water, it is a good idea to try these ones first. The well-tolerated brands are Malvern, Buxton and Evian. Carbonation – adding carbon dioxide to water to make it fizzy – has no effect on people's tolerance of bottled water.

If you are very sensitive to plastic, try to obtain bottled water in glass bottles. Evian is not generally available in glass; it is worth trying in plastic since even very sensitive people are often unaffected by it.

TIP

If you or your family and friends drink a lot of bottled water, it may be worth buying wholesale. Suma, wholefood wholesalers, stock a number of brands. Natural Foods deliver bottled waters in the London Area. Addresses in FOOD AND DRINK. Malvern is sold by wholesalers supplying the pub trade, and Buxton and Evian are sold by wholesalers and cash and carry merchants supplying grocers, confectioners and newsagents. Look for these in Yellow Pages.

If you react even to these brands, or to reverse osmosis water (see page 444), you can try rotating waters. Set up a four-day rotation for waters, allocating one type or brand of water to each day, Brand One to Day One and so on. Use just that water for drinking and cooking on that day, and change waters on each of the four days. >FOOD AND DRINK for a full explanation of the principle of rotation. Some people find this can help them tolerate water.

Neutralisation, a form of de-sensitisation, can sometimes be effective with bottled water. It can help if you are desperate. >MEDICAL HELP for more information.

TIP

Another method that sometimes helps is to pass bottled water through a jug filter. Again it is worth a try if you feel desperate.

If you are sensitive to tapwater, your symptoms should be clear or improve after four days. You may feel worse with withdrawal symptoms initially if you are extremely sensitive to water (>SYMPTOMS for details of possible withdrawal), but these will clear fast.

After four days, you can then test your tapwater to see if your symptoms return. Drink a glass of water, following the method of testing foods in FOOD AND DRINK. If your symptoms return on trying tapwater again, then you are sensitive to it.

How to Deal with Sensitivity to Water

If you find that you are sensitive to your tapwater, do not be daunted. It may not be as great a handicap or as difficult to deal with as it first appears. Unless you are exceptionally sensitive and very unlucky, it may be sufficient to take great care with water you swallow – for drinking, cooking and in dilute drinks and foods. For these, use a bottled water that you tolerate, or filtered or purified water.

TIP

Jug filters are reasonably effective at reducing chemical contaminants and are adequate for most sensitive people. Plumbed-in filter systems are more effective and convenient. For full advice on choosing, see page 443.

Take made-up drinks with you, or your own water, when going to work or school. Give toddlers and young children their own cup to take to nursery or playgroups. Take packed lunches if you are concerned about water used for cooking. If you have a sensitive baby, use bottled or filtered water to make up any feeds, boiling first and preparing feeds as usual. Avoid processed foods and drinks made up with water, as described in the detection programme above. You can make up your own fruit juices, for instance, by buying fruit juice concentrate (available from health food shops or direct from wholesaler Suma, see page 169 for address). You can make your own soya milk from soya flour (available from Green Farm Foodwatch, see page 168 for address). The soya milk recipe is on page 130.

On social occasions, arrange in advance to have a water you tolerate available, or take your own bottle if you have to. Friends, family, even restaurants, are usually very accommodating if you explain the situation. Bottled waters are now widely available at pubs and cafés. For children's parties, arrange in advance with hosts what your child will drink – if necessary, delivering a drink in advance so that your child does not appear too conspicuous.

If travelling or away from home, take a portable jug filter with you. Keep a jug filter at work, or take a flask of hot drink with you.

If You Are Highly Sensitive

If the above is not sufficient to relieve symptoms, then you may have to take greater precautions and limit your exposure to water generally as in the detection programme above. Try any or all of those avoidance measures and see how far you need to go.

If you are exceptionally sensitive, it may be worthwhile installing a plumbed-in filtering system of some kind (see below). Some people also find it helps to use a bottled water for cooking, washing vegetables and brushing teeth, although this is costly and inconvenient. Filtered or purified water is cheaper in the long run. If you are sensitive even to bottled waters, see page 441 for advice on how to cope.

TIP

Some people are very sensitive to the fumes of water when it first emerges from the tap or cistern. If this applies to you, try the following measures. Start the bath or basin filling, then leave the room while they fill, with the window open to ventilate. Return and turn off the taps. Leave the room again and leave the water to stand for a few minutes more if you need to. Avoid taking showers. The fumes are more concentrated in newly emerging water. Get someone to flush the lavatory for you, if you can. Keep the lid shut as it flushes.

Choosing a Water Treatment System

There is a bewildering array of competing systems for water treatment, purification and filtration on the market. They vary greatly in price, running costs, performance and capability. It is very difficult to compare like with like.

The main things you need to consider are:

- *Purity*
  How pure do you need the resulting water to be?

- *Initial Cost*
  How much do you want to pay to instal the system?
- *Running Costs*
  How much will it cost to run it over its life?
- *Coverage*
  What parts of your water system do you want to treat?
  Do you need just drinking water and cooking water, or do you want more coverage?
- *Convenience*
  Do you want a plumbed-in system?
  Do you want a system that requires frequent cartridge or membrane replacement?
  Do you object to a low flow-rate of water?
- *Taste*
  Do you mind a de-mineralised taste to your water?

The main types of purification and filtration methods are:

- Reverse Osmosis
- Kinetic Degradation Fluxion (KDF)
- Activated Carbon
- Distillation
- Softening

The way that these work and their principal benefits and drawbacks are explained below. The three methods which are useful for most chemically sensitive people's needs are reverse osmosis, KDF and activated carbon. All of these provide cheaper water than using bottled water.

Systems can be plumbed in variously, either undersink to supply one tap, or end of tap or showerhead to supply that outlet. Free-standing, or jug versions are available for some methods. Some methods are only suitable in certain variants – if you want a whole system version, or nitrate-reducing method, you only have limited choices.

Water Treatment Methods

Reverse Osmosis

Reverse Osmosis (RO) systems produce the purest water practicably available. They are purification systems, not filtering systems.

Independent tests have shown them to remove over 99 per cent of pesticide residues and chlorine, over 99 per cent of metals and 90 per cent of nitrates. They also remove most bacteria, parasites and viruses. Distillation systems are the only other water treatment systems which produce comparably pure water, but they have greater disadvantages.

RO systems work by forcing part of the water flow through a semipermeable membrane, combined usually with a sediment filter and an activated carbon filter (see below), which also absorbs contaminants. The water is stored in a small reservoir tank until needed.

The main benefit of RO systems is the purity of the water resulting. In addition, contaminants are washed away. They are not held in any treatment medium and cannot wash back into the system.

They have drawbacks, however. They have a very low flow-rate and need a high water pressure to work well. They are extremely wasteful of water. More than 75 per cent of the water used goes down the drain and this could be an important cost factor if water metering is introduced. Mineral salts are removed and the water has a bland, insipid taste which some people dislike.

Most of the reverse osmosis systems available are for plumbing in under a sink or basin with one tap outlet. A skilled DIYer could instal them, but many people will need a plumber's help. These undersink systems are also bulky and need a lot of space. They cost between £300 and £500, excluding any plumbing costs. The membranes need replacing every 18 months to three years and cost between £50 and £90. Carbon filter cartridges need replacing every six to twelve months and cost between £15 and £30.

A portable end-of-tap version is available at £90 (1992 prices), which is very convenient, and has the advantage that you can take it with you outside the home – to work, or on visits. See Table 17 for suppliers.

Firms will quote specially for installing reverse osmosis equipment to cover a whole water system. This will probably cost well over £1000 before plumbing costs, and the low flow-rate and water wastage would be very inconvenient in practice.

It has been known for some people – extremely isolated cases to react to RO water. However, it is the purest available and if you are unlucky enough to be that sensitive, it is probably still the best you can find. Manage your expectations if you are thinking of trying it though. Do not pin your hopes on it, just in case, if you have a history of exceptional sensitivity. Test it systematically before installing an expensive system. System suppliers can provide samples. >FOOD AND DRINK for how to test drinks.

Kinetic Degradation Fluxion

Kinetic Degradation Fluxion (KDF) treatment methods are based on the oxidation/reduction principle. These work through immersion of an alloy of copper and zinc in water. The two metals in the alloy have a different electrical potential and, in an electrically conductive fluid like water, this generates power like a battery, which starts a process of oxidation. This breaks down and modifies the structure of chemical contaminants, and kills bacteria. KDF filters are usually used in combination with sediment and activated carbon filters (see below).

Independent tests have shown that KDF filters remove over 90 per cent of metals, 100 per cent of chlorine, and reduce nitrates by over 75 per cent. Another benefit of KDF filters is that contaminants do not adhere to any filter medium as they do in activated carbon filters, and do not flush back into the system. Minerals are not removed, so that the water has a more acceptable taste than reverse osmosis water.

KDF filters can be plumbed in under a sink to supply one tap. They provide water at normal tap flow-rates, and, this plus the taste of the water, are a significant advantage over RO water. KDF filters can be installed by a skilled DIYer and can be bought at a price comparable to medium-range activated carbon filters – £105–165 before any plumbing. Cartridges need replacing every six to twelve months and cost between £25 and £50. An extra nitrate-reducing filter can be added to one version to remove virtually all nitrates.

There are no independent test results which compare KDF filtered water to activated carbon (AC) filtered water. Suppliers believe that KDF water is purer than AC water but have no precise evidence.

A showerhead version of a KDF filter is available for £50 which screws into the showerhead and needs replacing every 18 months or so. Chlorine is significantly reduced by this filter. It has no sediment or carbon filters.

Activated Carbon Filters

Activated Carbon (AC) filters are designed around activated carbon, a form of carbon which has been steam-treated. These work by adsorption, mopping up contaminant chemicals which pass through the filter and stick to the filter medium. They can absorb organic chemicals, pesticides and chlorine; many filter cartridges also contain ion exchange resins which reduce metals.

Suppliers will not make specific claims about the levels of contaminants which are reduced. A *Which?* report in August 1990 showed wide variations in the purity of results from comparable filters. But people who use them report significant improvement in their water quality and say they are worthwhile. People who use plumbed-in undersink or tap filters notice a marked improvement even over jug filters.

No AC filters kill bacteria. Filters containing silver are claimed to reduce bacterial growth in the system itself, although *Which?* tests did not demonstrate this. You need to take care, particularly with jug filters, not to allow bacteria to grow in standing water (see **Jug Filters**, below). If you are concerned about bacteria in a plumbed-in system, run the tap for a few minutes each morning, or after an absence from home, to allow fresh water from the mains to flow through the filter.

Minerals are not absorbed by AC filters, so tapwater retains an acceptable taste.

Undersink AC Filters

AC filters are plumbed in undersink to supply one tap, within the scope of the skilled DIYer. They cost between £50 and £200, before any plumbing costs. Most cost between £100 and £200. Replacement cartridges cost between £10 and £60, and it needs replacing every six to twelve months. Some systems offer filters which have indicators of when the cartridge needs replacing. Cartridges are generally slightly cheaper than KDF filters and the cost of water correspondingly lower. Nitrate-reducing versions of undersink filters are available. Tap-flow is not affected, unlike RO systems.

Contaminants can flush back into the system from the filter with some systems. Consult the latest *Which?* report to check which models do not do this. See also below for choice of system.

Compared to jug or end-of-tap filters, plumbed-in undersink filters are much more convenient to use and offer a higher level of purity. Depending on the model chosen, the cartridge costs are not necessarily more expensive than jug or tap filters, and the water can be comparable in cost.

Two makes of undersink filter, at the more expensive end of the range, performed particularly well in the *Which?* trials in terms of the purity of the water tested. These were the Everpure Citmart BW100 and the Ametek Fileder HM, priced at around £150–200. These systems did not flush back contaminants, and had indicators for cartridge change.

One smaller filter, the Berglen Tapmate AC 200, requiring more frequent cartridge replacement, also performed well in the *Which?* test and is priced at only £50. Cartridges cost £12 and need replacing monthly.

One undersink filter, the Opella Castalia, can be adapted to filter a whole house system. The system is designed primarily for use with a sediment filter, not a carbon filter, but a carbon filter can be used. This means that all your water, including toilet, bath and laundry, can be filtered. The disadvantage is that cartridges will need replacing monthly or every six weeks. This is costly – about £3.50 per week – and inconvenient. Some plumbing advisors also discourage using carbon filters in this way, since bacteria can grow in the system when chlorine has been removed.

Tap AC Filters

AC filters are available which fit on the end of a tap, or which are simple to plumb in to the sink top tap inlet pipe. They provide water on tap, at normal flow-rates. They are cheap, more convenient often than jug filters, and avoid any of the need to be careful about bacterial hygiene that jug filters involve. They are portable and can be taken with you if you go out or away. They cost between £11 and £90. Filters needs replacing every one to four months and cost between £8 and £19. They can be cheaper to run than jug filters. The quality of water is comparable to jug filters, and less pure generally than plumbed-in undersink AC or KDF filters.

Jug Filters

Jug filters cost between £10 and £20. A plastic container holding an activated carbon filter cartridge sits on a glass or plastic jug. You pour water through the tap container and it collects in the jug below.

Jug filters reduce the level of chemicals and metals in tapwater. They do not remove them completely, but people using them say that they do make a real difference.

You need to change the filter cartridge frequently – every 60–110 litres (13–24 gallons), or every month or so. If you live in a hard-water area, it will last less long than if you live in a soft-water area. Some jugs have a change-filter indicator to remind you when to change. The replacement cartridges cost between £2.50 and £3.50 (at 1992 prices). This can mean an annual running cost of £30–40, which is much cheaper than buying bottled water.

You need to take care not to allow bacteria to grow in the jug. Jugs and reservoirs are best cleaned weekly; filtered water should be kept in a fridge (best decanted into a bottle to save space). If water has stood in a jug for some time, it should not be used or it should be boiled before use.

The advantages of jug filters are their low initial cost and their flexibility – you can take them with you to work or if you visit or travel. You can buy filter systems with glass jugs if you are sensitive to plastic, and some filters will reduce nitrates significantly, although, again, not completely.

Distillation

Water distillers purify water by boiling water and cooling it again. Gases evaporate, bacteria and viruses are killed, and almost every other chemical salt, mineral and contaminant is left in the boiling chamber. The condensed water is then passed through an activated carbon filter, which removes organic chemicals which have not been removed in the steam. The distilled water is collected in a storage chamber. The resulting water is extremely pure – comparable to reverse osmosis water.

Distillation units cost between £400 and £600. They can be plumbed in under a sink, or can be used on a worktop or table top. Apart from the de-mineralised taste, their other drawbacks include the expense of electricity costs, their low flow-rate, their need for regular cleaning, and their bulk. The resulting water is warm also, so usually needs cooling before drinking. Their major disadvantage for the chemically sensitive, however, is that the water, being de-ionised, absorbs chemicals very readily from its environment and, being usually stored or held initially in a plastic container, has been known to upset people sensitive to plastics. Although it is so pure, in practice chemically sensitive people often tolerate distilled water less well than other types of purified or filtered water.

If you do not want to instal a distiller but want to use distilled water, one company The Freshwater Company (address below) supplies distilled water in containers (plastic) in the London and Home Counties area for a cost of between 21p and 25p per litre (2 pints) at 1992 prices. Pharmacies also sell distilled water, usually in plastic containers. You need to check whether it has been distilled with an activated carbon filter distiller. Some distilled or de-mineralised water sold for steam irons or other uses has not been filtered with activated carbon and still contains organic solvents.

Softening

Water softeners do not filter nor purify water. They are a long-established technology based on ion exchange. Water is passed over salts which remove the salts which cause hard water and soften the water. Impurities and contaminants are not reduced.

Water softeners cost between £300 and £600. The softener is

usually plumbed in to the whole system. A hard-water tap is usually kept for drinking and cooking use, since the softened water has a poor flavour and also contains high levels of sodium. Soft water can sometimes be of real benefit to people with eczema and dermatitis, since it is gentler on the skin, but it is no benefit generally to the chemically sensitive because it is no purer than tapwater.

Water softeners are also only of benefit in certain areas of the country, mostly the south of England, where the water is harder. They can save money on detergent use, and on heating costs because of reduced scale in pipes. The salts need refilling every few months, and cost £1 per week or so.

Which Water Treatment Method is Best for You?

If your main criterion is purity, then there is no substitute for a reverse osmosis system, despite its cost, and the disadvantages of flow-rate and taste. If you are short of money, an end-of-tap version is available for around £90 (supplier: Environmental Water Supplies) which has the merit that you can carry it with you when you go out or travel.

If you are sensitive to nitrates, use a reverse osmosis system for preference. Alternatively, look for a nitrate-reducing version of KDF, AC and jug filters.

If you are very short of money, but want something more convenient and effective than a jug filter, then your best choice may be a smaller plumbed-in undersink activated carbon filter at around £50 before plumbing costs (supplier: Berglen), or an end-of-tap activated carbon filter which costs between £11 and £90.

If you are sensitive to water you wash with, a showerhead KDF filter at about £50 (supplier: Environmental Water Supplies) is a cost-effective way of reducing problems and inconvenience. Users report that these are not always effective, so may not be useful if you are very sensitive.

If you want a system for your whole house, there is currently no ideal solution. There is an activated carbon filter system available for about £100 which will serve (supplier: Opella), but it is not designed for that purpose, and is costly and inconvenient in terms of filter replacement. Some suppliers are now just introducing purpose-built all-house AC filters – keep an eye out for new products coming on to the markets.

If money is no object, suppliers will quote to plumb in RO, KDF or

Table 17: **Suppliers of Water Treatment Systems**

SUPPLIERS	Reverse osmoic under sink	Reverse osmoic end of tap	KDF under sink	KDF shower head	Activated carbon whole	Activated carbon under sink	Activated carbon end of tap	Activated carbon jug	Activated carbon glass jug	Nitrate reducing system	Distillers	Distilled water	Water softeners
Addis								●		●			
Aldous and Slamp	●	●				●				●			●
Aqua Cure	●									●			
Berglen						●							
Boots						●							
Briggs Enterprises													●
Brita								●	●				
Citmart						●							
Ecowater	●					●				●	●		●
Environmental Office Water Supplies	●	●	●	●		●				●	●		●
Europlan	●	●				●				●			●
Fileder	●					●				●			
Freshwater												●	
Healthy House	●					●	●						
Krandojac						●							
Leisure Care						●							
Opella					●	●							
Scandinavia Direct						●							
Waymaster								●		●			

AC systems to supply multiple or different parts of your system – for instance, drinking water and sink, laundry, bathroom, or even lavatory. This could easily cost you upwards of £1000, so you need to be really sure it's worth it.

If you are not short of money, and not so sensitive that you really need RO water, a compromise solution may work better – say, with a good quality KDF or AC plumbed-in filter in the kitchen for drinking and cooking water, with a portable tap filter or jug filter available for other situations, and a showerhead filter for showers. Coverage of this kind would be possible for between £300 and £400 (before plumbing costs).

TIP

Many new products are coming on the market all the time. Consult *Which?* for the latest independent report or phone *Good Housekeeping* advice line (0839 141414). Calls at 48p per minute (1992 prices).

Also consult The British Effluent and Water Association (BEWA); details on page 453. They have a list of reputable equipment suppliers.

Always compare cartridge and membrane replacement costs as well as initial equipment costs. These vary widely and a cheaper model may be more expensive to run over the years.

Addresses of Suppliers

Addis Ltd
Ware Road
Hertford SG13 7HL
Tel: 0992 584221

Aldous & Stamp Ltd
86–90 Avenue Road
Beckenham
Kent BR3 4SA
Tel: 081–659 1833

Aqua Cure plc
Aqua Cure House
Hall Street
Southport PR9 0SE
Tel: 0704 501616

Berglen Group Ltd
Masons House
Kingsbury Road
London NW9 9NQ
Tel: 081–205 1133

Boots plc
1 Thane Road West
Nottingham NG2 3AA
Tel: 0602 506111

Briggs Enterprises
North Marston
Buckinghamshire MK18 3PD
Tel: 0296 67351

British Effluent & Water
Association
5 Castle Street
High Wycombe
Buckinghamshire HP13 6RZ
Tel: 0494 444544

Brita (UK) Ltd
Brita House
62–64 Bridge Street
Walton-on-Thames
Surrey KT12 1AP
Tel: 0932 228348

Citmart Ltd
Lympne Industrial Park
Hythe
Kent CT21 4LT
Tel: 0303 262211

Ecowater Systems Ltd
Unit 1
The Independent Business Park
Mill Road
Stokenchurch
Buckinghamshire HP14 3TP
Tel: 0494 484000

Environmental Office Water
Supplies
Waveney House
Victoria Road
Diss
Norfolk IP22 3JG
Tel: 0379 642525

Europlan Water Ltd
Euro House
Essex Court
Ashton Road
Romford RM3 8UF
Tel: 04023 81538

Fileder Filter Systems Ltd
Orchard Business Centre
20/20 Maidstone
Kent ME16 0JZ
Tel: 0622 691886

The Freshwater Company
64 Hadley Street
London NW1 8TA
Tel: 071–267 4919

The Healthy House
Cold Harbour
Ruscombe
Stroud
Gloucestershire GL6 4DA
Tel: 0453 752216

Krandojac Agents
Station Farmhouse
Thuxton
Norfolk NR9 4QJ
Tel: 0362 850320

Leisure Care Products Ltd
Samuel Whites House
Medina Road
Cowes
Isle of Wight PO31 7LP
Tel: 0983 299119

Opella Ltd
Rotherwas Industrial Estate
Hereford HR2 6JR
Tel: 0432 357331

Scandinavia Direct Ltd
18/19 Millbrook Business Park
Crowborough
East Sussex TN6 3JZ
Tel: 0892 663312

Waymaster Ltd
Meadow Road
Reading
Berkshire RG1 8LB
Tel: 0734 599444

PART 6
WHAT HELP IS AVAILABLE?

Medical Help

This section deals with information on medical treatments available, particularly

- Drug treatments
- Emollients and moisturisers
- Desensitisation and neutralisation

It also contains information on precautions to take with vaccination, anaesthetics and dental treatment. Finally, it provides information on societies of doctors who specialise in allergy, immunology and in environmental medicine.

If you are sensitive to antibiotics, >MOULDS for more advice.

This section is intended to give a brief explanation for the lay-person of the main types of treatment available. For full explanation, you should always consult a doctor.

For advice on emergency treatment, >EMERGENCY INFORMATION.

Drug Therapy

Drugs can be invaluable in treating reactions and people often have to take them for long periods to control severe symptoms. Some drugs have relatively few side effects, but others are potent and can have serious side effects. Avoidance of things which cause your reactions can mean in some cases that you no longer need drug treatment. For other people, particularly severe asthmatics, drugs may still be necessary even with strict avoidance, but the dosage required is usually much less and you are much more in control of your situation.

TIP

If you are chemically sensitive or food sensitive, you may perhaps have problems with excipients (e.g. colourings, sweetenings, grains, powders) with which drugs are formulated. Consult your doctor for the least troublesome form of drug.

The various types of drugs which can be used in treatment are:

- Anti-histamines
- Sodium cromoglycate
- Decongestants
- Steroids
- Bronchodilators and anti-cholinergics

Anti-histamines

Anti-histamine drugs work by blocking the action of histamine, a chemical released from cells during an allergic reaction and responsible for most of the unpleasant symptoms. They can be very effective against true allergic reactions – particularly so against itchiness, hay fever and rhinitis – but not against food intolerance or chemical sensitivity (>DEFINING ALLERGY). They are relatively simple drugs, with few side effects and are not addictive. They can be bought 'over the counter' but are best taken with medical advice.

Earlier types of anti-histamine, such as Piriton, cause drowsiness as a side effect and cannot be combined with alcohol. Other more modern drugs, such as Triludan, do not cause drowsiness.

Some people find that the effectiveness of anti-histamines wears off after a while. There are six separate classes of anti-histamine from different chemical groups and it can often work to try a drug from another class if one drug has ceased to be effective. A drug that has lost its effectiveness often regains it if you take another one for a while and then return to it.

Anti-histamines can be taken in tablets or syrups. Syrups are available without colouring and with the minimum of sugars for highly sensitive children (or indeed adults). Anti-histamines are also available as creams to apply to the skin, but you can become sensitive to preservatives and other substances in the cream, and their use is best kept to the absolute essential.

The anti-histamine drugs which have a sedative effect can be very useful if you have a child who is distressed by itchy skin or hives at night, in helping them to sleep through the discomfort.

Sodium Cromoglycate

Sodium cromoglycate is a drug which works by stabilising the mast cells which are the cells primarily responsible for releasing histamine and other chemicals during an allergic reaction. Stabilising the mast cells reduces the amount of histamine released. It works best for people who have true allergy (>DEFINING ALLERGY) but can be effective sometimes in cases of food intolerance or chemical sensitivity. It is almost totally free of side effects. Adverse reactions to it are extremely rare.

The drug can be given as eye-drops for conjunctivitis (e.g. Opticrom), as a nasal spray (e.g. Rynacrom) or in a spinhaler or pressurised aerosol for asthma (e.g. Intal). It can take from a few days to several weeks for the drug to take effect and needs to be taken continuously during the period of exposure.

It can be taken as a powder by mouth with water to block food sensitivity reactions (e.g. Nalcrom). Large doses of the drug may be needed to make this effective. It can also take a time of experimenting with Nalcrom to find the right dose (usually 6–10 capsules 30 minutes to an hour before a meal) as individuals vary in the dosage that they need. So most people who take it reserve its use for special occasions – for children to go to birthday parties for instance, for family celebrations, or for meals out. It is not usually prescribed for anyone who has had a violent, immediate allergic reaction to a food, who should avoid that food completely. The risks of the drug not working are very slight but not worth taking in these situations.

In clearly allergic cases, sodium cromoglycate is usually tried before steroid drugs are, and is effective in most cases, avoiding the need for steroids (see below).

Decongestants

Decongestants work by shrinking blood vessels, thereby relieving the effects of an allergic reaction, particularly in the mucus membranes of the nose. They can be taken as tablets or as nasal sprays (e.g. Otrivine, Afrazine and Sudafed). They can be effective against hay fever and rhinitis, but their major drawback is that they lose their effectiveness as time goes on. Moreover, they can actually make symptoms worse when their use is stopped. The blood vessels react to this cessation by expanding again, which causes congestion once more, even if the allergen is absent and you are not reacting.

The best advice is not to use decongestants continuously for more than three to five days, and to avoid prolonged use. You should use them on doctor's advice rather than buy them over the counter.

Some decongestants are combined with anti-histamines (e.g. Congesteeze, Haymine, Sudafed Plus).

Decongestants can be dangerous if you have a history of high blood pressure or heart disease. Consult your doctor.

Steroids

Steroids are very powerful and potentially dangerous drugs which are used to prevent the inflammatory reactions that accompany allergic reactions. They are used particularly in more serious cases and are very effective.

For serious conditions, steroids may need to be taken for long periods at higher dosages, with the risk of inducing side effects which may not be readily reversible. If you have an alternative, such as avoiding the substances or foods which are triggering the disease, this is clearly better. If there is no alternative, then it is necessary to weigh up the advantages of the steroids against their risks. Ask your doctor to discuss it with you openly, so that you can make an informed decision. If you have serious disease or disability, do not refuse steroids without understanding the consequences.

Steroids should not be stopped suddenly if they have been taken for more than a few days, because they depress the natural production of steroids by the body, which must be given a chance to recover.

The worst side effects of steroids are mostly associated with prolonged oral treatments, or repeated injections, though if you use steroid creams or ointments too lavishly (particularly the stronger ones) you can absorb enough to have general effects. Side effects include facial swelling, obesity, brittle bones, high blood pressure, cataracts, diabetes, peptic ulceration, changes in mental state, and slowing the growth of children. Local effects include thinning of the skin and mucus membrane, nosebleeds, and reduced resistance to infections.

Very few people experience side effects from short courses of steroids or from the regular use of steroid inhalers, and this is the treatment of choice for moderate or severe asthma which cannot be controlled by avoiding allergens or other triggers.

Steroid inhalers (e.g. Becotide, Becloforte, Pulmicort) have less side effects than using tablets. (Sodium cromoglycate inhalers, see above, are usually tried before steroids because they can be effective, particularly with allergic asthma.) As a side effect, steroid inhalers can cause candidiasis (thrush) in the throat. This can be reduced by using a spacer, or by gargling with water after each use.

Steroid nasal sprays (e.g. Beconase, Syntaris, Rhinocort) are often prescribed for pollen allergy and are best used for the pollen season, and a short while in advance only. For grass pollen allergy, use is recommended from early May to the end of grass pollen season (mid to end July). For tree pollen allergy, use is often recommended from

February, depending on the pollens which affect you (>POLLENS). Nose bleeds sometimes result from use of nasal sprays.

Steroids are sometimes given as short courses of treatment for severe seasonal rhinitis as tablets (e.g. Prednisolone) or by injection (e.g. Kenalog).

Steroid eye drops should only be used under the direction of an eye specialist. They can have serious effects if not used appropriately.

Steroid creams and ointments (e.g. hydrocortisone creams or Tinnocort, Betnovate, Dermovate) are very commonly prescribed for eczema and dermatitis. If too much is used, the steroids are absorbed through the skin and can result in the general side effects described above. It is unwise to use steroid creams and ointments lavishly, to smother a child or adult in them, however badly affected, or to use them continuously over a long period. Always consult your doctor about the best way to use these and other medication.

Bronchodilators and Anti-cholinergics

Bronchodilators are used in the control of asthma by making the bronchial muscles relax. There are two types of drugs used as bronchodilators – beta-adrenoceptor agonists, and xanthine drugs.

Beta adrenoceptor agonists can be given in aerosol, powder or tablets. They relax the muscles around the lung airways and are primarily used to *relieve*, not prevent, bronchospasm; they are sometimes taken before steroid inhalers to free the airways so that the steroids penetrate throughout the lungs. The effectiveness of an inhaled dose lasts for up to six hours. Slow-release tablets or syrup can be useful overnight. They may cause side effects, but usually only briefly if used in excessive doses; these include tremors, palpitations, and headaches. The beneficial effects of the drugs cease once use is stopped.

At present, it appears wiser to *prevent* asthma using avoidance, desensitisation and, if necessary, inhaled steroids so that relief medication of this kind is not required too frequently, as there is some evidence that prolonged regular use may increase the twitchiness of the airways. Some doctors prefer prevention of asthma to prescribing these drugs indefinitely.

The most commonly used types are as follows:

- Salbutamol: Ventolin, Ventodisks, Volmax, Cobutolin, Salbulin, Salbuvent, Asmaven, Aerolin-Auto
- Terbutaline: Bricanyl, Monovent
- Fenoterol: Berotec

- Pirbuterol: Exirel
- Reproterol: Bronchodil
- Rimiterol: Pulmadil

For people sensitive to excipients – other ingredients used in preparing the drug – the powder form of an inhaler is usually well tolerated.

One of the most important elements in the effectiveness of these drugs lies in operating the inhaler properly so that the right amount of drug reaches the affected parts. Many inhalers now have metered doses – in forms of turbohaler, diskhaler, or rotohaler.

It is particularly important for children to learn to operate an inhaler properly on their own. Many GPs now run asthma clinics and can advise. The National Asthma Campaign (address in CHARITIES) also offers advice and local support groups.

If a child has problems using an inhaler, bronchodilator drugs can be given as slow-release tablets or in syrups. If the child is highly sensitive to many things, however, a powder inhaler is probably the best alternative.

TIP

Make sure that staff at school understand when and how your child may need his or her inhaler, and that it is available for use whenever necessary.

Remember that children's muscles tire easily – never take your child's asthma for granted. If the child does not respond to his or her reliever medicine or inhaler, call your doctor urgently or take the child to the hospital where they will have a nebuliser that delivers the reliever medicine more efficiently.

Xanthine bronchodilators (such as Phyllocontin, Nuelin, Uniphyllin) have a different chemical effect from beta-adrenoceptor agonists, although they too relax the muscles around the airways. At the correct dose for the individual, they cause no side effects; your doctor will need to adjust the dosage should they cause known side effects of stomach upsets, palpitations, sleep disturbance, or epileptic fits. These are not permanent effects. These drugs are given as tablets or suppositories and can be useful for slow release overnight to avoid waking to use an inhaler.

Anti-cholinergics are drugs which control the width of the airways of the lung. They work by blocking the contraction of muscle around the airways. A modern version of the drug called Atrovent can be used as an aerosol and inhaled. Its side effects are rare except at high doses; they include a dry mouth, constipation and finding passing urine difficult.

Emollients and Moisturisers

Emollients and moisturisers are used in a variety of ways to help relieve the distress of eczema and dermatitis. Their main functions are both to soothe the skin and to protect it against things touching or entering.

It is possible to become sensitive to creams and ointments used in this way, which can aggravate the condition. Sensitivity is moreover highly personal – one person will tolerate one product but not another – so it is difficult to give general advice about what to use, or how and when.

Aqueous cream is used for moisturising and soothing. It is not occlusive, i.e. it does not shut out or prevent anything entering or touching the affected site. 'Simple aqueous cream' contains only phenoxyethanol held in boiled and cooled purified water: ask a pharmacist for this. Some aqueous creams contain wool fat, including lanolin, and preservatives which cause some people to react. These may suit you but Patch Test (>CHEMICALS for method) before widespread use.

Occlusive ointments usually have a greasy ingredient, such as soft paraffin, to put a film over the affected skin and protect it. Some such as Unguentum Merck wash off readily in water.

Some creams and ointments come in combinations of emollient and moisturiser, and some can be used in the bath to soothe.

The National Eczema Society offers an excellent advisory service for choosing emollients and moisturisers, together with a computerised database of product ingredients, if you know you react to a specific chemical. Their address and telephone number are in CHARITIES.

Ultraviolet light treatment can also help eczema, as can a stay at the seaside. Trials are under way of therapy with evening primrose oil, and of traditional Chinese herbal remedies which have shown results in some people with eczema.

Desensitisation and Neutralisation

Treatment of allergies and sensitivity by immunotherapy – stimulating the immune system in some way to stop the allergic reaction – is practised in three main forms – desensitisation, neutralisation, and enzyme-potentiated desensitisation. These are controversial – partly because the mechanisms are not entirely understood, and partly because they do not work equally well on everybody. They are not alternative or complementary medicine techniques. When properly applied, the techniques can be very effective and they offer a drug-free and relatively simple solution. They all work best when combined with avoidance measures.

Desensitisation

Desensitisation (also called immunotherapy or hyposensitisation) is carried out by giving a series of injections, into tissue beneath the skin, of the substance to which the person is allergic, over a period of months or years. The first injection is dilute, but may still cause a local reaction or a mild general reaction. Provided the reaction is mild, the next injection is stronger, and the injections continue to increase, week by week. On each occasion the individual must be watched for two hours, because very rarely the injections can cause a more severe reaction. This method is now only used in hospitals, and is mainly used to protect people who get serious reactions to bee and wasp stings, for which it is the only effective protection and can be life-saving.

Courses of injections are usually given in the three to six months before the start of seasonal exposure: in some people, two or three courses may result in marked improvement in symptoms lasting for many years. Not everybody manages to tolerate the treatment.

If desensitisation works for you and you stay the course, it can be a very convenient and straightforward therapy. Desensitisation is known to be most effective against bee and wasp stings, and inhalant allergens such as grass pollens and house dust mites; and for symptoms such as hay fever and asthma. It is not usually very effective against food allergy. For seasonal allergens, such as moulds or pollens, it is best carried out before the season starts.

Neutralisation

Neutralisation is also known as the Miller technique. It has some similarities to desensitisation but is carried out in a different way and does not carry the same risks. A small amount of a dilute allergen extract – foods or inhalants – is injected intra-dermally (between the two layers of skin) in a small weal – a bubble of liquid. If the person is allergic to the substance, the weal will grow to form a sharp edge and harden. Sometimes there will also be a flare – red, itchy skin – around the weal. Some people also produce symptoms, brought on by the specific allergen. If at the end of ten minutes, there is no change to the weal, and no flare, the reaction is negative.

The aim of the neutralisation testing is to find the strongest extract which does not cause a reaction in the skin – that is, that does not result in an increase in the size of the weal. After a positive reaction, a weaker dilution is tried, using the same procedure. If that is positive, the process continues using weaker and weaker doses until a negative reaction is found. That dilution is called the endpoint – the strongest dose that fails to produce a positive reaction. In practice, most people find that this endpoint – specific to them – turns off their symptoms, and they can encounter an allergen or eat a food without reacting to it.

The person is given either drops (to take under the tongue) or vaccine (to inject themselves) with their own endpoints which, used regularly, will protect them and control their symptoms. Multiple extracts can be included in one vial so that only one drop or vaccine is required to cover the various allergens. The neutralisation effect is not permanent – the drops or vaccine need to be taken regularly to prevent reactions. The intervals at which they need to be taken depend on the individual and the severity of their reactions. The effects of drops wear off after a few hours and are most convenient for foods eaten irregularly or substances not encountered every day. Injected vaccines have a longer lasting effect and, while most people need to inject once every two days, others need only to inject once or twice a week.

Neutralisation is most effective for inhaled allergens (such as moulds, dust mites and pollens) but it also works for food allergy and intolerance, and for chemical sensitivity. (Neutralisation for chemical sensitivity is usually done by placing drops of extract under the tongue and monitoring symptoms: when symptoms are relieved, the endpoint is found.)

When neutralisation works, the effect, like desensitisation, can be magical. Symptoms melt away and it can be a boon for people with multiple allergies and sensitivity. If on a very restricted diet, it can actually enable you to eat trigger foods with virtually no problems.

Neutralisation has its drawbacks, however. Many people do not reproduce symptoms on testing with inhalant allergens, but if you do, the process of testing can be tiring and painful. Occasionally people's symptoms do not 'turn off' at the strongest negative dilution and for them, it is necessary to continue testing until the symptoms disappear.

It can also take a while for the endpoint to become effective. The neutralising effects of the endpoint do not always work fully at first and it can take a few weeks for the effect to build up. It can be a confusing and difficult time to experience.

Many people find that they do not need the neutralising endpoints permanently. Combined with avoidance, their system recovers sufficiently to cope without, and usually within eighteen months to two years, neutralisation is no longer necessary. In a minority of people, endpoints may shift from time to time within that period (often as the individual gets better), and the vaccines need retesting. It can be tiresome and time-consuming to retest, especially if you have many allergies, but it is worthwhile to have the endpoint right again.

Neutralisation is only available on the NHS at one or two centres in the UK. It is a relatively safe procedure – no fatal nor near-fatal reactions have ever been recorded. Like desensitisation, some people do not respond to it at all, but for those who do (particularly those with multiple sensitivity, with very severe reactions, or people intolerant of drugs), it can be one of their few means of relief.

Enzyme-Potentiated Desensitisation (EPD)

In Enzyme-Potentiated Desensitisation (EPD), an enzyme β-glucuronidase is used in combination with allergen extracts to enhance the desensitising effect. A wide range of extracts of allergens, foods and chemicals is mixed with the enzyme which is held by a small plastic cup against a scrape on the skin for 24–48 hours, or injected into the skin. Symptoms usually show some improvement within a week, lasting two to three months at first. Treatment is repeated about once every three months, for between one and two years.

The same mixture of extract at the same dose is given to everyone, so there is no need for individual, time-consuming testing. Elimination diets or challenge testing are less important (these are usually necessary with neutralisation) but best results are obtained if these are carried out in conjunction with treatment.

Developed by Dr Len McEwen at St Mary's Hospital, Paddington, this method works very well for some people, although some do get worse before they improve.

EPD is a less costly and less disruptive form of desensitisation and has achieved some impressive results. For more information, contact the National Society for Research into Allergy which has a leaflet on the subject, and Action Against Allergy (addresses in CHARITIES).

Vaccination

Some people react to the sera on which immunising vaccines are cultivated. These have been greatly purified and refined, and adverse reactions are rare, but it is worth asking your doctor what the base of any vaccine is before it is given. Horse serum and eggs are sometimes used, for instance, and might affect you if you are sensitive to these. For advice on babies and immunisation, >BABYCARE.

Anaesthetics

It is known for people to have adverse reactions to anaesthetics more commonly to general anaesthetics than to local anaesthetics. A surgeon or anaesthesist will usually check with you before any procedure whether you have any history of allergy or sensitivity, but make sure they know if you have such a history. Local anaesthetics are less hazardous – opt for a local, rather than general, anaesthetic if a choice is offered. If you have already had an adverse reaction, you can be tested in advance of any operation to see what chemical you react to, and a more appropriate mix of drugs chosen for you. Your GP can contact the National Adverse Reaction Consultancy Service (NARCOS) which is a specialist advisory service.

NARCOS
Royal Hallamshire Hospital
Glossop Road
Sheffield
South Yorkshire S10 2JF
Tel: 0942 766222

Dental Treatment

Anaesthetising injections used in dental treatment are relatively simple chemicals given locally and reaction is rare. If you are concerned, try to avoid having injections unless absolutely essential. If you have had adverse reactions, >**Anaesthetics** (above). If sensitive to water and disinfectants, take your own water with you for rinsing your mouth.

Some people are affected by the mercury in amalgam fillings. Replacement or new fillings of material other than amalgam can be paid for under usual NHS funding if your dentist is willing to do it, but it requires a special letter from your doctor saying that the work is essential. Consult your dentist and doctor.

Other materials used in dental treatment very rarely cause problems, or are used only fleetingly (e.g. in making moulds for braces or dentures). If you think you have become sensitive to your dentures, try changing your denture cleaning material first (>PERSONAL HYGIENE). If you are sensitive to plastic materials, it is possible to have metal dentures made.

Doctors' Organisations

If you want to find a doctor who specialises in allergy and sensitivity, there are two specialist societies who may be able to advise you of doctors convenient for you:

The British Society for Allergy and Environmental Medicine
Acorns
Romsey Road
Southampton SO4 2NN

British Society for Allergy and Clinical Immunology
Department of Respiratory Medicine
St Bartholomew's Hospital
London EC1A 7BE

Complementary Therapy

Many people with allergy and sensitivity find real benefit from various kinds of complementary therapy. This section describes the main types, and sets out any areas of treatment where people with allergies and sensitivity may need to take extra care.

This section looks in particular at:

- Acupuncture
- Homeopathy
- Reflexology
- Aromatherapy

It also discusses other types of therapy, such as naturopathy and herbalism, plus healing, psychotherapy, growth and relaxation therapies.

Whatever type of complementary therapy you might try, it is important to *go to a qualified and reputable practitioner*. Check what training and qualifications practitioners have and get a personal reference from one of their clients if you can. Some less reputable practitioners make inflated claims about what they can achieve – multiple allergy and sensitivity can be difficult to sort out and can take time, even for the experienced; unless you have relatively straightforward problems, you should be wary of anyone who offers an instant, or one-answer solution.

Using complementary therapy may not remove the need for carrying out avoidance techniques – you may still have to take care with diet or other measures. Treat any therapy as another weapon in your armoury, not your only route to wellbeing.

If you are extremely sensitive to chemicals or foods, or have multiple sensitivity, you should take extra care with any therapy that involves using chemicals (even if natural, such as oils or herbs); that involves special diets, or taking herbal, plant or other remedies (such as homeopathy). See below for advice on individual therapies.

Acupuncture

Acupuncture is a sophisticated therapy, based on Chinese traditional methods, in which fine needles are inserted at specific points in the body, to stimulate energy flow and to restore equilibrium in the body. The theory of acupuncture is that the lifeforce functions through the flow of energy through certain channels in the body and if there is a blockage, illness results. Diagnosis is based, not on organic dysfunction and specific symptoms, as in Western medicine, but on a wide-ranging appraisal of the individual's character, temperament, constitution and life situation. Allergies and sensitivity in this system are a specific manifestation of the disequilibrium of the individual.

Acupuncture is taken very seriously as a therapy now in certain quarters of Western medicine and is used for anaesthesia; for pain relief; and for complementary treatment by a number of general practices. For people with allergies and sensitivity, acupuncture treatment can be very helpful and many people respond to a course of treatment. It can be relaxing and invigorating, even if specific symptoms do not respond straightaway. The only materials used are the fine needles inserted in the skin, so the therapy does not cause reactions in itself.

Homeopathy

Homeopathy can be a powerful and effective treatment for allergies and sensitivity. It is best to go to a practitioner for treatment if you can, rather than to treat yourself with over-the-counter remedies. People sensitive to one substance or a small number often respond rapidly and extremely well to a short course of treatment. If you have more complicated problems, or are extremely sensitive, it is particularly important to go to a qualified practitioner experienced in the field of allergy and sensitivity. Homeopathy can have quite a powerful impact if you have multiple sensitivity, and you can be made more unwell before you get better. An experienced practitioner will understand this hypersensitivity and will take care accordingly.

Homeopathy works on the principle of treating like with like. Specific symptoms are seen as the manifestation of the body's own natural striving to rid itself of disorders – be they infections, viruses, genetic disorders, emotional stress or whatever. The remedies which are given are based on substances which, in a healthy person, replicate the ill person's symptoms – as if the remedy is giving a nudge to the healing system of the body, helping it to throw off and shed the stresses upon it.

Remedies are chosen either for specific symptoms or as a constitutional remedy which fits the person's temperament, constitution and nature. The constitutional remedy works at a much deeper level, often more slowly, sometimes clearing symptoms and unresolved ill-health which has been with the individual for a long time.

If you consult a homeopath, he or she may give you a specific remedy for your pressing symptoms, and/or a constitutional remedy. The substances on which the remedies are based are natural or mineral substances, such as plants or naturally occuring chemicals. They are given at minute, almost unidentifiable dilutions. Scientific tests have shown that traces of the dilutions can be detected as electrical charges, but not by chemical means.

You can become worse when you first take a remedy, as the body clears old symptoms, especially if you take a constitutional remedy. But improvement can come rapidly – most people can expect benefits within months, although if you have many problems, it can take longer.

Homeopathic treatment for pollen allergy can be very effective. This is done either with a remedy based on a pollen mixture, or on a remedy to relieve specific symptoms. Therapy is most effective if started in advance of the pollen season. >POLLENS for details of timing of tree, grass and other pollens.

If you are extremely sensitive to foods or chemicals, you may need to take care in how you take a remedy. Most are tableted with lactose or sugar. You can have remedies dispensed in distilled water and this may be a better way to take them. Distilled water remedies are also better for giving to children or babies – they can be given as drops under the tongue.

Ainsworths Pharmacy will make up remedies in distilled water by mail order:

Ainsworths Homeopathic Pharmacy
38 New Cavendish Street
London W1M 7LH
Tel: 071–935 5330

Some people with allergies and sensitivity find homeopathic creams and tinctures very useful for certain kinds of first aid (>FIRST AID AND HOME MEDICINE). Some of the creams are alcohol-based, contain

TIP

If you are very sensitive, you may also react to the remedy itself, even if it is the right one for you. Try it at different dilutions to find a dilution which does not upset you. This should then work well.

preservatives and do not suit the very sensitive. Tinctures are usually based on purified water and are often well tolerated.

Reflexology

Reflexology is a form of foot massage which claims to alleviate and resolve illness. There are various systems of reflexology, but all have in common that they divide the foot into zones which correspond to organs or systems of the body. Reflexologists claim that massage of specific areas of the foot, and of the feet in general, addresses organic disorders and restores overall equilibrium.

Some people with allergies and sensitivity find reflexology very helpful, in particular finding it relaxing and invigorating. It is non-invasive and requires taking no remedies, oils or creams. It rarely causes adverse reaction. Some practitioners use special talcum powder. If this upsets you, ask for massage to be done without, or to use magnesium carbonate powder (available from pharmacies).

Aromatherapy

Aromatherapy is a form of therapy which combines massage with the application of oils from plants. The oils are chosen for their ability to stimulate certain systems of the body, and to alleviate specific symptoms.

Aromotherapy can be relaxing and helpful if you have mild sensitivity, but it can sometimes be troublesome if you have skin problems, and if you are chemically sensitive. The oils used, although from natural sources, are complex chemicals and can cause or aggravate chemical sensitivity. You should do a Patch Test or Sniff Test (>CHEMICALS on how to do these) on individual oils before using them. Only use oils which do not upset you and make sure the practitioner knows that you are prone to allergy and sensitivity. It is probably best not to use the oils on a highly sensitive baby or child. >also PLANTS AND TREES and CHEMICALS if you want to know more about sensitivity to natural chemicals.

Naturopathy and Herbalism

Naturopathic and herbalist therapies rely on various combinations of diet cleansing the system, and administration of natural or herbal remedies to alleviate symptoms. They, like other complementary therapies, look at the individual in the round, taking into account the person's temperament, constitution and life situation.

Therapies of this kind can be extremely effective against allergies and sensitivity. (A form of Chinese herbal treatment for eczema is currently undergoing medical trials in the UK by doctors to assess how widespread its effectiveness is.)

If you have food and chemical sensitivity, you may need to take care with any special diet proposed (including special drinks or infusions), or with taking herbal remedies. If you have a pre-disposition to food or chemical sensitivity, you may become intolerant of, and start to react to, components of the diet or remedies. If you start to feel ill on a special regime, test out whether you are sensitive to remedies, drinks or herbs, using the protocol in FOOD AND DRINK (page 126). Again, take extra care if these therapies are used on a highly sensitive child. Do not give to a baby.

Healing, Psychotherapeutic, Growth and Relaxation Therapies

Healing, personal growth and relaxation therapies of all kinds can be very beneficial. Stress – conscious or unconscious, resulting from the illness itself or from other areas of life – plays an important role in allergies and sensitivity; most people recognise that their symptoms worsen noticeably at times of strain and stress. Learning to relax, using breathing and other techniques, dealing with unfinished business or confronting problem areas of your life can help enormously and improve your wellbeing.

Emergency Information

The danger signs in any reaction are swelling of the lips, mouth and throat, and constriction in breathing caused by these, as well as pallor and collapse. Always ring a doctor immediately or seek emergency help if you have any suspicion of a shock reaction. It is better to be safe than sorry. Full symptoms of shock reactions are given in SYMP-TOMS.

If you have a history of shock or near-fatal reaction, your doctor may prescribe for you adrenalin which you can carry with you in a syringe. This is to be used only in life-threatening situations with medical supervision and you will be given precise instructions on when and how to administer it.

If you have had a shock or near-fatal reaction in the past, you should get a doctor's advice before you carry out any of the home test procedures in this book. If he or she see no danger, then carry out the tests but

- Have any emergency kit prescribed (such as an adrenalin syringe) to hand
- Never do a test without someone else being present or close at hand for the period of testing and a few hours afterwards.

To protect you in emergencies, it may be useful for you to register with Medic-Alert, if you have a history, for instance, of anaphylactic shock, or of life-threatening asthma attack, or if you are allergic to drugs or anaesthetics. Medic-Alert is a charity that keeps a register of personal medical information and can be contacted by doctors anywhere in the world, in case of emergency or accident. You wear a disc round your neck or wrist which carries short medical details and a contact telephone number. It costs a minimum of £26 to register (at 1992).

Medic-Alert Foundation
12 Bridge Wharf
156 Caledonian Road
London N1 9UU
Tel: 071–833 3034

Alternatively, you can buy from jewellers an SOS Talisman locket, which does not provide a central register of information but rather key information held in the locket. The SOS symbol is widely known and recognised.

If you do not carry these, make sure that you carry details of allergy or sensitivity on your person – say in a diary or wallet. For a child at school or nursery, make sure their details are held by the institution where they can be consulted quickly if needed.

For precautions to take if you have had an adverse reaction to anaesthetics, >MEDICAL HELP.

Charities

There are a number of charities which can offer you support and advice on living with allergy and sensitivity. Some charities concentrate on particular diseases linked to allergy or intolerance, such as asthma, eczema, coeliac disease, colitis and Crohn's disease or myalgo-encephalomyelitis (ME). Some of these can put you in touch with local support groups and give you practical advice. There are also charities which exist to raise money for research, and to give counselling on preconceptual care.

Details of Charities

Action Against Allergy (AAA) offers help and advice to individuals, and campaigns for increased medical provision and research into allergy. Its quarterly newsletter has tips and advice on living with allergy. AAA can also give you individual counselling and advice, or put you in touch with members who live near you if you want to meet fellow sufferers. They have a subsidiary company, Merton Books, which sells a wide range of books on allergy.

> Action Against Allergy
> 24–26 High Street
> Hampton Hill
> Middlesex TW12 1PD
> (No telephone)

The British Allergy Foundation campaigns to increase public awareness of allergy and to advance knowledge and research.

> The British Allergy Foundation
> St Bartholomew's Hospital
> West Smithfield
> London EC1A 7BE
> Tel: 071–600 6127

For sufferers of *coeliac disease*:

> Coeliac Society
> PO Box 220
> High Wycombe
> Buckinghamshire HP11 2HY
> Tel: 0494 437278

The Environmental Medicine Foundation funds research into illness caused by environmental factors:

> Environmental Medicine Foundation
> Symondsbury House
> Bridport
> Dorset DT6 6HB
> Tel: 0308 22956

Foresight gives advice and counselling on preconceptual care.

> Foresight
> The Old Vicarage
> Church Lane
> Witley
> Godalming
> Surrey GU8 5PN
> Tel: 0483 427839

Hyperactivity (or hyperkinesis) in children is sometimes linked to hypersensitivity and allergy (>CHILDCARE). *The Hyperactive Children's Support Group* have local support groups. It can be contacted at:

> 71 Whyke Lane
> Chichester
> West Sussex PO19 2LD
> Tel: 0903 725182

For sufferers of myalgic-encephalomyelitis (ME):

> Myalgic-Encephalomyelitis (ME) Association
> Stanhope House
> High Street
> Stanford-le-Hope
> Essex SS17 0HA
> Tel: 0375 642466

For sufferers of colitis and Crohn's disease:

National Association for Colitis & Crohn's Disease
98A London Road
St Albans
Hertfordshire AL1 1NX
Tel: 0727 44296

The National Asthma Campaign offers information and support for asthma sufferers, and funds medical research projects. They have a series of pamphlets and guides on aspects of asthma. They can put you in contact with local branches and have a quarterly newspaper. They have a Helpline telephone number, charged at local call rates.

National Asthma Campaign
Providence House
Providence Place
London N1 0NT
Tel: 071–226 2266
Helpline: 0345 010203

The National Eczema Society (NES) offers a wide range of help and information, including a quarterly magazine and information packs. It has local branches which offer support and advice. It has a computer database which, with the co-operation of many manufacturers, can help you to identify products which do not contain allergens which upset you. If you know which substances you are sensitive to, the NES can search the database, check the ingredients of products you are currently using, and give you a list of products whose ingredients you may tolerate better. Their database covers:

• Emollients
• Steroids
• Foods
• Skincare products
• Cosmetics
• Laundry products

While not all manufacturers participate in the database, the coverage is wide and it is a good starting-point for your own searches. The service is available to any member of the public, not just to NES members, and no fee is charged, although donations, if you can afford them, are appreciated. The address is:

The National Eczema Society
Tavistock House East
Tavistock Square
London WC1H 9SR
Tel: 071–388 4097

The National Society for Research into Allergy (NSRA) offers advice on detection of allergy and sensitivity, and expertise in avoidance. The NSRA offers dietary advice and has some pamphlets on treatment and diets. It also has some local support groups.

National Society for Research into Allergy
PO Box 45
Hinckley
Leicestershire LE10 1JY
(No telephone)

Support Groups

Of the major national charities, The National Asthma Campaign and the National Eczema Society have local branches which provide support and advice. Action Against Allergy, The Hyperactive Children's Support Group and the National Society for Research into Allergy all have local groups or individual contacts around the country who can provide support and counselling.

Addresses and contact numbers for all these charities are to be found in CHARITIES.

There are independent local support and self-help groups in Bedford, Hertfordshire, Lancaster, Lothian and Sussex. The contacts are as follows:

Bedford Support Group 54 Bedford Road Houghton Conquest Bedford MK45 3NE	Sue Matthews 0234 740375 Ros Stephenson 0234 342276 Franca Garrick 0234 360941
Hertfordshire Support Group 20 Westbury Close Hitchin Hertfordshire SG5 2NE	Jacky Parvin 0462 432804
Lancaster Support Group 4 Church Brow Bolton-Le-Sands Carnforth Lancashire LA5 8DY	May Lea 0524 824077
Lothian Support Group 55 Manor Place Edinburgh EH3 7EG	Fabienne Smith 031–225 7503

Sussex Support Group
Flat 3
28 Egremont Road
Brighton
East Sussex BN2 2GA

Eva March
0903 208722

Sue Kett
0903 265258

TIP

If you are thinking of setting up a self-help group in your area, The Self-Help Centre can provide basic information on how to go about it.

The Self-Help Centre
Regents Wharf
8 All Saints Street
London N1 9RL
071–713 6161

Financial Help

Very limited financial help is available to people who are severely affected by allergies or sensitivity.

Local Authority Grants

If you are registered disabled, you can apply to your local authority for grants towards the cost of any alterations you need to make to your home. These grants are made under the 1987 Local Government Housing Act.

The grants are means-tested, however, so if you have any savings, you may not get one. In addition, there is often a long waiting list for grants which are usually dealt with in date order of receipt, rather than any other priority. The waiting list is often months or years long.

Charitable Grants

Around the country, there are many small local charities giving out small amounts of money to people in need. These have often been set up as family trusts, and sometimes have very specific categories of need to which they can give help. It is worth investigating any local trusts to see if your needs might fit into their categories. In your local reference library, you will find the Directory of Grant-Making Trusts – a reference book listing trusts which give out money to individuals, and the conditions of grants.

Social Security

Some people who are on special diets and on social security benefits have been able to make a case, and receive extra funding, for the extra expense of a medically prescribed diet. This is usually at the discretion of a local office.

Send In Your Ideas!

Do you have any tips and advice, or details of products that you have found worked for you? If you would like to share them, please write them down and send them in:

_____

_____

_____

_____

_____

_____

_____

_____

Your Name _____ Telephone _____

Address _____

_____

_____

SEND TO: The Allergy Survival Guide
           PO Box 37
           SKIPTON
           North Yorkshire BD23 1QX

Further Reading

General

Allergy: A Guide to Coping
Dr Jonathan Maberly and Dr Honor Anthony (1989)

The Complete Guide to Food Allergy and Intolerance
Dr Jonathan Brostoff and Linda Gamlin (1989)

Allergy: The Facts
Robert Davies and Susan Ollier (1989)

Not All In The Mind
Dr Robert Mackarness (1976)

Photosensitivity

Photosensitivity
Allergy Survival Guide (1993)
(Available from:
  The Allergy Survival Guide
  PO Box 37
  Skipton
  North Yorkshire BD23 1QX)

Contact Dermatitis
Alexander A. Fisher (ed.) (1983)

Allergy: The Facts
Robert Davies and Susan Ollier (1989)

Seasonal Affective Disorder (SAD)

Daylight Robbery
Dr Damien Downing

Sick Building Syndrome

Sick Building Syndrome: Causes, Effects and Control
London Hazards Centre Handbook (1990)

(Available from:
The London Hazards Centre

Headland House
308 Gray's Inn Road
London WC1X 8DS
Tel: 071–837 5605)

Chemicals

C for Chemicals
Michael Birkin and Brian Price (1989)

Contact Dermatitis
Alexander A. Fisher (ed.) (1986)

The Penguin Dictionary of Chemistry
D. W. A. Sharp (ed.) (1983)

Food Families

Coping With Your Allergies
Natalie Golos and Frances Golbitz (1986)

Chemical Victims
Dr Richard Mackarness (1980)

Food Family List
Allergy Survival Guide (1993)
(available as shown left)

Food Combining

Food Combining for Health
Doris Grant and Jean Joice (1984)

Food Combining for Vegetarians
Jackie Le Tissier (1992)

The Food Combining Cookbook
Erwina Lidolt (1987)

Nutrition

Nutritional Medicine
Dr Stephen Davies and Dr Alan Stewart (1987)

The Vegetarian Mother and Baby Book
Rose Elliot (1984)

Cookbooks

The Foodwatch Alternative Cookbook
Foodwatch (1984)

The Allergy Diet
Elizabeth Workman, Dr V. A. Jones and Dr J. Hunter (1988)

Food Adulteration and Additives

Food Adulteration
The London Food Commission (1988)

Additives
Felicity Lawrence (1986)

(Both available from:
The Food Commission
102 Gloucester Place
London W1H 3DA
Tel: 071–935 9078)

Organic Foods

The New Organic Food Guide
Alan Gear (1987)

Identifying Pollens

Britain's Wildlife, Plants and Flowers
Reader's Digest (1987)

Trees in Britain
Roger Phillips (1978)

Wild Flowers in Britain
Roger Phillips (1977)

Hyperactivity

Allergies and the Hyperactive Child
Doris J. Rapp (1979)

Natural Contraception

Green Babies
Dr Penny Stanway (1990)

The Billings Method of Natural Family Planning
Dr Evelyn Billings and Ann Westmore (1980)

Index